Pub
82-

MAY 2014

Teen Health Series

Mental Health Information For Teens, Fourth Edition

Mental Health Information For Teens, Fourth Edition

Health Tips About Mental Wellness And Mental Illness

Including Facts About Recognizing And Treating Mood, Anxiety, Personality, Psychotic, Behavioral, Impulse Control, And Addiction Disorders

Edited by Lisa Bakewell

Omnigraphics

155 W. Congress, Suite 200
Detroit, MI 48226

Bibliographic Note

Because this page cannot legibly accommodate all the copyright notices, the Bibliographic Note portion of the Preface constitutes an extension of the copyright notice.

Edited by Lisa Bakewell

Teen Health Series

Karen Bellenir, *Managing Editor*
David A. Cooke, M.D., *Medical Consultant*
Elizabeth Collins, *Research and Permissions Coordinator*
EdIndex, *Services for Publishers, Indexers*

* * *

Omnigraphics, Inc.
Matthew P. Barbour, *Senior Vice President*
Kevin M. Hayes, *Operations Manager*

* * *

Peter E. Ruffner, *Publisher*
Copyright © 2014 Omnigraphics, Inc.
ISBN 978-0-7808-1321-2
E-ISBN 978-0-7808-1322-9

Library of Congress Cataloging-in-Publication Data

Mental health information for teens : health tips about mental wellness and mental illness, including facts about recognizing and treating mood, anxiety, personality, psychotic, behavioral, impulse control, and addiction disorders / edited by Lisa Bakewell. -- Fourth edition.
    pages cm. -- (Teen health series)
 Includes bibliographical references and index.
 Summary: "Provides basic consumer health information about the causes, warning signs, and symptoms of mental health disorders, along with facts about treatment approaches and tips for teens on coping with stress, building self-esteem, and maintaining mental wellness. Includes a further reading list, a directory of crisis helplines and related organizations, and an index"-- Provided by publisher.
 ISBN 978-0-7808-1321-2 (hardcover : alk. paper) 1. Teenagers--Mental health. 2. Adolescent psychology. 3. Child mental health. I. Bakewell, Lisa.
 RJ499.M419 2014
 616.89'140835--dc23   616.89
                                                              M
                                                                        2013042664

Table of Contents

Preface

Part Three: Personality And Psychotic Disorders

Part Four: Behavioral, Impulse Control, And Addiction Disorders

Part Five: Other Situations And Disorders With Mental Health Consequences

Part Six: Mental Health Treatments

Part Seven: Mental Wellness Topics For Teens

Part Eight: If You Need More Information

Preface

About This Book

Adolescence is difficult. Not only are teens under stress to be liked, to do well in school, and to get along with their families, they also have big decisions to make while hormones are running rampant. Most of the time stressors such as these are normal, but teens sometimes find themselves feeling very sad, hopeless, overwhelmed, or worthless. These situations are possible signs of debilitating mental health problems, and teens experiencing them are not alone. Mental health disorders are common among adolescents in the United States, and according to the Centers for Disease Control and Prevention (CDC) an estimated 13–20 percent of the nation's youth experience a mental disorder in any given year.

Mental Health Information For Teens, Fourth Edition offers updated information on mental health and its importance. It presents facts about the causes, warning signs, and diagnosis of mental illnesses, and it explains how the adolescent brain differs from the adult brain. Some of the specific disorders described in detail include anxiety, depression, eating disorders, posttraumatic stress disorder, psychoses, schizophrenia, and impulse control disorders. Mental health therapies—both traditional and alternative—are discussed, and the consequences of not receiving treatment are addressed. A section on mental wellness provides tips for building healthy self-esteem, coping with stress and disaster, getting along with family and friends, and dealing with challenges such as divorce, abuse, grief, and thoughts of suicide. For readers seeking more information, the book concludes with suggestions for additional reading, a list of crisis lines, and a directory of mental health organizations.

How To Use This Book

This book is divided into parts and chapters. Parts focus on broad areas of interest; chapters are devoted to single topics within a part.

Part One: Mental Health And Mental Illness offers information on understanding mental health, its overall effect on well-being, and how resilience plays a vital role in mental wellness. Mental illness is defined, and its possible causes and warning signs are described. A chapter on the developing adolescent brain and how it differs from the adult brain is also included.

Part Two: Mood And Anxiety Disorders discusses an array of disorders that alter emotional and fear responses. These include depression, premenstrual syndrome, seasonal affective disorder, bipolar disorder, generalized anxiety disorder, social anxiety disorder, obsessive-compulsive disorder, post-traumatic stress disorder, panic disorder, and phobias.

Part Three: Personality And Psychotic Disorders describes mental illnesses that affect how people perceive reality. These include antisocial disorders, borderline personality disorder, factitious disorders, and dissociative disorders, as well as psychosis and schizophrenia.

Part Four: Behavioral, Impulse Control, And Addiction Disorders explores mental illnesses that influence how people act and possibly disregard societal norms. Examples include eating disorders, body dysmorphic disorder, impulse control disorder, conduct disorder, and oppositional defiant disorders.

Part Five: Other Situations And Disorders With Mental Health Consequences provides information on adolescent circumstances that may impact mental wellbeing. These include puberty, child abuse, bullying, violence, and self-harm. Chronic disorders that may impact mental health, including autism spectrum disorder, attention deficit hyperactivity disorder (ADHD), and Tourette syndrome, are also discussed.

Part Six: Mental Health Treatments explains how mental illness is diagnosed and discusses the consequences of not receiving treatment. It explores the ways in which the treatment of children with mental illness can differ from that of adults. Various common approaches to mental health care—including psychotherapy, the use of medications, and complementary and alternative medicine practices—are also described.

Part Seven: Mental Wellness Topics For Teens offers information on coping with challenges that can arise during adolescence. It provides tips for building a healthy self-esteem, improving mental health, dealing with depression, and coping with stress. It also offers strategies for handling traumatic events, important relationships, and thoughts of suicide.

Part Eight: If You Need More Information offers suggestions for additional reading, a list of crisis helplines and hotlines, and a directory of organizations able to provide further materials about adolescent mental health.

Bibliographic Note

This volume contains documents and excerpts from publications issued by the following government agencies: Centers for Disease Control and Prevention (CDC); GirlsHealth.gov; Health Resources and Services Administration (HRSA); National Center for Complementary and Alternative Medicine (NCCAM); National Institutes of Health (NIH); National Institute of Mental Health (NIMH); National Institute of Neurological Disorders and Stroke (NINDS); National Institute on Drug Abuse (NIDA); National Library of Medicine; Office on Women's Health; StopBullying.gov; Substance Abuse and Mental Health Services Administration (SAMHSA); U.S. Department of Food and Drug Administration (FDA); and the U.S. Department of Health and Human Services (HHS).

In addition, this volume contains copyrighted documents and articles produced by the following organizations: A.D.A.M., Inc.; Biological Sciences Curriculum Study (BSCS); Cleveland Clinic Foundation; Helpguide; NAMI, the National Alliance on Mental Illness; Nemours Foundation; and PsychCentral.

The photograph on the front cover is © Elena Rostunova/Shutterstock.

Full citation information is provided on the first page of each chapter. Every effort has been made to secure all necessary rights to reprint the copyrighted material. If any omissions have been made, please contact Omnigraphics to make corrections for future editions.

Acknowledgements

In addition to the organizations listed above, special thanks are due to Bonnie L. Stafford, best cheerleader ever; Liz Collins, research and permissions coordinator; Karen Bellenir, managing editor; and WhimsyInk, prepress services provider.

About The *Teen Health Series*

At the request of librarians serving today's young adults, the *Teen Health Series* was developed as a specially focused set of volumes within Omnigraphics' *Health Reference Series*. Each volume deals comprehensively with a topic selected according to the needs and interests of people in middle school and high school.

Teens seeking preventive guidance, information about disease warning signs, medical statistics, and risk factors for health problems will find answers to their questions in the *Teen Health Series*. The *Series*, however, is not intended to serve as a tool for diagnosing illness, in prescribing treatments, or as a substitute for the physician/patient relationship. All people concerned about medical symptoms or the possibility of disease are encouraged to seek professional care from an appropriate health care provider.

If there is a topic you would like to see addressed in a future volume of the *Teen Health Series*, please write to:

Editor
Teen Health Series
Omnigraphics, Inc.
155 West Congress, Suite 200
Detroit, MI 48226

A Note About Spelling And Style

Teen Health Series editors use *Stedman's Medical Dictionary* as an authority for questions related to the spelling of medical terms and the *Chicago Manual of Style* for questions related to grammatical structures, punctuation, and other editorial concerns. Consistent adherence is not always possible, however, because the individual volumes within the *Series* include many documents from a wide variety of different producers and copyright holders, and the editor's primary goal is to present material from each source as accurately as is possible following the terms specified by each document's producer. This sometimes means that information in different chapters or sections may follow other guidelines and alternate spelling authorities. For example, occasionally a copyright holder may require that eponymous terms be shown in possessive forms (Crohn's disease *vs.* Crohn disease) or that British spelling norms be retained (leukaemia *vs.* leukemia).

Locating Information Within The *Teen Health Series*

The *Teen Health Series* contains a wealth of information about a wide variety of medical topics. As the *Series* continues to grow in size and scope, locating the precise information needed by a specific student may become more challenging. To address this concern, information about books within the *Teen Health Series* is included in *A Contents Guide to the Health Reference Series*. The *Contents Guide* presents an extensive list of more than 16,000 diseases, treatments, and other topics of general interest compiled from the Tables of Contents and major index headings from the books of the *Teen Health Series* and *Health Reference Series*. To access *A Contents Guide to the Health Reference Series*, visit www.healthreferenceseries.com.

Our Advisory Board

We would like to thank the following advisory board members for providing guidance to the development of this *Series*:

Dr. Lynda Baker, Associate Professor of Library and Information Science, Wayne State University, Detroit, MI

Nancy Bulgarelli, William Beaumont Hospital Library, Royal Oak, MI

Karen Imarisio, Bloomfield Township Public Library, Bloomfield Township, MI

Karen Morgan, Mardigian Library, University of Michigan-Dearborn, Dearborn, MI

Rosemary Orlando, St. Clair Shores Public Library, St. Clair Shores, MI

Medical Consultant

Medical consultation services are provided to the *Teen Health Series* editors by David A. Cooke, MD. Dr. Cooke is a graduate of Brandeis University, and he received his MD degree from the University of Michigan. He completed residency training at the University of Wisconsin Hospital and Clinics. He is board-certified in internal medicine. Dr. Cooke currently works as part of the University of Michigan Health System and practices in Ann Arbor, MI. In his free time, he enjoys writing, science fiction, and spending time with his family.

Part One
Mental Health And Mental Illness

Chapter 1

Understanding Mental Health

Often people are afraid to talk about mental health because there are many misconceptions about mental illnesses. It's important to learn the facts to stop discrimination and to begin treating people with mental illnesses with respect and dignity. Following are answers to common questions about mental health.

Is there hope for people with mental illnesses?

Yes. There are more treatments, strategies, and community supports than ever before, and even more are on the horizon. People with mental illnesses lead active, productive lives.

What can I do for someone with mental health needs?

You can do a lot, starting with the way you act and how you speak. You can nurture an environment that builds on people's strengths and promotes good mental health. For example:

- Avoid labeling people with words like "crazy," "wacko," "loony," or by their diagnosis. Instead of saying someone is a "schizophrenic" say "a person with schizophrenia."

- Learn the facts about mental health and share them with others, especially if you hear something that is untrue.

- Treat people with mental illnesses with respect and dignity, as you would anybody else.

- Respect the rights of people with mental illnesses and don't discriminate against them when it comes to housing, employment, or education. Like other people with disabilities, people with mental health needs are protected under Federal and State laws.

About This Chapter: Excerpted from "Myths and Facts About Mental Health," Substance Abuse and Mental Health Services Administration Center for Mental Health Services (www.samhsa.gov), June 2012.

Are people with mental illnesses violent?

Not usually. The vast majority of people who have mental health needs are no more violent than anyone else. You probably know someone with a mental illness and don't even realize it.

Is mental illness common?

Yes. Mental illnesses are surprisingly common. They affect almost every family in America. Mental illnesses do not discriminate—they can affect anyone.

Is mental illness the same as mental retardation?

No, the two are distinct disorders. A mental retardation diagnosis is characterized by limitations in intellectual functioning and difficulties with certain daily living skills. In contrast, people with mental illnesses—health conditions that cause changes in a person's thinking, mood, and behavior—have varied intellectual functioning, just like the general population.

Is mental illnesses brought on by a weakness of character?

No. Mental illnesses are a product of the interaction of biological, psychological, and social factors. Research has shown genetic and biological factors are associated with schizophrenia,

---

Mental Health

Mental health includes our emotional, psychological, and social wellbeing. It affects how we think, feel, and act as we cope with life. It also helps determine how we handle stress, relate to others, and make choices. Mental health is important at every stage of life, from childhood and adolescence through adulthood.

Mental illnesses are serious disorders which can affect your thinking, mood, and behavior. There are many causes of mental disorders. Your genes and family history may play a role. Your life experiences, such as stress or a history of abuse, may also matter. Biological factors can also be part of the cause. Mental disorders are common, but treatments are available.

Source: Excerpted from "Mental Health," U.S. National Library of Medicine, National Institutes of Health (www.nlm.nih .gov), February 2013.

depression, and alcoholism. Social influences, such as loss of a loved one or a job, can also contribute to the development of various disorders.

Can people with mental illnesses tolerate the stress of holding down a job?

Of course! In essence, all jobs are stressful to some extent. Productivity is maximized when there is a good match between the employee's needs and working conditions, whether or not the individual has mental health needs.

Are people with mental health needs poor workers?

Not necessarily. Employers who have hired people with mental illnesses report good attendance and punctuality, as well as motivation, quality of work, and job tenure on par with (or greater than) other employees. Studies by the National Institute of Mental Health (NIMH) and the National Alliance for the Mentally Ill (NAMI) show that there are no differences in productivity when people with mental illnesses are compared to other employees.

Do people recover from mental illness?

It's possible. Studies show that most people with mental illnesses get better, and many recover completely. Recovery refers to the process in which people are able to live, work, learn, and participate fully in their communities. For some individuals, recovery is the ability to live a fulfilling and productive life. For others, recovery implies the reduction or complete remission of symptoms. Science has shown that having hope plays an integral role in an individual's recovery.

Is therapy a waste of time?

No. Therapy can be very helpful, because treatment varies depending on the individual. A lot of people work with therapists, counselors, their peers, psychologists, psychiatrists, nurses, and social workers in their recovery process. They also use self-help strategies and community supports. Often these methods are combined with some of the most advanced medications available.

Do kids experience mental illnesses?

Yes. A report from the President's New Freedom Commission on Mental Health showed that in any given year 5–9 percent of children experience serious emotional disturbances. Just like adult mental illnesses, these are clinically diagnosable health conditions that are a product of the interaction of biological, psychological, social, and sometimes even genetic factors.

Do kids misbehave or fail in school just to get attention?

It depends. Behavior problems can be symptoms of emotional, behavioral, or mental disorders, rather than merely attention-seeking devices. These children can succeed in school with appropriate understanding, attention, and mental health services.

Chapter 2

The Teen Brain: Still Under Construction

One of the ways that scientists have searched for the causes of mental illness is by studying the development of the brain from birth to adulthood. Powerful new technologies have enabled them to track the growth of the brain and to investigate the connections between brain function, development, and behavior.

The research has turned up some surprises, among them the discovery of striking changes taking place during the teen years. These findings have altered long-held assumptions about the timing of brain maturation. In key ways, the brain doesn't look like that of an adult until the early 20s.

An understanding of how the brain of an adolescent is changing may help explain a puzzling contradiction of adolescence: Young people at this age are close to a lifelong peak of physical health, strength, and mental capacity, and yet, for some, this can be a hazardous age. Mortality rates jump between early and late adolescence. Rates of death by injury between ages 15–19 are about six times that of the rate between ages 10–14. Crime rates are highest among young males and rates of alcohol abuse are high relative to other ages. Even though most adolescents come through this transitional age well, it's important to understand the risk factors for behavior that can have serious consequences. Genes, childhood experience, and the environment in which a young person reaches adolescence all shape behavior. Adding to this complex picture, research is revealing how all these factors act in the context of a brain that is changing, with its own impact on behavior.

The more we learn, the better we may be able to understand the abilities and vulnerabilities of teens, and the significance of this stage for life-long mental health.

About This Chapter: Excerpted from "The Teen Brain: Still Under Construction," National Institute of Mental Health (www.nimh.nih.gov), May 2012.

The "Visible" Brain

A clue to the degree of change taking place in the teen brain came from studies in which scientists did brain scans of children as they grew from early childhood through age 20. The scans revealed unexpectedly late changes in the volume of gray matter, which forms the thin, folding outer layer or cortex of the brain. The cortex is where the processes of thought and memory are based. Over the course of childhood, the volume of gray matter in the cortex increases and then declines. A decline in volume is normal at this age and is in fact a necessary part of maturation.

The assumption for many years had been that the volume of gray matter was highest in very early childhood, and gradually fell as a child grew. The more recent scans, however, revealed that the high point of the volume of gray matter occurs during early adolescence.

While the details behind the changes in volume on scans are not completely clear, the results push the timeline of brain maturation into adolescence and young adulthood. In terms of the volume of gray matter seen in brain images, the brain does not begin to resemble that of an adult until the early 20s.

The scans also suggest that different parts of the cortex mature at different rates. Areas involved in more basic functions mature first: those involved, for example, in the processing of information from the senses, and in controlling movement. The parts of the brain responsible for more "top-down" control, controlling impulses, and planning ahead—the hallmarks of adult behavior—are among the last to mature.

What's Gray Matter?

The details of what is behind the increase and decline in gray matter are still not completely clear. Gray matter is made up of the cell bodies of neurons, the nerve fibers that project from them, and support cells. One of the features of the brain's growth in early life is that there is an early blooming of synapses—the connections between brain cells or neurons—followed by pruning as the brain matures. Synapses are the relays over which neurons communicate with each other and are the basis of the working circuitry of the brain. Already more numerous than an adult's at birth, synapses multiply rapidly in the first months of life. A 2-year-old has about half again as many synapses as an adult. (For an idea of the complexity of the brain: A cube of brain matter, one millimeter on each side, can contain between 35 and 70 million neurons and an estimated 500 billion synapses.)

Scientists believe that the loss of synapses as a child matures is part of the process by which the brain becomes more efficient. Although genes play a role in the decline in synapses, animal research has shown that experience also shapes the decline. Synapses "exercised" by experience survive and are strengthened, while others are pruned away. Scientists are working to determine to what extent the changes in gray matter on brain scans during the teen years reflect growth and pruning of synapses.

A Spectrum Of Change

Research, using many different approaches, is showing that more than gray matter is changing in adolescence. Other changes include:

- Connections between different parts of the brain increase throughout childhood and well into adulthood. As the brain develops, the fibers connecting nerve cells are wrapped in a protein that greatly increases the speed with which they can transmit impulses from cell to cell. The resulting increase in connectivity—a little like providing a growing city with a fast, integrated communication system—shapes how well different parts of the brain work in tandem. Research is finding that the extent of connectivity is related to growth in intellectual capacities such as memory and reading ability.

- Several lines of evidence suggest that the brain circuitry involved in emotional responses is changing during the teen years. Functional brain imaging studies, for example, suggest that the responses of teens to emotionally loaded images and situations are heightened relative to younger children and adults. The brain changes underlying these patterns involve brain centers and signaling molecules that are part of the reward system with which the brain motivates behavior. These age-related changes shape how much different parts of the brain are activated in response to experience, and in terms of behavior, the urgency and intensity of emotional reactions.

- Enormous hormonal changes take place during adolescence. Reproductive hormones shape not only sex-related growth and behavior, but overall social behavior. Hormone systems involved in the brain's response to stress are also changing during the teens. As with reproductive hormones, stress hormones can have complex effects on the brain, and as a result, behavior.

- In terms of sheer intellectual power, the brain of an adolescent is a match for an adult's. The capacity of a person to learn will never be greater than during adolescence. At the same time, behavioral tests, sometimes combined with functional brain imaging, suggest differences in how adolescents and adults carry out mental tasks. Adolescents and adults seem to engage different parts of the brain to different extents during tests requiring calculation and impulse control, or in reaction to emotional content.

- Research suggests that adolescence brings with it brain-based changes in the regulation of sleep that may contribute to teens' tendency to stay up late at night. Along with the obvious effects of sleep deprivation, such as fatigue and difficulty maintaining attention, inadequate sleep is a powerful contributor to irritability and depression. Studies of children and adolescents have found that sleep deprivation can increase impulsive behavior; some researchers report finding that it is a factor in delinquency. Adequate sleep is central to physical and emotional health.

The Changing Brain And Behavior In Teens

One interpretation of all these findings is that in teens, the parts of the brain involved in emotional responses are fully online, or even more active than in adults, while the parts of the brain involved in keeping emotional, impulsive responses in check are still reaching maturity. Such a changing balance might provide clues to a youthful appetite for novelty, and a tendency to act on impulse—without regard for risk.

While much is being learned about the teen brain, it is not yet possible to know to what extent a particular behavior or ability is the result of a feature of brain structure—or a change in brain structure. Changes in the brain take place in the context of many other factors, among them, inborn traits, personal history, family, friends, community, and culture.

Teens And The Brain: More Questions For Research

Scientists continue to investigate the development of the brain and the relationship between the changes taking place, behavior, and health. The following questions are among the important ones that are targets of research:

- How do experience and environment interact with genetic preprogramming to shape the maturing brain, and as a result, future abilities and behavior? In other words, to what extent does what a teen does and learns shape his or her brain over the rest of a lifetime?

- In what ways do features unique to the teen brain play a role in the high rates of illicit substance use and alcohol abuse in the late teen to young adult years? Does the adolescent capacity for learning make this a stage of particular vulnerability to addiction?

- Why is it so often the case that, for many mental disorders, symptoms first emerge during adolescence and young adulthood?

This last question has been the central reason to study brain development from infancy to adulthood. Scientists increasingly view mental illnesses as developmental disorders that have their roots in the processes involved in how the brain matures. By studying how the circuitry of the brain develops, scientists hope to identify when and for what reasons development goes off track. Brain imaging studies have revealed distinctive variations in growth patterns of brain tissue in youth who show signs of conditions affecting mental health. Ongoing research is providing information on how genetic factors increase or reduce vulnerability to mental illness; and how experiences during infancy, childhood, and adolescence can increase the risk of mental illness or protect against it.

The Adolescent And Adult Brain

It is not surprising that the behavior of adolescents would be a study in change, since the brain itself is changing in such striking ways. Scientists emphasize that the fact that the teen brain is in transition doesn't mean it is somehow not up to par. It is different from both a child's and an adult's in ways that may equip youth to make the transition from dependence to independence. The capacity for learning at this age, an expanding social life, and a taste for exploration and limit testing may all, to some extent, be reflections of age-related biology.

Understanding the changes taking place in the brain at this age presents an opportunity to intervene early in mental illnesses that have their onset at this age. Research findings on the brain may also serve to help adults understand the importance of creating an environment in which teens can explore and experiment while helping them avoid behavior that is destructive to themselves and others.

Alcohol And The Teen Brain

Adults drink more frequently than teens, but when teens drink they tend to drink larger quantities than adults. There is evidence to suggest that the adolescent brain responds to alcohol differently than the adult brain, perhaps helping to explain the elevated risk of binge drinking in youth. Drinking in youth, and intense drinking are both risk factors for later alcohol dependence. Findings on the developing brain should help clarify the role of the changing brain in youthful drinking, and the relationship between youth drinking and the risk of addiction later in life.

Chapter 3

Why Is Mental Health Important?

Your mental health is very important. You will not have a healthy body if you don't also take care of your mind. People depend on you. It's important for you to take care of yourself so that you can do the important things in life—whether it's working, learning, volunteering, enjoying the outdoors, or whatever is important to you.

Good mental health helps you enjoy life and cope with problems. It offers a feeling of well-being and inner strength. Just as you take care of your body by eating right and exercising, you can do things to protect your mental health. In fact, eating right and exercising can help maintain good mental health. You don't automatically have good mental health just because you don't have mental health illness. You have to work to keep your mind healthy.

Nutrition And Mental Health

The food you eat can have a direct effect on your energy level, physical health, and mood. A "healthy diet" is one that has enough of each essential nutrient, contains many foods from all of the basic food groups, provides the right amount of calories to maintain a healthy weight, and does not have too much fat, sugar, salt, or alcohol.

By choosing foods that can give you steady energy, you can help your body stay healthy. This may also help your mind feel good. The same diet doesn't work for every person. In order to find the best foods that are right for you, talk to your health care professional.

Some vitamins and minerals may help with the symptoms of depression. Experts are looking into how a lack of some nutrients—including folate, vitamin B12, calcium, iron, selenium,

About This Chapter: Excerpted from "Good Mental Health," U.S. Department of Health and Human Services, Office on Women's Health (www.womenshealth.gov), April 2013.

zinc, and omega-3—may contribute to depression in new mothers. Ask your doctor or another health care professional for more information.

Visit choosemyplate.gov to help find personalized eating plans and other interactive tools to help you make good food choices.

Exercise And Mental Health

Regular physical activity is important to the physical and mental health of almost everyone, including older adults. Being physically active can help you continue to do the things you enjoy and stay independent as you age. Regular physical activity over long periods of time can produce long-term health benefits. That's why health experts say that everyone should be active every day to maintain their health.

If you are diagnosed with depression or anxiety, your doctor may tell you to exercise in addition to taking any medications or receiving counseling. This is because exercise has been shown to help with the symptoms of depression and anxiety. Your body makes certain chemicals, called endorphins, before and after you work out. They relieve stress and improve your mood. Exercise can also slow or stop weight gain, which is a common side effect of some medications used to treat mental health disorders.

Sleep And Mental Health

Your mind and body will feel better if you sleep well. Your body needs time every day to rest and heal. If you often have trouble sleeping—either falling asleep or waking during the night and being unable to get back to sleep—one or several of the following ideas might be helpful to you:

- Go to bed at the same time every night and get up at the same time every morning. Avoid "sleeping in" (sleeping much later than your usual time for getting up). It will make you feel worse.

- Establish a bedtime "ritual" by doing the same things every night for an hour or two before bedtime so your body knows when it is time to go to sleep.

- Avoid caffeine, nicotine, and alcohol.

- Eat on a regular schedule and avoid a heavy meal prior to going to bed. Don't skip any meals.

- Eat plenty of dairy foods and dark green leafy vegetables.

- Exercise daily, but avoid strenuous or invigorating activity before going to bed.

- Play soothing music on a tape or CD that shuts off automatically after you are in bed.

- Try a turkey sandwich and a glass of milk before bedtime to make you feel drowsy.

- Try having a small snack before you go to bed, something like a piece of fruit and a piece of cheese, so you don't wake up hungry in the middle of the night. Have a similar small snack if you awaken in the middle of the night.

- Take a warm bath or shower before going to bed.

- Place a drop of lavender oil on your pillow.

- Drink a cup of herbal chamomile tea before going to bed.

You need to see your doctor if:

- You often have difficulty sleeping and the solutions listed previously are not working for you

- You awaken during the night gasping for breath

- Your breathing stops when you are sleeping

- You snore loudly

- You wake up feeling like you haven't been asleep

- You fall asleep often during the day

Stress And Mental Health

Stress can happen for many reasons. Stress can be brought about by a traumatic accident, death, or emergency situation. Stress can also be a side effect of a serious illness or disease.

There is also stress associated with daily life, school, and family responsibilities. It's hard to stay calm and relaxed in our hectic lives. With all we have going on in our lives, it seems almost impossible to find ways to de-stress. But it's important to find those ways. Your health depends on it.

Common symptoms include:

- Headache

- Sleep disorders

- Difficulty concentrating

- Short temper

- Upset stomach

- Dissatisfaction

- Low morale

- Depression

- Anxiety

Remember to always make time for you. It's important to care for yourself. Think of this as an order from your doctor, so you don't feel guilty! No matter how busy you are, you can try to set aside at least 15 minutes each day in your schedule to do something for yourself, like taking a bubble bath, going for a walk, or calling a friend.

Chapter 4

Resilience: A Vital Component Of Mental Health

What is resilience?

Resilience refers to the ability of an individual, family, organization, or community to cope with adversity and adapt to challenges or change. It is an ongoing process that requires time and effort and engages people in taking a number of steps to enhance their response to adverse circumstances. Resilience implies that, after an event, a person or community may not only be able to cope and recover, but also change to reflect different priorities arising from the experience and prepare for the next stressful situation. Resilience is the ability to:

- Bounce back

- Take on difficult challenges and still find meaning in life

- Respond positively to difficult situations

- Rise above adversity

- Cope when things look bleak

- Tap into hope

- Transform unfavorable situations into wisdom, insight, and compassion

- Endure

Resilience is the most important defense people have against stress, and research has shown that resilience is ordinary, not extraordinary. People regularly demonstrate this ability.

About This Chapter: Excerpted from "Resilience and Stress Management: Resilience," Substance Abuse and Mental Health Services Administration (www.samhsa.gov), 2012.

It is important to build and foster resilience to be ready for future challenges to enable the development of a reservoir of internal resources to draw upon during stressful situations. Keep in mind:

- Resilience is not a trait that people either have or do not have.

- Resilience involves behaviors, thoughts, and actions that can be learned and developed in anyone.

- Resilience is tremendously influenced by a person's environment.

Resilience changes over time. It fluctuates depending on how much a person nurtures internal resources or coping strategies. Some people are more resilient in work life, while others exhibit more resilience in their personal relationships. People can build resilience and promote the foundations of resilience in any aspect of life they choose.

What is individual or personal resilience?

Individual resilience is a person's ability to positively cope after failures, setbacks, and losses. Developing resilience is a personal journey. Individuals do not react the same way to traumatic or stressful life events. An approach to building resilience that works for one person might not work for another. People use varying strategies to build their resilience. Because resilience can be learned, it can be strengthened. Personal resilience is related to many factors, including: individual health and well-being; factors with and into which a person is born; life history and experience; and social support.

What is family resilience?

Family resilience is the coping process in the family as a functional unit. Crisis events and persistent stressors affect the whole family, posing risks not only for individual dysfunction, but also for relational conflict and family breakdown. Family processes mediate the impact of stress for all of its members and relationships, and the protective processes in place foster resilience by buffering stress and facilitating adaptation to current and future events. The three key factors in family resilience are:

- Family belief systems foster resilience by making meaning in adversity, creating a sense of coherence, and providing a positive outlook.

- Family organization promotes resilience by facilitating flexibility, capacity to adapt, connectedness and cohesion, emotional and structural bonding, and access to resources.

- Family communication enhances resilience by involving clear communication, open and emotional expressions, trust and collaborative problem solving, and conflict management.

Factors That Influence Health And Well-Being

Birth Traits

- Personality
- Cultural background
- Ethnicity
- Economic background

Life History And Experience

Past events and relationships that influence how people approach current stressors include:

- Family history
- Previous mental health
- Past social experiences
- Previous physical health
- Trauma history
- Past cultural experiences

Social Support

Support systems, provided by family, friends, and members of the community, work, or school environments, include:

- Feeling connected to others
- Feeling connected to resources
- A sense of security

Information about birth traits, life history and experience, and social support was adapted from Simon, J., Murphy, J., & Smith, S. (2008). Building resilience: Appreciate the little things in life. *British Journal of Social Work*, 38, 218–235.

Resilience Also Includes These Attributes

Along with the factors listed above, there are several attributes that have been correlated with building and promoting resilience. The American Psychological Association reports that resilience includes the following attributes:

- The capacity to make and carry out realistic plans
- Communication and problem-solving skills
- A positive or optimistic view of life
- Confidence in personal strengths and abilities
- The capacity to manage strong feelings, emotions, and impulses

For more information from the American Psychological Association about the topic of resilience, visit http://www.apa.org/helpcenter/road-resilience.aspx.

Source: SAMHSA, 2012.

What is community resilience?

Community resilience is the individual and collective capacity to respond to adversity and change. A resilient community is one that takes intentional action to enhance the personal and collective capacity of its citizens and institutions to respond to and influence the course of social and economic change. For a community to be resilient, its members must put into practice early and effective actions so that they can respond to change. When responding to stressful events, a resilient community will be able to strengthen community bonds, resources, and the capacity to cope. Systems involved with building and maintaining community resilience must work together.

How does culture influence resilience?

Cultural resilience refers to a culture's capacity to maintain and develop cultural identity and critical cultural knowledge and practices. Along with an entire culture fostering resilience, the interaction of culture and resilience for an individual also is important. An individual's culture will have an impact on how the person communicates feelings and copes with adversity. Cultural parameters are often embedded deep in an individual. A person's cultural background may deeply influence in how he or she responds to different stressors. Assimilation could be a factor in cultural resilience, as it could be a positive way for a person to manage his/her environment. However, assimilation could create conflict between generations, so it could be seen as positive or negative depending on the individual and culture. Because of this, coping strategies are going to be different. With growing cultural diversity, the public has greater access to a number of different approaches to building resilience. It is something that can be built using approaches that make sense within each culture and are tailored to each individual.

What factors promote resilience?

Resilience involves the modification of a person's response to a potentially risky situation. People who are resilient are able to maintain high self-esteem and self-efficacy in spite of the challenges they face. By fostering resilience, people are building psychological defenses against stress. The more resources and defenses available during a time of struggle, the better able to cope and bounce back from adverse circumstances people will be. A person's ability to regain a sense of normalcy or define a new normalcy after adverse circumstances will be partially based on the resources available to him/her. Resilience building can begin at any time. Table 4.1 contains information regarding types of resilience, the qualities of which each type consists, factors that can inhibit or enhance resilience, and people who help facilitate the growth of individual resilience. Table 4.2 contains the same types of information for community resilience.

Table 4.1. Types, Qualities, Factors, And Facilitators Of Individual Resilience

Individual resilience is the ability for an individual to cope with adversity and change.

Signs Of This Type of Resilience	Vulnerability Factors Inhibiting Resilience	Protective Factors Enhancing Resilience	Facilitators of Resilience
Optimism	Poor social skills	Social competence	Individuals
Flexibility	Poor problem solving	Problem-solving skills	Parents
Self-confidence	Lack of empathy	Good coping skills	Grandparents
Competence	Family violence	Empathy	Caregivers
Insightfulness	Abuse or neglect	Secure or stable family	Children
Perseverance	Divorce or partner breakup	Supportive relationships	Adolescents
Perspective		Intellectual abilities	Friends
Self-control	Death or loss	Self-efficacy	Partners
Sociability	Lack of social support	Communication skills	Teachers
			Faith Community

Source: SAMHSA, 2012.

Table 4.2. Types, Qualities, Factors, And Facilitators Of Community Resilience

Community resilience is the ability for an individual and the collective community to respond to adversity and change.

Signs Of This Type of Resilience	Vulnerability Factors Inhibiting Resilience	Protective Factors Enhancing Resilience	Facilitators of Resilience
Connectedness	Lack of support services	Access to support services	Community leaders
Commitment to community	Social discrimination	Community networking	Faith-based organizations
Shared values	Cultural discrimination	Strong cultural identity	Volunteers
Structure, roles, and responsibilities exist throughout community	Norms tolerating violence	Strong social support systems	Nonprofit organizations
Supportive	Deviant peer group	Norms against violence	Churches/houses of worship
Good communication	Low socioeconomic status	Identification as a community	Support services staff
Resource sharing	Crime rate	Cohesive community leadership	Teachers
Volunteerism	Community disorganization		Youth groups
Responsive organizations	Civil rivalry		Boy/Girl Scouts
Strong schools			Planned social networking events

Source: SAMHSA, 2012.

How is personal resilience built?

Developing resilience is a personal journey. People do not react the same way to traumatic events. Some ways to build resilience include the following actions:

- Making connections with others

- Looking for opportunities for self-discovery

- Nurturing a positive view of self

- Accepting that change is a part of living

- Taking decisive actions

- Learning from the past

The ability to be flexible is a great skill to obtain and facilitates resilience growth. Getting help when it is needed is crucial to building resilience. It is important to try to obtain information on resilience from books or other publications, self-help or support groups, and online resources.

What can be done to promote family resilience?

Developing family resilience, like individual resilience, is different for every family. The important idea to keep in mind is that an underlying stronghold of family resilience is cohesion, a sense of belonging, and communication. It is important for a family to feel that when their world is unstable they have each other. This sense of bonding and trust is what fuels a family's ability to be resilient. Families that learn how to cope with challenges and meet individual needs are more resilient to stress and crisis. Healthy families solve problems with cooperation, creative brainstorming, openness to others, and emphasis on the role of social support and connectedness (versus isolation) in family resiliency. Resilience is exercised when family members demonstrate behaviors such as confidence, hard work, cooperation, and forgiveness. These are factors that help families withstand stressors throughout the family lifecycle.

How is community resilience fostered?

Fostering community resilience will greatly depend on the community itself and involves the community working as a whole toward preparedness. It is the capacity for the collective to take preemptive action toward preparedness. Community resilience involves the following factors:

- Connection and caring

- Collective resources

- Critical analysis of the community

- Skill building for community members

- Prevention, preparedness, and response to stressful events

Resilience is exercised when community members demonstrate behaviors such as confidence, hard work, cooperation, resourcefulness, and support of those who have needs during particular events. These are factors that help communities withstand challenging circumstances.

Developing resilience is a personal journey. All people do not react identically to traumatic and stressful life events. An approach to building resilience that works for one person might not work for another. People use varying strategies. Resilience involves maintaining flexibility and balance in life during stressful circumstances and traumatic events. Being resilient does not mean that a person does not experience difficulty or distress. Emotional pain and sadness are common in people who have suffered major adversity or trauma in their lives. Stress can be dealt with proactively by building resilience to prepare for stressful circumstances, while learning how to recognize symptoms of stress. Fostering resilience or the ability to bounce back from a stressful situation is a proactive mechanism to managing stress.

Chapter 5

Defining Mental Illness

We can all be "sad" or "blue" at times in our lives. We have all seen movies about the madman and his crime spree, with the underlying cause of mental illness. We sometimes even make jokes about people being crazy or nuts, even though we know that we shouldn't. We have all had some exposure to mental illness, but do we really understand it or know what it is? Many of our preconceptions are incorrect. A mental illness can be defined as a health condition that changes a person's thinking, feelings, or behavior (or all three) and that causes the person distress and difficulty in functioning. As with many diseases, mental illness is severe in some cases and mild in others. Individuals who have a mental illness don't necessarily look like they are sick, especially if their illness is mild. Other individuals may show more explicit symptoms such as confusion, agitation, or withdrawal. There are many different mental illnesses, including depression, schizophrenia, attention deficit hyperactivity disorder (ADHD), autism, and obsessive-compulsive disorder. Each illness alters a person's thoughts, feelings, and/or behaviors in distinct ways. In this chapter, we will discuss mental illness in general terms. Depression, schizophrenia, and ADHD will be presented in greater detail than other mental illnesses.

Not all brain diseases are categorized as mental illnesses. Disorders such as epilepsy, Parkinson disease, and multiple sclerosis are brain disorders, but they are considered neurological diseases rather than mental illnesses. Interestingly, the lines between mental illnesses and these other brain or neurological disorders is blurring somewhat. As scientists continue to investigate the brains of people who have mental illnesses, they are learning that mental illness is associated with changes in the brain's structure, chemistry, and function and that mental illness does indeed have a biological basis. This ongoing research is, in some ways, causing scientists to minimize the distinctions between mental illnesses and these other brain disorders. In this curriculum supplement, we will restrict our discussion of mental illness to those illnesses that are traditionally classified as mental illnesses.

Mental Illness In The Population

Many people feel that mental illness is rare, something that only happens to people with life situations very different from their own, and that it will never affect them. Studies of the epidemiology of mental illness indicate that this belief is far from accurate. In fact, the surgeon general reports that mental illnesses are so common that few U.S. families are untouched by them.

Mental Illness In Children And Adolescents

Mental illness is not uncommon among children and adolescents. Approximately 12 million children under the age of 18 have mental disorders. The National Mental Health Association has compiled some statistics about mental illness in children and adolescents:

- Mental health problems affect one in every five young people at any given time.

- An estimated two-thirds of all young people with mental health problems are not receiving the help they need.

- Less than one-third of the children under age 18 who have a serious mental health problem receive any mental health services.

- As many as one in every 33 children may be depressed. Depression in adolescents may be as high as one in eight.

- Suicide is the third leading cause of death for 15- to 24-years-olds and the sixth leading cause of death for 5- to 15-year-olds.

- Schizophrenia is rare in children under age 12, but it occurs in about three of every 1,000 adolescents.

- Between 118,700 and 186,600 youths in the juvenile justice system have at least one mental illness.

- Of the 100,000 teenagers in juvenile detention, an estimated 60 percent have behavioral, cognitive, or emotional problems.

Warning Signs For Mental Illness

Each mental illness has its own characteristic symptoms. However, there are some general warning signs that might alert you that someone needs professional help. Some of these signs include:

- A marked personality change

- An inability to cope with problems and daily activities

- Strange or grandiose ideas

- Excessive anxieties

- Prolonged depression and apathy

- Marked changes in eating or sleeping patterns

- Thinking or talking about suicide or harming oneself

- Extreme mood swings—high or low

- Abuse of alcohol or drugs

- Excessive anger, hostility, or violent behavior

A person who shows any of these signs should seek help from a qualified health professional.

Diagnosing Mental Illness

Mental Health Professionals

To be diagnosed with a mental illness, a person must be evaluated by a qualified professional who has expertise in mental health. Mental health professionals include psychiatrists, psychologists, psychiatric nurses, social workers, and mental health counselors. Family doctors, internists, and pediatricians are usually qualified to diagnose common mental disorders such as depression, anxiety disorders, and attention deficit hyperactivity disorder (ADHD). In many cases, depending on the individual and his or her symptoms, a mental health professional who is not a psychiatrist will refer the patient to a psychiatrist. A psychiatrist is a medical doctor (MD) who has received additional training in the field of mental health and mental illnesses. Psychiatrists evaluate the person's mental condition in coordination with his or her physical condition and can prescribe medication. Only psychiatrists and other MDs can prescribe medications to treat mental illness.

Mental Illnesses Are Diagnosed By Symptoms

Unlike some disease diagnoses, doctors can't do a blood test or culture some microorganisms to determine whether a person has a mental illness. Maybe scientists will develop discrete physiological tests for mental illnesses in the future; until then, however, mental health professionals will have to diagnose mental illnesses based on the symptoms that a person has. Basing a diagnosis on symptoms and not on a quantitative medical test, such as a blood chemistry test, a throat swab, X-rays, or urinalysis, is not unusual. Physicians diagnose many diseases, including migraines, Alzheimer disease, and Parkinson disease based on their symptoms alone. For other diseases, such as asthma or mononucleosis, doctors rely on analyzing symptoms to get a good idea of what the problem is and then use a physiological test to provide additional information or to confirm their diagnosis.

When a mental health professional works with a person who might have a mental illness, he or she will, along with the individual, determine what symptoms the individual has, how long the symptoms have persisted, and how his or her life is being affected. Mental health professionals often gather information through an interview during which they ask the patient about his or her symptoms, the length of time that the symptoms have occurred, and the severity of the symptoms. In many cases, the professional will also get information about the patient from family members to obtain a more comprehensive picture. A physician likely will conduct a physical exam and consult the patient's history to rule out other health problems.

Mental health professionals evaluate symptoms to make a diagnosis of mental illness. They rely on the criteria specified in the *Diagnostic and Statistical Manual of Mental Disorders* (*DSM-5* currently, the fifth edition), published by the American Psychiatric Association, to diagnose a specific mental illness. For each mental illness, the *DSM-5* gives a general description of the disorder and a list of typical symptoms. Mental health professionals refer to the *DSM-5* to confirm that the symptoms a patient exhibits match those of a specific mental illness. Although the *DSM-5* provides valuable information that helps mental health professionals diagnose mental illness, they realize it is important to observe patients over a period of time to understand the individual's mental illness and its effects on his or her life.

Mental Illness And The Brain

The term mental illness clearly indicates that there is a problem with the mind. But is it just the mind in an abstract sense, or is there a physical basis to mental illness? As scientists continue to investigate mental illnesses and their causes, they learn more and more about how the biological processes that make the brain work are changed when a person has a mental illness.

The Basics Of Brain Function

Before thinking about the problems that occur in the brain when someone has a mental illness, it is helpful to think about how the brain functions normally. The brain is an incredibly complex organ. It makes up only two percent of our body weight, but it consumes 20 percent of the oxygen we breathe and 20 percent of the energy we take in. It controls virtually everything we as humans experience, including movement, sensing our environment, regulating our involuntary body processes (such as breathing), and controlling our emotions. Hundreds of thousands of chemical reactions occur every second in the brain; those reactions underlie the thoughts, actions, and behaviors with which we respond to environmental stimuli. In short, the brain dictates the internal processes and behaviors that allow us to survive.

How does the brain take in all this information, process it, and cause a response? The basic functional unit of the brain is the neuron. A neuron is a specialized cell that can produce different actions because of its precise connections with other neurons, sensory receptors, and muscle cells. Neurons communicate using both electrical signals and chemical messages.

The nervous system uses a variety of neurotransmitter molecules, but each neuron specializes in the synthesis and secretion of a single type of neurotransmitter. Some of the predominant neurotransmitters in the brain include glutamate, gamma-aminobutyric acid (GABA), serotonin, dopamine, and norepinephrine. Each of these neurotransmitters has a specific distribution and function in the brain.

Investigating Brain Function

Mental health professionals base their diagnosis and treatment of mental illness on the symptoms that a person exhibits. The goal for these professionals in treating a patient is to relieve the symptoms that are interfering with the person's life so that the person can function well. Research scientists, on the other hand, have a different goal. They want to learn about the chemical or structural changes that occur in the brain when someone has a mental illness. If scientists can determine what happens in the brain, they can use that knowledge to develop better treatments or find a cure.

The techniques that scientists use to investigate the brain depend on the questions they are asking. For some questions, scientists use molecular or biochemical methods to investigate specific genes or proteins in the neurons. For other questions, scientists want to visualize changes in the brain so that they can learn more about how the activity or structure of the brain changes. Historically, scientists could examine brains only after death, but new imaging procedures enable scientists to study the brain in living animals, including humans. It is important to realize that these brain imaging techniques are not used for diagnosing mental illness. Mental illnesses are diagnosed by the set of symptoms that an individual exhibits. Scientists believe that mental illnesses result from problems with the communication system in the brain.

The Causes Of Mental Illnesses

At this time, scientists do not have a complete understanding of what causes mental illnesses. If you think about the structural and organizational complexity of the brain together with the complexity of effects that mental illnesses have on thoughts, feelings, and behaviors, it is hardly surprising that figuring out the causes of mental illnesses is a daunting task. The fields of neuroscience, psychiatry, and psychology address different aspects of the relationship between the biology of the brain and individuals' behaviors, thoughts, and feelings, and how their actions sometimes get out of control. Through this multidisciplinary research, scientists are trying to find the causes of mental illnesses. Once scientists can determine the causes of a mental illness, they can use that knowledge to develop new treatments or to find a cure.

The Biology Of Mental Illnesses

Most scientists believe that mental illnesses result from problems with the communication between neurons in the brain (neurotransmission). For example, the level of the neurotransmitter serotonin is lower in individuals who have depression. This finding led to the development of certain medications for the illness. Selective serotonin reuptake inhibitors (SSRIs) work by reducing the amount of serotonin that is taken back into the presynaptic neuron. This leads to an increase in the amount of serotonin available in the synaptic space for binding to the receptor on the postsynaptic neuron. Changes in other neurotransmitters (in addition to serotonin) may occur in depression, thus adding to the complexity of the cause underlying the disease.

Scientists believe that there may be disruptions in the neurotransmitters dopamine, glutamate, and norepinephrine in individuals who have schizophrenia. One indication that dopamine might be an important neurotransmitter in schizophrenia comes from the observation that cocaine addicts sometimes show symptoms similar to schizophrenia. Cocaine acts on dopamine-containing neurons in the brain to increase the amount of dopamine in the synapse.

Risk Factors For Mental Illnesses

Although scientists at this time do not know the causes of mental illnesses, they have identified factors that put individuals at risk. Some of these factors are environmental, some are genetic, and some are social. In fact, all these factors most likely combine to influence whether someone becomes mentally ill.

Environmental factors such as head injury, poor nutrition, and exposure to toxins (including lead and tobacco smoke) can increase the likelihood of developing a mental illness.

Genes also play a role in determining whether someone develops a mental illness. The illnesses that are most likely to have a genetic component include autism, bipolar disorder, schizophrenia, and ADHD. For example, the observation that children with ADHD are much more likely to have a sibling or parent with ADHD supports a role for genetics in determining whether someone is at risk for ADHD. In studies of twins, ADHD is significantly more likely to be present in an identical twin than a fraternal twin. The same can be said for schizophrenia and depression. Mental illnesses are not triggered by a change in a single gene; scientists believe that the interaction of several genes may trigger mental illness. Furthermore, the combination of genetic, environmental, and social factors might determine whether a case of mental illness is mild or severe.

Social factors also present risks and can harm an individual's, especially a child's, mental health. Social factors include:

- Severe parental discord

- Death of a family member or close friend

- Parent's mental illness

- Parent's criminality

- Overcrowding

- Economic hardship

- Abuse

- Neglect

- Exposure to violence

Treating Mental Illnesses

At this time, most mental illnesses cannot be cured, but they can usually be treated effectively to minimize the symptoms and allow the individual to function in work, school, or social environments. To begin treatment, an individual needs to see a qualified mental health professional. The first thing that the doctor or other mental health professional will do is speak with the individual to find out more about his or her symptoms, how long the symptoms have lasted, and how the person's life is being affected. The physician will also do a physical examination to determine whether there are other health problems. For example, some symptoms (such as emotional swings) can be caused by neurological or hormonal problems associated with chronic illnesses such as heart disease, or they can be a side effect of certain medications. After the individual's overall health is evaluated and the condition diagnosed, the doctor will develop a treatment plan. Treatment can involve both medications and psychotherapy, depending on the disease and its severity.

Medications

Medications are often used to treat mental illnesses. Through television commercials and magazine advertisements, we are becoming more aware of those medications. To become fully effective, medications for treating mental illness must be taken for a few days or a few weeks. When a patient begins taking medication, it is important for a doctor to monitor the patient's health. If the medication causes undesirable side effects, the doctor may change the dose or switch to a different medication that produces fewer side effects. If the medication does not relieve the symptoms, the doctor may prescribe a different medication.

Sometimes, individuals who have a mental illness do not want to take their medications because of the side effects. It is important to remember that all medications have both positive and negative effects. For example, antibiotics have revolutionized treatment for some bacterial diseases. However, antibiotics often affect beneficial bacteria in the human body, leading to side effects such as nausea and diarrhea. Psychiatric drugs, like other medications, can alleviate symptoms of mental illness but can also produce unwanted side effects. People who take a medication to treat an illness, whether it is a mental illness or another disease, should work with their doctors to understand what medication they are taking, why they are taking it, how to take it, and what side effects to watch for.

Occasionally, the media reports stories in which the side effects of a psychiatric medication are tied to a potentially serious consequence, such as suicide. In these cases, it is usually very difficult to determine how much suicidal behavior was due to the mental disorder and what the role of the medication might have been. Medications for treating mental illness can, like other medications, have side effects. The psychiatrist or physician can usually adjust the dose or change the medication to alleviate side effects.

Psychotherapy

Psychotherapy is a treatment method in which a mental health professional (psychiatrist, psychologist, or other mental health professional) and the patient discuss problems and feelings. This discussion helps patients understand the basis of their problems and find solutions. Psychotherapy may take different forms. The therapy can help patients:

- Change thought or behavior patterns
- Understand how past experiences influence current behaviors
- Solve other problems in specific ways
- Learn illness self-management skills

Psychotherapy may occur between a therapist and an individual; a therapist and an individual and his or her family members; or a therapist and a group. Often, treatment for mental illness is most successful when psychotherapy is used in combination with medications. For severe mental illnesses, medication relieves the symptoms and psychotherapy helps individuals cope with their illness.

Just as there are no medications that can instantly cure mental illnesses, psychotherapy is not a one-time event. The amount of time a person spends in psychotherapy can range from a few visits to a few years, depending on the nature of the illness or problem. In general, the more severe the problem, the more lengthy the psychotherapy should be.

The Stigma Of Mental Illness

"The last great stigma of the twentieth century is the stigma of mental illness."—Tipper Gore, wife of the former U.S. Vice President

"Mentally ill people are nuts, crazy, wacko." "Mentally ill people are morally bad." "Mentally ill people are dangerous and should be locked in an asylum forever." "Mentally ill people need somebody to take care of them." How often have we heard comments like these or seen these types of portrayals in movies, television shows, or books? We may even be guilty of making comments like them ourselves. Is there any truth behind these portrayals, or is that negative view based on our ignorance and fear?

Stigmas are negative stereotypes about groups of people. Common stigmas about people who are mentally ill are:

- Individuals who have a mental illness are dangerous.
- Individuals who have a mental illness are irresponsible and can't make life decisions for themselves.
- People who have a mental illness are childlike and must be taken care of by parents or guardians.
- People who have a mental illness should just get over it.

Each of those preconceptions about people who have a mental illness is based on false information. Very few people who have a mental illness are dangerous to society. Most can hold jobs, attend school, and live independently. A person who has a mental illness cannot simply decide to get over it any more than someone who has a different chronic disease such as diabetes, asthma, or heart disease can. A mental illness, like those other diseases, is caused by a physical problem in the body.

Stigmas against individuals who have a mental illness lead to injustices, including discriminatory decisions regarding housing, employment, and education. Overcoming the stigmas commonly associated with mental illness is yet one more challenge that people who have a mental illness must face. Indeed, many people who successfully manage their mental illness report that the stigma they face is in many ways more disabling than the illness itself. The stigmatizing attitudes toward mental illness held by both the public and those who have a mental illness lead to feelings of shame and guilt, loss of self-esteem, social dependence, and a sense of isolation and hopelessness. One of the worst consequences of stigma is that people who are struggling with a mental illness may be reluctant to seek treatment that, in most cases, would significantly relieve their symptoms.

Providing accurate information is one way to reduce stigmas about mental illness. Advocacy groups protest stereotypes imposed upon those who are mentally ill. They demand that the media stop presenting inaccurate views of mental illness and that the public stops believing these negative views. A powerful way of countering stereotypes about mental illness occurs when members of the public meet people who are effectively managing a serious mental illness: holding jobs, providing for themselves, and living as good neighbors in a community. Interaction with people who have mental illnesses challenges a person's assumptions and changes a person's attitudes about mental illness.

Attitudes about mental illness are changing, although there is a long way to go before people accept that mental illness is a disease with a biological basis. A survey by the National Mental Health Association found that 55 percent of people who have never been diagnosed with depression recognize that depression is a disease and not something people should "snap out of." This is a substantial increase over the 38 percent of survey respondents in 1991 who recognized depression as a disease.

Chapter 6

Causes And Warning Signs Of Mental Illness

Like adults, adolescents can have mental health or substance use problems that interfere with the way they think, feel, and act. Such problems—if not addressed—may interfere with learning and the ability to form and sustain friendships, contribute to disciplinary problems and family conflicts, and increase risky behaviors.

Possible Causes Of Mental Illness

Serious mental health problems often are a factor in drug abuse and suicide. Early use of alcohol is a risk factor for developing alcohol problems; in addition, motor vehicle collisions related to teen alcohol use are among the most common causes of teen death.

Adolescents whose family members are living with conditions such as depression or other mental health disorders may have a higher risk of developing similar conditions. Youths with developmental disabilities and chronic medical conditions also can have a co-occurring mental health condition or can develop a substance use problem. For example, youths with asthma are at higher risk of developing depression than those who do not have asthma.

Adolescents who are questioning their sexual identity or becoming aware of the possibility that they may be gay, lesbian, bisexual, or transgender can be at high risk for certain mental health disorders and misuse of substances. Adolescents in the juvenile justice system—especially girls—have been found to have a very high incidence of mental health and substance abuse disorders.

About This Chapter: Excerpted from "Identifying Mental Health and Substance Use Problems of Children and Adolescents," Substance Abuse and Mental Health Services Administration (www.samhsa.gov), 2012.

Protective factors such as family stability, supportive and nurturing relationships, a strong community, and faith organizations can help prevent certain kinds of problems from developing in adolescents. These protective factors also can be a source of support that helps adolescents cope with mental health and substance use problems if such problems develop.

Stress and psychological trauma are among a number of environmental risk factors that can contribute to the development of mental health or substance use problems in adolescents and also can increase the severity of such problems. Psychological trauma occurs when a youth experiences an intense event that threatens or causes harm to his or her emotional and physical well-being. A range of physiological and psychological behaviors can provide signs that the youth is having difficulty dealing with a traumatic event. However, these reactions are the body's normal response when confronted by danger. Some adolescents who have experienced a traumatic event will have longer lasting reactions that can interfere with their physical and emotional health, such as:

- Adolescents in families that have experienced significant losses may face greater challenges to healthy development than those without such losses.

- Adolescents from poor families have increased rates of developmental problems, stress, and uncertainty, which—along with other factors associated with poverty—can trigger behavioral health problems.

- Psychological trauma can trigger mental health and substance use problems. Adolescents who have been abused or neglected are at a higher risk of having mental health or substance use problems.

- Adolescents who were exposed to chronic violence at home or in their communities or who experienced a natural disaster or school violence are at heightened risk for mental health or substance use problems.

The Value Of Early Identification

Caregivers are usually the first to recognize early signs of problems in their children. Medical providers, teachers, or direct care workers in children's programs also are well positioned to improve the identification of mental health and substance use problems among the adolescents they serve. Just as schools screen for vision and hearing problems before such problems interfere with learning, service providers can develop early identification programs for mental health and substance use problems.

As children grow older, events in their lives may put them at risk for various problems. For adolescents who show clear signs of a mental health or substance use problem, a discrete identification process may not be necessary; instead, these youths can be referred directly for assessment.

Caregivers and personnel serving children may find it helpful to learn some of the commons signs of mental health and substance use problems and use these signs to help evaluate whether a youth's behavior indicates possible problems that warrant further assessment.

Assessment

An assessment is conducted by a qualified, experienced mental health or substance abuse professional who gathers more information about the youth to determine whether an identified possible condition is, in fact, present. In addition to speaking with or observing the youth, the professional also should talk to parents or caregivers and—with the consent of parents or caregivers—to teachers or others who know the youth well. This step may involve determining whether a youth meets specific, defined criteria for a diagnosis according to a formal classification system in the *Diagnostic and Statistical Manual of Mental Disorders, 4th edition* (*DSM-IV*).

The professional also will collect information that is helpful in working with the child or adolescent and his or her family to develop a plan to address the problem. Because no screening or identification process is perfect, some children and adolescents may be incorrectly found to not have a mental health or substance use problem—when, in fact, they actually have one; or they incorrectly may be found to have a mental health or substance use problem when, in fact, they actually do not have one.

Intervention And/Or Treatment

The goal of identifying adolescents with a high likelihood of having mental health and substance use problems is to provide an appropriate intervention or to connect the youths and their families with assessment and treatment resources. Even when an organization can offer an intervention, it must be prepared for the possibility that a youth's problem may warrant additional, different, or more specialized services.

Methods To Identify Adolescents Who May Have Mental Illness

People who are not mental health or substance abuse professionals can employ two basic methods to identify children and adolescents who may have a mental health or substance use problem:

- Become familiar with signs of mental health and substance use problems
- Administer a scientifically validated screening tool

Become Familiar With Signs Of Mental Illness

Often, an adolescent's behavior or appearance can provide signs of a mental health or substance use problem. These signs warrant action by caregivers and adults who work with the youth and can reliably identify the indicators so that the problem is assessed further and the child or adolescent has the opportunity to receive appropriate treatment.

Signs of some problems—such as depression, bulimia, or early stages of substance use—either may be actively concealed from adults or may not be readily apparent. Research has shown that these types of problems are difficult to identify. The National Institute of Mental Health (NIMH) and the Substance Abuse and Mental Health Services Administration (SAMHSA) sponsored a research group of scientists and physicians to identify signs that indicate the need to take action and address mental health conditions in adolescents.

Higher risk populations among adolescents can be identified in a number of ways. Here are some common examples of their attributes:

- **Behavior Or Functioning:** Adolescents may demonstrate disciplinary problems; declining academic performance; or a marked change in behavior, mood, or functioning. However, some behavior signs are subtle and easily missed.

- **Illnesses Or Disabilities:** Adolescents with certain health problems are at higher risk for depression and other mental health problems. Adolescents serving as caretakers for ill or disabled parents or caregivers also are at high risk.

- **Environmental Stress:** Adolescents living in a community with a high rate of poverty or violence are at increased risk of being identified with problems such as substance use or suicide, as compared to adolescents in other communities.

Identification Is Not Diagnosis

The goal in identifying adolescents with possible mental health or substance use problems is to provide the option for further assessment. Such identification does not involve reaching a diagnosis of a particular condition. Only mental health, substance abuse, or medical professionals (as determined by each state's licensing laws) are qualified to make a diagnosis. Neither action signs nor screening tools provide sufficient information to reach a diagnosis.

Source: SAMSHA, 2012.

- **High-Risk Life Situations:** Adolescents—particularly those who were prenatally exposed to drugs and alcohol—who come to the attention of child welfare systems or who are in homeless or domestic violence shelters are at high risk for mental health and substance use problems. Adolescents involved with the juvenile justice system also are associated with a much higher risk of mental health and substance use problems than adolescents in the general population.

- **Stressful Events:** Stressful events or transitions that are the result of becoming homeless or entering into the child welfare system or juvenile detention involve significant losses and create considerable uncertainty for children and adolescents. Already vulnerable, these youths become even more so. Others caring for these adolescents not only must safeguard the individual from harming himself or herself but also must ensure that the youth does not harm others.

- **Traumatic Events:** Adolescents not otherwise at risk may be exposed to an incident of violence or a natural disaster that warrants an effort to identify those who need assistance.

- **Age Groups:** Certain ages or developmental stages might be prioritized for identification because of the high value of identifying problems or the low likelihood that problems will be identified elsewhere. For example, screening preschool children presents an early opportunity for intervention and has great value in preventing a problem or minimizing its impact on the child's future school performance and overall functioning. Screening teens in high school—a time when they no longer may see a primary care physician on a regular basis—has the potential to identify problems less likely to be identified elsewhere. Natural but stressful events associated with specific ages, such as the transition from elementary to middle school, also present potentially useful points of intervention.

- **Sexual Orientation:** Adolescents questioning their sexual orientation or gender identity and those who identify as gay, lesbian, bisexual, transgender, queer, intersex, or two-spirit may have an elevated risk of mental health and substance use problems.

Administer A Scientifically Validated Screening Tool

The specific questions (items) included in a validated screening tool were tested on a large number of youths and were found to most accurately identify adolescents with a high likelihood of having mental health or substance use problems. Because different conditions are prone to arise at different stages of development or manifest differently at different ages, screening tools are designed for specific age ranges. Different tools or versions of a tool have been designed and tested to identify different conditions and to be answered by different informants. Informants can be physicians, parents or other caregivers, teachers, or other child service providers who are able to observe the youth; the informant also can be the adolescent if he or she is able to understand and answer the questions.

A number of studies have shown that such screening tools are better than the interviewing process used by primary care physicians or a clinical assessment conducted by mental health clinicians at identifying children and adolescents with mental health and substance use problems. The research results for the tested tools indicate the rate and type of problems found in different populations. Screening tools are the best brief method available for those who are not mental health or substance abuse professionals to identify adolescents at risk of mental health and substance use problems; but, like any medical test, no screening tool is correct all of the time.

Part Two
Mood And Anxiety Disorders

Chapter 7

Depression

Depression can occur during adolescence, a time of great personal change. You may be facing changes in where you go to school, your friends, your after-school activities, as well as in relationships with your family members. You may have different feelings about the type of person you want to be, your future plans, and may be making decisions for the first time in your life.

Many students don't know where to go for mental health treatment or believe that treatment won't help. Others don't get help because they think depression symptoms are just part of the typical stresses of school or being a teen. Some students worry what other people will think if they seek mental health care.

This chapter addresses common questions about depression and how it can affect high school students.

What is depression?

Depression is a common but serious mental illness typically marked by sad or anxious feelings. Most students occasionally feel sad or anxious, but these emotions usually pass quickly—within a couple of days. Untreated depression lasts for a long time and interferes with your day-to-day activities.

What are the symptoms of depression?

Different people experience different symptoms of depression. If you are depressed, you may feel:

About This Chapter: Excerpted from "Depression and High School Students," National Institute of Mental Health (www.nimh.nih.gov), 2012.

- Sad

- Anxious

- Empty

- Hopeless

- Guilty

- Worthless

- Helpless

- Irritable

- Restless

You may also experience one or more of the following symptoms:

- Loss of interest in activities you used to enjoy

- Lack of energy

- Problems concentrating, remembering information, or making decisions

- Problems falling sleep, staying asleep, or sleeping too much

- Loss of appetite or eating too much

- Thoughts of suicide or suicide attempts

- Aches, pains, headaches, cramps, or digestive problems that do not go away

Depression in adolescence frequently co-occurs with other disorders such as anxiety, disruptive behavior, eating disorders, or substance abuse. It can also lead to increased risk for suicide.

Are there different types of depression?

Yes. The most common depressive disorders are:

- **Major Depressive Disorder:** Also called major depression, the symptoms of major depressive disorder are disabling and interfere with everyday activities such as studying, eating, and sleeping. People with this disorder may have only one episode of major depression in their lifetimes. But more often, depression comes back repeatedly.

- **Dysthymic Disorder:** Also called dysthymia, dysthymic disorder is mild, chronic depression. The symptoms of dysthymia last for a long time—2 years or more. Dysthymia is less severe than major depression, but it can still interfere with everyday activities.

People with dysthymia may also experience one or more episodes of major depression during their lifetimes.

• **Minor Depression:** Similar to major depression and dysthymia, symptoms of minor depression are less severe and/or are usually shorter term. Without treatment, however, people with minor depression are at high risk for developing major depressive disorder.

Study Reveals New Clues To How Depression May Develop

Depression is one of the most studied mental disorders, with research honing in on brain structures, circuits, and biochemical processes critical to the development of the disorder. Many questions remain, however, about how changes in the brain result in the symptoms and behaviors associated with depression.

To advance the science in this area, researchers explored the role and connectivity of neurons in the lateral habenula (LHb) in rats that showed learned helplessness (a set of behaviors similar to symptoms of depression in people). The LHb is associated with how humans and animals experience disappointment or anticipate negative outcomes.

The researchers found that LHb neurons receive input from many different brain regions involved in responding to stress. LHb neurons also connect out to many brain regions, such as the ventral tegmental area (VTA), which helps to control reward-seeking behavior and may have a role in depression and other mood disorders.

LHb neurons in helpless rats were more responsive, such that communication signals to the VTA were more likely to be transmitted in the helpless rats than in control rats. In an attempt to moderate this phenomenon, the researchers tested the effects of deep brain stimulation (DBS), a surgical procedure currently being tested in humans for treatment-resistant depression. Applying continuous electrical stimulation directly to the LHb resulted in greatly reduced transmission to the VTA and a marked reduction in helpless behavior. The effects on transmission lasted only as long as the stimulation lasted. More intense stimulation resulted in stronger behavioral effects.

Although LHb activity was previously unstudied in the context of mood disorders, these findings suggest that this brain structure may actually play a central role in the development of depression.

Further studies focusing on the molecular processes and signals underlying LHb activity in depression may reveal new targets for treatment development, according to the researchers. Such new treatments also may be able to reverse some forms of depressive disorders.

Source: Excerpted from "Study Reveals New Clues to How Depression May Develop," National Institutes of Mental Health (www.nimh.nih.gov), February 2013.

Other types of depression include:

- **Psychotic Depression:** Severe depression accompanied by some form of psychosis, such as hallucinations and delusions.

- **Seasonal Affective Disorder:** Depression that begins during the winter months and lifts during spring and summer.

What causes depression?

Depression does not have a single cause. Several factors can lead to depression. Some people carry genes that increase their risk of depression. But not all people with depression have these genes, and not all people with these genes have depression. Environment—your surroundings and life experiences—also affects your risk for depression. Any stressful situation may trigger depression. And high school students encounter a number of stressful situations.

How can I find out if I have depression?

The first step is to talk with your parents or a trusted adult who can help you make an appointment to speak with a doctor or mental health care provider. Your family doctor or school counselor may also be able to help you find appropriate care.

The doctor or mental health care provider can do an exam to help determine if you have depression or if you have another health or mental health problem. Some medical conditions or medications can produce symptoms similar to depression. The doctor or mental health care provider will ask you about:

- Your symptoms
- Your history of depression
- Your family's history of depression
- Your medical history
- Alcohol or drug use
- Any thoughts of death or suicide

How is depression treated?

A number of very effective treatments for depression are available. The most common treatments are antidepressants and psychotherapy. A clinical trial of 439 teens with major depression, funded by National Institute of Mental Health (NIMH), found that a combination of medication and psychotherapy was the most effective treatment option. A doctor or mental health care provider can help you find the treatment that's right for you.

What are antidepressants?

Antidepressants work on brain chemicals called neurotransmitters, especially serotonin and norepinephrine. Other antidepressants work on the neurotransmitter dopamine. Scientists have found that these particular chemicals are involved in regulating mood, but they are unsure of the exact ways that they work.

If a doctor prescribes an antidepressant, how long will I have to take it?

You will need to take regular doses of antidepressants for 4–6 weeks before you feel the full effect of these medicines. Some people need to take antidepressants for a short time. If your depression is long lasting or comes back again and again, you may need to take antidepressants longer.

What is psychotherapy?

Psychotherapy involves talking with a mental health care professional to treat a mental illness. Types of psychotherapy that have been shown to be effective in treating depression include:

- **Cognitive-Behavioral Therapy (CBT),** which helps people change negative styles of thinking and behavior that may contribute to depression
- **Interpersonal Therapy (IPT),** which helps people understand and work through troubled personal relationships that may cause or worsen depression.

Depending on the type and severity of your depression, a mental health professional may recommend short-term therapy, lasting 10–20 weeks, or longer-term therapy.

How can I help myself if I am depressed?

If you have depression, you may feel exhausted, helpless, and hopeless. But it is important to realize that these feelings are part of the depression and do not reflect your real circumstances. Treatment can help you feel better. To help yourself feel better:

- Give treatment a fair chance—attend sessions and follow your doctor's or therapist's advice, including advice about specific exercises or "homework" to try between appointments.
- Engage in mild physical activity or exercise.

- Participate in activities that you used to enjoy.

- Break up large projects into smaller tasks and do what you can.

- Spend time with or call your friends and family.

- Expect your mood to improve gradually with treatment.

Remember that positive thinking will replace negative thoughts as your depression responds to treatment.

How can I help a friend who is depressed?

If you think a friend may have depression, you can help him or her get diagnosed and treated. Make sure he or she talks to an adult and gets evaluated by a doctor or mental health provider. If your friend seems unable or unwilling to seek help, offer to go with him or her and tell your friend that his or her health and safety is important to you.

Encourage your friend to stay in treatment or seek a different treatment if he or she does not begin to feel better after 6–8 weeks. You can also:

- Offer emotional support, understanding, patience, and encouragement.

- Talk to your friend, not necessarily about depression, and listen carefully.

- Never discount the feelings your friend expresses, but point out realities and offer hope.

- Never ignore comments about suicide.

- Report comments about suicide to your friend's parents, therapist, or doctor.

- Invite your friend out for walks, outings, and other activities—keep trying if your friend declines, but don't push him or her to take on too much too soon.

- Remind your friend that with time and treatment, the depression will lift.

What if I or someone I know is in crisis?

If you are thinking about harming yourself or having thoughts of suicide, or if you know someone who is, seek help right away.

- Call your doctor or mental health care provider.

- Call 911 or go to a hospital emergency room to get immediate help, or ask a friend or family member to help you do these things.

- Call your campus suicide or crisis hotline.

- Call the National Suicide Prevention Lifeline's toll-free, 24-hour hotline at 1-800-273-TALK (1-800-273-8255) or TTY: 1-800-799-4TTY (1-800-799-4889) to talk to a trained counselor.

- If you are in crisis, make sure you are not left alone.

- If someone else is in crisis, make sure he or she is not left alone.

What efforts are underway to help high school students who have depression?

Researchers continue to study new ways to diagnose and treat depression in high school age students. Some scientists are also looking into different ways to classify symptoms, which may provide new clues about how the disorder develops and which treatments are most effective. Increasing the early detection and treatment of depression can help more students succeed academically and achieve their goals in school and after graduation.

You can find more information about the causes, diagnosis, and treatment of depression, including research related to adolescents and young adults, on the National Institute of Mental Health (NIMH) website (http://www.nimh.nih.gov/health/topics/depression/index.shtml). You can also connect with NIMH through social media:

- NIMH Facebook: http://www.facebook.com/nimhgov

- NIMH Twitter: http://twitter.com/nimhgov

- NIMH YouTube: http://www.youtube.com/nimhgov

Chapter 8

Premenstrual Syndrome And Premenstrual Dysphoric Disorder

Premenstrual dysphoric disorder (PMDD) is a condition in which a woman has severe depression symptoms, irritability, and tension before menstruation. The symptoms of PMDD are more severe than those seen with premenstrual syndrome (PMS).

PMS refers to a wide range of physical or emotional symptoms that typically occur about 5–11 days before a woman starts her monthly menstrual cycle. The symptoms usually stop when, or shortly after, her period begins.

Causes

The causes of PMS and PMDD have not been found. Hormone changes that occur during a woman's menstrual cycle may play a role. PMDD affects between 3% and 8% of women during the years when they are having menstrual periods. Many women with this condition have:

- Anxiety
- Severe depression
- Seasonal affective disorder (SAD)

Other factors that may play a role include:

- Alcohol abuse
- Being overweight

About This Chapter: Information in this chapter is from "Premenstrual Dysphoric Disorder, © 2013 A.D.A.M., Inc. Reprinted with permission.

- Drinking large amounts of caffeine

- Having a mother with a history of the disorder

- Lack of exercise

Symptoms

The symptoms of PMDD are similar to those of PMS. However, they are generally more severe and debilitating and include a least one mood-related symptom. Symptoms occur during the week just before menstrual bleeding and usually improve within a few days after the period starts.

Five or more of the following symptoms must be present to diagnose PMDD, including one mood-related symptom:

- No interest in daily activities and relationships

- Fatigue or low energy

- Feeling of sadness or hopelessness, possible suicidal thoughts

- Feelings of tension or anxiety

- Feeling out of control

- Food cravings or binge eating

- Mood swings with periods of crying

- Panic attacks

- Irritability or anger that affects other people

- Physical symptoms, such as bloating, breast tenderness, headaches, and joint or muscle pain

- Problems sleeping

- Trouble concentrating

Exams And Tests

No physical examination or lab tests can diagnose PMDD. A complete history, physical examination (including a pelvic exam), and psychiatric evaluation should be done to rule out other conditions.

Keeping a calendar or diary of symptoms can help women identify the most troublesome symptoms and the times when they are likely to occur. This information may help the health care provider diagnose PMDD and determine the best treatment.

Treatment

A healthy lifestyle is the first step to managing PMDD. Eat healthy foods with more whole grains, vegetables, fruit, and little or no salt, sugar, alcohol, and caffeine [and] get regular aerobic exercise throughout the month to reduce the severity of PMS symptoms. If you have problems sleeping, try changing your sleep habits before taking medicines for insomnia.

Keep a diary or calendar to record the type of symptoms you are having, how severe they are, [and] how long they last.

Antidepressants may be helpful. The first option is usually an antidepressant known as a selective serotonin-reuptake inhibitor (SSRI). You can take SSRIs in the second part of your cycle up until your period starts, or for the whole month. Ask your doctor.

Cognitive behavioral therapy (CBT) may be used either with, or instead of, antidepressants. During CBT, you have about 10 visits with a mental health professional over several weeks. Other treatments that may help include:

- Birth control pills may decrease or increase PMS symptoms, including depression.
- Diuretics may be useful for women who gain a lot of weight from fluid retention.
- Nutritional supplements—such as vitamin B6, calcium, and magnesium—may be recommended.
- Other medicines (such as Depo-Lupron) suppress the ovaries and ovulation.
- Pain relievers such as aspirin or ibuprofen may be prescribed for headache, backache, menstrual cramping, and breast tenderness.

Outlook (Prognosis)

After proper diagnosis and treatment, most women with PMDD find that their symptoms go away or drop to tolerable levels.

Possible Complications

PMDD symptoms may be severe enough to interfere with a woman's daily life. Women with depression may have worse symptoms during the second half of their cycle and may need changes in their medication.

Some women with PMDD have had suicidal thoughts. Suicide in women with depression is more likely to occur during the second half of the menstrual cycle.

PMDD may be associated with eating disorders and smoking.

When To Contact A Medical Professional

Call 911 or a local crisis line right away if you are having thoughts of suicide. Call for an appointment with your health care provider if symptoms do not improve with self-treatment [and/or] symptoms interfere with your daily life.

Alternative Names

PMDD; Severe PMS

Chapter 9

Seasonal Affective Disorder

What is seasonal affective disorder (SAD)?

The symptoms of depression are very common. Some people experience these only at times of stress, while others may experience them regularly at certain times of the year. Seasonal affective disorder (SAD) is characterized by recurrent episodes of depression, usually in late fall and winter, alternating with periods of normal or high mood the rest of the year.

Whether SAD is a distinct mental illness or a specific type of major depressive disorder is a topic of debate in the scientific literature. Researchers at the National Institute of Mental Health (NIMH) first posited [theorized] the condition [was] a response to decreased light, and pioneered the use of bright light to address the symptoms. It has been suggested that women are more likely to have this illness than men and that SAD is less likely in older individuals. SAD can also occur in children and adolescents.

Scientists have identified that the neurotransmitter serotonin may not be working optimally in many patients with SAD. The role of hormones and sleep-wake cycles (called circadian rhythms) during the changing seasons is still being studied in people with SAD. Some studies have also shown that SAD is more common in people who live in northern latitudes.

What are the patterns of SAD?

In SAD, the seasonal variation in mood states is the key factor to understand. Symptoms of SAD usually begin in October or November and subside in March or April. Some patients

About This Chapter: Excerpted from "Seasonal Affective Disorder (SAD) Fact Sheet," December 2012, © NAMI, the National Alliance on Mental Illness, www.nami.org.

begin to "slump" as early as August, while others remain well until January. Regardless of the time of onset, most patients don't feel fully "back to normal" until early May.

Depressions are usually mild to moderate, but they can be severe. Treatment planning needs to match the severity of the condition for the individual. Although some individuals do not necessarily show these symptoms, the classic characteristics of recurrent winter depression include oversleeping, daytime fatigue, carbohydrate craving, and weight gain. Additionally, many people may experience other features of depression including decreased sexual interest, lethargy, hopelessness, suicidal thoughts, lack of interest in normal activities, and decreased socialization.

In a minority of cases, symptoms occur in the summer rather than winter. During that period, the depression is more likely to be characterized by insomnia, decreased appetite, weight loss, and agitation or anxiety. In still fewer cases, a patient may experience both winter and summer depressions, while feeling fine each fall and spring, around the equinoxes. Many people with SAD also report that their depression worsens or reappears whenever there is "less light around."

Some people with bipolar disorder can also have seasonal changes in their mood and experience acute episodes in a recurrent fashion at different times of the year.

How is SAD treated?

Many people with SAD will find that their symptoms respond to a very specific treatment called light therapy. For people who are not severely depressed and are unable—or unwilling—to use antidepressant medications, light therapy may be the best initial treatment. Light therapy consists of regular, daily exposure to a "light box," which artificially simulates high-intensity sunlight. Practically, this means that a person will spend approximately 30 minutes sitting in front of this device shortly after they awaken in the morning. Side effects of light therapy are uncommon and usually reversible when the intensity of light therapy is decreased. The most commonly experienced side effects include irritability, eyestrain, headaches, nausea, and fatigue.

Scientific studies have shown light therapy to be effective when compared to placebo and as effective as antidepressants in many cases of non-severe SAD. Light therapy may also work faster than antidepressants for some people, with notable effects beginning with in a few days of starting treatment. Other people may find that it takes a few weeks. Antidepressant medications have also been found to be useful in treating people with SAD.

Some people may require treatment of their symptoms only for the period of the year in which they experience symptoms. Other people may elect for year-round treatment or prophylactic [preventative] treatment that begins prior to the onset of the season in which their symptoms are most severe. This is yet another reason to discuss treatment options with one's physicians. While not explicitly studied for the treatment of SAD, psychotherapy, such as cognitive behavioral therapy (CBT), is likely a useful additional option.

What should I do if I think I have SAD?

Any person experiencing significant symptoms of depression should feel comfortable discussing their concerns with their doctors. Some primary care doctors (e.g., pediatricians and general practitioners) may be experienced in treating SAD and will feel comfortable treating this illness. Other doctors may want to refer people with SAD to a psychiatrist for treatment of this illness. This is more common in people with complex psychiatric illnesses or more severe symptoms. Before starting any treatment for SAD, a person should make sure to meet with their doctor to discuss the benefits and risks of treatment. Friends and family members of people with SAD may be appropriately concerned for the well-being of their loved one.

Chapter 10

Bipolar Disorder

In the last decade, the number of children receiving the diagnosis of bipolar disorder, sometimes, called manic-depressive illness, has grown substantially. But what does the diagnosis really mean for a teen? This chapter discusses bipolar disorder in children and teens.

What is bipolar disorder?

Bipolar disorder, also known as manic-depressive illness, is a brain disorder that causes unusual shifts in mood, energy, and activity levels. It can also make it hard to carry out day-to-day tasks, such as going to school or hanging out with friends. Symptoms of bipolar disorder can be severe. They are different from the normal ups and downs that everyone goes through from time to time. Bipolar disorder symptoms can result in damaged relationships, poor school performance, and even suicide. But bipolar disorder can be treated, and many people with this illness can lead full and productive lives.

Symptoms of bipolar disorder often develop in the late teens or early adult years, but some people have their first symptoms during childhood. At least half of all cases start before age 25.

Bipolar disorder tends to run in families. Children with a parent or sibling who has bipolar disorder are up to six times more likely to develop the illness, compared with children who do not have a family history of bipolar disorder. However, most children with a family history of bipolar disorder will not develop the illness.

About This Chapter: Excerpted from "Bipolar Disorder in Children and Adolescents," National Institute of Mental Health (www.nimh.nih.gov), 2012.

What are the signs and symptoms of bipolar disorder in adolescents?

Youth with bipolar disorder experience unusually intense emotional states that occur in distinct periods called "mood episodes." The extreme highs and lows of mood are accompanied by extreme changes in energy, activity, sleep, and behavior. Each mood episode represents a drastic change from a person's usual mood and behavior.

An overly joyful or overexcited state is called a manic episode. An extremely sad or hopeless state is called a depressive episode. Sometimes, a mood episode includes symptoms of both mania and depression. This is called a mixed state. People with bipolar disorder also may be explosive and irritable during a mood episode.

Symptoms of bipolar disorder are described in Table 10.1. It's normal for almost every child or teen to show some of these behaviors sometimes. These passing changes should not be confused with bipolar disorder.

Table 10.1. Symptoms Comparison: Bipolar Disorder And Depression

Mania Symptoms	**Depression Symptoms**
Mood Changes	*Mood Changes*
Being in an overly silly or joyful mood that's unusual (different from times when just being silly and having fun)	Being in a sad mood that lasts a long time
Having an extremely short temper and unusual irritability	Losing interest in activities once enjoyed
	Feeling worthless or guilty
Behavioral Changes	*Behavioral Changes*
Sleeping little but not feeling tired	Complaining about pain more often, such as headaches, stomach aches, and muscle pains
Talking a lot and having racing thoughts	Eating a lot more or less and gaining or losing a lot of weight
Having trouble concentrating or paying attention, jumping from one thing to the next in an unusual way	Sleeping or oversleeping when these were not problems before
Talking and thinking about sex more often than usual	Losing energy
Behaving in risky ways more often, seeking pleasure a lot, and doing more activities than usual	Recurring thoughts of death or suicide

Source: National Institute of Mental Health (www.nimh.nih.gov), 2012.

Symptoms of bipolar disorder are not like the normal changes in mood and energy that everyone has. Bipolar symptoms are more extreme and tend to last for most of the day, nearly every day, for at least one week. Also, depressive or manic episodes include moods very different from a child's normal mood, and the behaviors described in Table 10.1 generally all come on at the same time. Sometimes the symptoms of bipolar disorder are so severe that the child needs to be treated in a hospital.

Bipolar disorder can be present even when mood swings are less extreme. For example, sometimes a child may have more energy and be more active than normal, but not show the severe signs of a full-blown manic episode. This is called hypomania. It generally lasts for at least four days in a row. Hypomania causes noticeable changes in behavior, but does not harm a child's ability to function in the same way that mania does.

How does bipolar disorder affect adolescents differently than adults?

Bipolar disorder that starts during childhood or the early teen years is called early-onset bipolar disorder, and seems to be more severe than the forms that first appear in older teens and adults. Youth with bipolar disorder are different from adults with bipolar disorder. Young people with the illness appear to have more frequent mood switches, are sick more often, and have more mixed episodes.

Watch out for any sign of suicidal thinking or behaviors. Take these signs seriously. On average, people with early-onset bipolar disorder are at greater risk for attempting suicide than those whose symptoms start in adulthood. One large study on bipolar disorder in children and teens found that more than one-third of study participants made at least one serious suicide attempt. Some suicide attempts are carefully planned and others are not. Either way, it is important to understand that suicidal feelings and actions are symptoms of an illness that must be treated.

How is bipolar disorder detected in adolescents?

No blood tests or brain scans can diagnose bipolar disorder. However, a doctor or health care provider may use tests like these to help rule out other possible causes for a child's symptoms. In addition, they may recommend testing for problems in learning, thinking, or speech and language. A careful medical exam may also detect problems that commonly co-occur with bipolar disorder and need to be treated, such as substance abuse.

Health care professionals who have experience with diagnosing early-onset bipolar disorder will ask questions about changes in your mood. They will also ask about sleep patterns, activity or energy levels, and if you have had any other mood or behavioral disorders. They may also ask whether there is a family history of bipolar disorder or other psychiatric illnesses, such as depression or alcoholism.

Doctors diagnose bipolar disorder using guidelines from the *Diagnostic and Statistical Manual of Mental Disorders* (*DSM*). To be diagnosed, the symptoms must be a major change from the teen's normal mood or behavior. There are four basic types of bipolar disorder:

- **Bipolar I Disorder:** This type is defined by manic or mixed episodes that last at least seven days, or by manic symptoms that are so severe that the person needs immediate hospital care. Usually, depressive episodes occur as well, typically lasting at least two weeks.

- **Bipolar II Disorder:** This type is defined by a pattern of depressive episodes shifting back and forth with hypomanic episodes, but no full-blown manic or mixed episodes.

- **Bipolar Disorder Not Otherwise Specified (BP-NOS):** BP-NOS is diagnosed when a person has symptoms of the illness that do not meet diagnostic criteria for either bipolar I or II. However, the symptoms are clearly out of the person's normal range of behavior.

- **Cyclothymic Disorder:** Cyclothymic disorder, which is also called cyclothymia, is a mild form of bipolar disorder. People with cyclothymia have episodes of hypomania as well as mild depression for at least two years. However, the symptoms do not meet the diagnostic requirements for any other type of bipolar disorder.

When children have manic symptoms that last for less than four days, experts may diagnose BP-NOS. Some evidence indicates that many of these young people will develop longer episodes within a few years and then meet the criteria for bipolar I or II.

What illnesses often co-exist with bipolar disorder in adolescents?

People with bipolar disorder may develop other mental illnesses as well, including:

- **Alcoholism:** Adults with bipolar disorder are at very high risk of developing a substance abuse problem. Young people with bipolar disorder may have the same risk.

- **Attention-Deficit Hyperactivity Disorder (ADHD):** Mania and ADHD share some symptoms, such as distractibility, hyperactivity, and the tendency to engage in impulsive and risky behavior. However, mania is episodic, and the behaviors are uncharacteristic—starting at a [specific] time, with a dramatic change in mood. In contrast, ADHD symptoms are persistent and typical, although they may wax and wane to a certain degree. Many children with bipolar disorder also have a history of ADHD.

How does the rate of teen bipolar disorder symptoms compare adult symptoms?

The rate of bipolar symptoms among U.S. teens is nearly as high as the rate found among adults, according to research funded by National Institute of Mental Health (NIMH). Nationally representative data indicate that about 3.9 percent of adults meet criteria for bipolar disorder in their lifetime, but limited data exist on the rates of bipolar disorder among adolescents—despite strong evidence indicating that bipolar disorder tends to emerge in adolescence or early adulthood.

Recently, researchers analyzed data from the NIMH-funded National Comorbidity Survey-Adolescent Supplement (NCS-A), a nationally representative, face-to-face survey of more than 10,000 teens ages 13–18. Using criteria established by the *American Psychiatric Association's Diagnostic and Statistical Manual (DSM-IV)*, the researchers assessed teens for the hallmark symptoms of bipolar disorder—mania and depression. They also examined the rates of teens who showed evidence of mania alone.

The researchers found that 2.5 percent of youth met criteria for bipolar disorder in their lifetime and about 1.7 percent reported having mania alone within their lifetime. Researcher found that rates increased with age—about 2 percent of younger teens reported bipolar disorder symptoms, whereas 3.1 percent of older teens did.

These findings reveal that the prevalence of bipolar disorder in adolescents approaches that of adults, underscoring the widely held belief that the disorder first appears in youth. In addition, the presence of mania alone suggests that mania without depression should receive greater attention when evaluating mood disorders in teens, especially since it may precede or be associated with behavioral problems such as substance use disorders and attention deficit hyperactivity disorder, according to the researchers.

Source: Excerpted from "Science Update: Rate of Bipolar Symptoms Among Teens Approaches That of Adults," National Institute of Mental Health (www.nimh.nih.gov), June 2012.

- **Anxiety Disorder:** Anxiety disorders, such as separation anxiety and generalized anxiety disorder, also commonly co-occur with bipolar disorder.

- **Other Mental Disorders:** Some mental disorders cause symptoms similar to bipolar disorder. One example is major depression, sometimes called unipolar depression. Sometimes, it is extremely difficult to tell the difference between major depression and a depressive episode in bipolar disorder. For this reason, if a child has bipolar disorder and becomes depressed, be sure that the doctor is aware of any past manic symptoms or episodes.

What treatments are available for adolescents with bipolar disorder?

Currently, there is no cure for bipolar disorder. However, treatment with medications, psychotherapy, or both may help people recover from their episodes, and may help to prevent future episodes.

To treat children and teens with bipolar disorder, doctors often rely on information about treating adults. This is because there haven't been many studies on treating young people with the illness.

One large study with adults funded by NIMH was the Systematic Treatment Enhancement Program for Bipolar Disorder (STEP-BD). This study found that treating adults with medications and intensive psychotherapy for about nine months helped them get better. These adults got better faster and stayed well longer than adults treated with less intensive psychotherapy for six weeks. Combining medication treatment and psychotherapies may help young people with early-onset bipolar disorder, as well. However, children sometimes respond differently to psychiatric medications than adults.

What medications are used in treating bipolar disorder?

Before starting medication, your doctor will want to determine your physical and mental health. This is called a "baseline" assessment. You will need regular follow-up visits to monitor treatment progress and side effects. Most children with bipolar disorder will also need long-term or even lifelong medication treatment. This is often the best way to manage symptoms and prevent relapse, or a return of symptoms.

It's better to limit the number and dose of medications. A good way to remember this is to "start low, go slow." Talk to the doctor about using the smallest amount of medication that helps relieve your symptoms. To judge a medication's effectiveness, you may need to take a medication for several weeks or months. The doctor or specialist needs this time to decide whether the medication is working or if they need to switch to a different medication. Because children's symptoms are usually complex, they commonly need more than one type of medication.

Keep a daily log of your most troublesome symptoms. Doing so can make it easier for you and your doctor to decide whether a medication is helpful. Also, be sure to tell your doctor about all other prescription drugs, over-the-counter medications, or natural supplements you are taking. Combining certain medications and supplements may cause unwanted or dangerous side effects.

Mood Stabilizers: Mood stabilizers, such as lithium, are usually the first choice to treat bipolar disorder. Lithium is approved for the treatment and prevention of manic symptoms in children ages 12 and older. In addition, lithium might act as an antidepressant and help prevent suicidal behavior. However, FDA's approval of lithium was based on treatment studies in adults, not children.

Lithium Poisoning

Early signs of lithium poisoning include:

- Diarrhea
- Muscle weakness
- Drowsiness
- Lack of coordination
- Vomiting

Go to the emergency room if you are taking lithium and have these symptoms. The risk of lithium poisoning goes up when a child or adolescent becomes dehydrated. Make sure you have enough to drink when you have a fever or you sweat a lot during very active play or work.

Source: National Institute of Mental Health (www.nimh.nih.gov), 2012.

Anticonvulsant Medications: Anticonvulsant medications, originally developed to treat seizures, are also sometimes used as mood stabilizers. They are not approved by the FDA for treating bipolar disorder in children, but your doctor may prescribe one on an "off label" basis. They may be very helpful for difficult-to-treat bipolar episodes. For some children, anticonvulsants may work better than lithium. Examples of anticonvulsant medications include valproic acid or divalproex sodium (Depakote) and lamotrigine (Lamictal).

Atypical Antipsychotics: Atypical antipsychotics are sometimes used to treat symptoms of bipolar disorder. Those approved by the FDA to treat youth with bipolar disorder are risperidone (Risperdal), aripiprazole (Abilify), quetiapine (Seroquel), and olanzapine (Zyprexa). Short-term treatment with risperidone can help reduce symptoms of mania or mixed mania in children ages 10 and up. Some research has indicated that risperidone is more effective in treating mania in young children than other medications. Aripiprazole and quetiapine are approved to treat mania symptoms in children 10–17 years old who have bipolar I, while olanzapine is approved for use in children ages 13–17.

Should girls take valproic acid?

Valproic acid may increase levels of testosterone (a male hormone) in teenage girls. It could lead to a condition called polycystic ovarian syndrome (PCOS) in women who begin taking the medication before age 20. PCOS can cause obesity, excess body hair, an irregular menstrual cycle, and other serious symptoms. Most of these symptoms will improve after stopping treatment with valproic acid. Young girls and women taking valproic acid should be monitored carefully by a doctor.

Source: National Institute of Mental Health (www.nimh.nih.gov), 2012.

What role does psychotherapy play in treating bipolar disorder?

In addition to medication, psychotherapy can be an effective treatment for bipolar disorder. When treating bipolar disorder, psychotherapy is usually prescribed in combination with medication. Studies in adults show that it can provide support, education, and guidance to people with bipolar disorder and their families. Psychotherapy may also help children continue taking their medications to stay healthy and prevent relapse.

Some psychotherapy treatments used for bipolar disorder include:

- **Cognitive Behavioral Therapy (CBT):** CBT helps young people with bipolar disorder learn to change harmful or negative thought patterns and behaviors.

- **Family-Focused Therapy:** This type of therapy includes a child's family members. It helps enhance family coping strategies, such as recognizing new episodes early and helping their child. It also improves communication and problem-solving.

- **Interpersonal And Social Rhythm Therapy:** This type of therapy helps children and teens with bipolar disorder improve their relationships with others and manage their daily routines. Regular daily routines and sleep schedules may help protect against manic episodes.

- **Psychoeducation:** Psychoeducation teaches young people with bipolar disorder about the illness and its treatment. This treatment helps people recognize signs of an impending relapse, allowing them time to seek treatment early, before a full-blown episode occurs.

Other types of therapies may be tried as well, or used along with those mentioned. The number, frequency, and type of psychotherapy sessions should be based on your treatment needs.

A licensed psychologist, social worker, or counselor typically provides these therapies. He or she should work with your doctor to monitor care. In addition to getting therapy to help

Sexual Activity, Pregnancy, And Adolescents With Bipolar Disorder

Many teens make risky choices about sex. But having bipolar disorder is also linked with impulsive and risky choices. Teenage girls with bipolar disorder who are pregnant or may become pregnant face special challenges because medications for the illness may have harmful effects on a developing fetus or nursing infant. Specifically, lithium and valproic acid should not be used during pregnancy. Also, some medications may reduce the effectiveness of birth control pills.

Source: National Institute of Mental Health (www.nimh.nih.gov), 2012.

reduce symptoms of bipolar disorder, children and teens may also benefit from therapies that address problems at school, work, or in the community. Such therapies may target communication skills, problem-solving skills, or skills for school or work. Other programs (such as, those provided by social welfare programs or support and advocacy groups) can help, as well.

Some children with bipolar disorder may also have learning disorders or language problems. Your school may need to make accommodations that reduce the stresses of a school day and provide proper support or interventions.

What can adolescents with bipolar disorder expect from treatment?

There is no cure for bipolar disorder, but it can be treated effectively over the long term. Your doctor should keep track of your symptoms and treatment effects to decide whether changes to the treatment plan are needed. One way to do this is by creating a mood or daily life chart, where you and the doctor can track your moods, treatments, sleep patterns, and life events. The chart can help you track and treat the illness more effectively. Be sure to work closely with your treatment providers. Talk openly and frequently with them about treatment choices.

Sometimes a child may switch from one type of bipolar disorder to another. This calls for a change in treatment. Because different medications may be more helpful for one type of symptom than another (manic or depressive), you may need to change medications or try different treatments if your symptoms change.

Where can I go for help?

If you are unsure where to go for help, ask your family doctor. Others who can help are:

- Mental health specialists, such as psychiatrists, psychologists, social workers, or mental health counselors

- Health maintenance organizations

- Community mental health centers

- Hospital psychiatry departments and outpatient clinics

- Mental health programs at universities or medical schools

- State hospital outpatient clinics

- Family services, social agencies, or clergy

- Peer support groups

- Private clinics and facilities

- Employee assistance programs

- Local medical and/or psychiatric societies

You can also check the phone book under "mental health," "health," "social services," "hotlines," or "physicians" for phone numbers and addresses. An emergency room doctor can also provide temporary help and can tell you where and how to get further help.

Chapter 11

Generalized Anxiety Disorder: When Worry Gets Out Of Control

Uncontrolled Worry

Are you extremely worried about everything in your life, even if there is little or no reason to worry? Are you very anxious about just getting through the day? Are you afraid that everything will always go badly? If so, you may have an anxiety disorder called generalized anxiety disorder (GAD).

What is GAD?

All of us worry about things like health, money, or family problems, but people with GAD are extremely worried about these and many other things—even when there is little or no reason to worry about them. They are very anxious about just getting through the day. They think things will always go badly. At times, worrying keeps people with GAD from doing everyday tasks.

GAD develops slowly. It often starts during the teen years or young adulthood. Symptoms may get better or worse at different times, and often are worse during times of stress.

People with GAD may visit a doctor many times before they find out they have this disorder. They ask their doctors to help them with headaches or trouble falling asleep, which can be symptoms of GAD, but they don't always get the help they need right away. It may take doctors some time to be sure that a person has GAD instead of something else.

About This Chapter: This chapter begins with excerpts from "Generalized Anxiety Disorder: When Worry Gets Out Of Control," National Institute of Mental Health (www.nimh.nih.gov), March 2012. It ends with excerpts from "Computer-Based Treatment Eases Anxiety Symptoms in Children: Small Clinical Trial Supports Larger Scale Testing," National Institute of Mental Health (www.nimh.nih.gov), March 2012.

What are the signs and symptoms of GAD?

A person with GAD may:

- Worry very much about everyday things

- Have trouble controlling their constant worries

- Know that they worry much more than they should

- Not be able to relax

- Have a hard time concentrating

- Be easily startled

- Have trouble falling asleep or staying asleep

Generalized Anxiety Disorder (GAD)

People with generalized anxiety disorder (GAD) go through the day filled with exaggerated worry and tension, even though there is little or nothing to provoke it. They anticipate disaster and are overly concerned about health issues, money, family problems, or difficulties at school. Sometimes just the thought of getting through the day produces anxiety.

GAD is diagnosed when a person worries excessively about a variety of everyday problems for at least six months. People with GAD can't seem to get rid of their concerns, even though they usually realize that their anxiety is more intense than the situation warrants. They can't relax, startle easily, and have difficulty concentrating. Often they have trouble falling asleep or staying asleep. Physical symptoms that often accompany the anxiety include fatigue, headaches, muscle tension, muscle aches, difficulty swallowing, trembling, twitching, irritability, sweating, nausea, lightheadedness, having to go to the bathroom frequently, feeling out of breath, and hot flashes.

When their anxiety level is mild, people with GAD can function socially and hold down a job. Although they don't avoid certain situations as a result of their disorder, people with GAD can have difficulty carrying out the simplest daily activities if their anxiety is severe.

GAD affects about 6.8 million American adults, including twice as many women as men. The disorder develops gradually and can begin at any point in the life cycle, although the years of highest risk are between childhood and middle age. There is evidence that genes play a modest role in GAD.

Other anxiety disorders, depression, or substance abuse, often accompany GAD, which rarely occurs alone. GAD is commonly treated with medication or cognitive-behavioral therapy, but co-occurring conditions must also be treated using the appropriate therapies.

Source: Excerpted from "Anxiety Disorders," National Institute of Mental Health (www.nimh.nih.gov), December 17, 2012.

What is it like to have GAD?

"I was worried all the time about everything. It didn't matter that there were no signs of problems, I just got upset. I was having trouble falling asleep at night, and I couldn't keep my mind focused at work. I felt angry at my family all the time.

"I saw my doctor and explained my constant worries. My doctor sent me to someone who knows about GAD. Now I am taking medicine and working with a counselor to cope better with my worries. I had to work hard, but I feel better. I'm glad I made that first call to my doctor."

Source: Excerpted from "Generalized Anxiety Disorder: When Worry Gets Out Of Control," National Institute of Mental Health (www.nimh.nih.gov), March 2012.

- Feel tired all the time

- Have headaches, muscle aches, stomach aches, or unexplained pains

- Have a hard time swallowing

- Tremble or twitch

- Be irritable, sweat a lot, and feel light-headed or out of breath

- Have to go to the bathroom a lot

What causes GAD?

GAD sometimes runs in families, but no one knows for sure why some people have it, while others don't. Researchers have found that several parts of the brain are involved in fear and anxiety. By learning more about fear and anxiety in the brain, scientists may be able to create better treatments. Researchers are also looking for ways in which stress and environmental factors may play a role.

How is GAD treated?

GAD is generally treated with psychotherapy, medication, or both. First, talk to your doctor about your symptoms. Your doctor should do an exam to make sure that another physical problem isn't causing the symptoms. The doctor may refer you to a mental health specialist.

Psychotherapy: A type of psychotherapy called cognitive behavior therapy is especially useful for treating GAD. It teaches a person different ways of thinking, behaving, and reacting to situations that help him or her feel less anxious and worried.

Medication: Doctors also may prescribe medication to help treat GAD. Two types of medications are commonly used to treat GAD—anti-anxiety medications and antidepressants. Anti-anxiety medications are powerful and there are different types. Many types begin working right away, but they generally should not be taken for long periods.

Antidepressants are used to treat depression, but they also are helpful for GAD. They may take several weeks to start working. These medications may cause side effects such as headache, nausea, or difficulty sleeping. These side effects are usually not a problem for most people, especially if the dose starts off low and is increased slowly over time. Talk to your doctor about any side effects that you may have.

It's important to know that although antidepressants can be safe and effective for many people, they may be risky for some, especially teens and young adults. A "black box" (the most serious type of warning that a prescription drug can have) has been added to the labels of antidepressant medications. These labels warn people that antidepressants may cause some people to have suicidal thoughts or make suicide attempts. Anyone taking antidepressants should be monitored closely, especially when they first start treatment with medications.

Some people do better with cognitive behavior therapy, while others do better with medication. Still others do best with a combination of the two. Talk with your doctor about the best treatment for you.

Computer-Based Treatment Eases Anxiety Symptoms In Children

A computer-based training method that teaches a person with anxiety to shift attention away from threatening images reduced symptoms of anxiety in a small clinical trial in children with the condition. The results of this first randomized clinical trial of the therapy in children with anxiety suggest that the approach warrants more extensive testing as a promising therapy.

As many as a quarter of 13- to 18-year-olds have met the criteria for an anxiety disorder at some point. Currently available treatments—including cognitive behavioral therapy and medication—relieve symptoms of anxiety in about 70 percent of children treated. Most children with clinical anxiety do not receive treatment, partly because of difficulties in access to care, including distance and financial resources. Scientists are searching for additional approaches, including therapies that do not involve medication with its associated side effects.

A treatment called attention bias modification (ABM) has emerged from the observation that people with anxiety unconsciously pay more attention than others to anything that seems threatening. One way of detecting such a bias is a dot probe test. In the test, people view a computer screen on which angry and neutral faces are flashed briefly, adjacent to each other. After the faces disappear, a test image of dots appears where either one or the other face was, and the person has to respond by pushing a button. People with anxiety consistently respond more quickly to dots that appear where the angry face was located.

ABM presents patients with an exercise similar to the dot probe test, but the dots always appear where the neutral face was, and thus consistently draw the attention of the participant to this non-threatening image. Recent meta-analyses of ABM in adults, by some of the same investigators who carried out this work, suggested its potential as a treatment.

Researchers at Tel Aviv University (TAU) in Israel carried out a clinical trial on ABM as an outcome of a three-year collaboration with scientists at the National Institute of Mental Health (NIMH) and the University of Maryland, College Park, Maryland. Yair Bar-Haim of TAU led the study, which appears in the *American Journal of Psychiatry*. The study enrolled 40 children, 8–14 years old, who had sought help for anxiety. For children receiving ABM, after faces appeared on a screen, two dots appeared on the screen; children had to determine whether the dots were side by side, or one above the other. In every case, dots appeared only where the neutral face had been. There were also two control groups: In the first group, dots appeared equally frequently where angry and neutral faces appeared; in the second, the only faces that appeared throughout were neutral, so the dots always appeared in the location of a neutral face. The object of the second control group was to help confirm that any therapeutic effect was from the ABM training, and not from desensitizing the children to threatening faces. Children in the study were randomly assigned to receive treatment, or to be in one of two control groups. All children had four training sessions over four weeks, with 480 dot-probe trials per session.

Although the trial was small, there was a "reasonably robust" decrease in the severity of anxiety, according to the authors. Following ABM, both the number and severity of symptoms were reduced.

An important feature of ABM, says NIMH author Daniel Pine, is that it addresses the fundamental neurological function underlying anxiety: attention. Changes in attention happen very quickly—in milliseconds. "We know from neuroscience that if you want to change behaviors that happen very quickly, you have to practice. You can't just tell someone how to drive or throw a ball. You have to practice," says Pine.

Longitudinal studies that follow children into adulthood suggest that most chronic mood and anxiety disorders in adults begin as high levels of anxiety in children. In fact, childhood anxiety is as important in predicting adult depression as it is for adult anxiety. The ability to influence attention biases early in development might provide a powerful means of prevention for both of these disorders later in life. The approach requires no medication and in practical terms, the computer-based nature of ABM lends itself to large-scale dissemination—in a medium that children are comfortable with. Larger-scale trials will be able to provide more information on the efficacy of the treatment in children and how it works to reduce symptoms of anxiety.

Chapter 12

Social Anxiety Disorder: Always Embarrassed

Are you afraid of being judged by others or of being embarrassed all the time? Do you feel extremely fearful and unsure around other people most of the time? Do these worries make it hard for you to do everyday tasks like run errands or talk to people at work or school? If so, you may have a type of anxiety disorder called social phobia, also called social anxiety disorder.

What is social phobia?

Social phobia is a strong fear of being judged by others and of being embarrassed. This fear can be so strong that it gets in the way of going to work or school or doing other everyday things.

Everyone has felt anxious or embarrassed at one time or another. For example, meeting new people or giving a public speech can make anyone nervous. But people with social phobia worry about these and other things for weeks before they happen.

People with social phobia are afraid of doing common things in front of other people. For example, they might be afraid to sign a check in front of a cashier at the grocery store, or they might be afraid to eat or drink in front of other people, or use a public restroom. Most people who have social phobia know that they shouldn't be as afraid as they are, but they can't control their fear. Sometimes, they end up staying away from places or events where they think they might have to do something that will embarrass them. For some people, social phobia is a problem only in certain situations, while others have symptoms in almost any social situation.

About This Chapter: Excerpted from "Social Phobia (Social Anxiety Disorder): Always Embarrassed," National Institute of Mental Health (www.nimh.nih.gov), June 2012.

Social phobia usually starts during youth. A doctor can tell that a person has social phobia if the person has had symptoms for at least six months. Without treatment, social phobia can last for many years or a lifetime.

What are the signs and symptoms of social phobia?

People with social phobia tend to:

- Be very anxious about being with other people and have a hard time talking to them, even though they wish they could

- Be very self-conscious in front of other people and feel embarrassed

- Be very afraid that other people will judge them

- Worry for days or weeks before an event where other people will be

- Stay away from places where there are other people

- Have a hard time making friends and keeping friends

- Blush, sweat, or tremble around other people

- Feel nauseous or sick to their stomach when with other people

What causes social phobia?

Social phobia sometimes runs in families, but no one knows for sure why some people have it, while others don't. Researchers have found that several parts of the brain are involved in fear and anxiety. By learning more about fear and anxiety in the brain, scientists may be able to create better treatments. Researchers are also looking for ways in which stress and environmental factors may play a role.

What is it like having social phobia?

"In school I was always afraid of being called on, even when I knew the answers. When I got a job, I hated to meet with my boss. I couldn't eat lunch with my co-workers. I worried about being stared at or judged, and I worried that I would make a fool of myself; my heart would pound, and I would start to sweat when I thought about meetings. The feelings got worse as the time of the event got closer. Sometimes I couldn't sleep or eat for days before a staff meeting.

I'm taking medicine and working with a counselor to cope better with my fears. I had to work hard, but I feel better. I'm glad I made that first call to my doctor."

Source: NIMH, June 2012.

How is social phobia treated?

First, talk to your doctor about your symptoms. Your doctor should do an exam to make sure that another physical problem isn't causing the symptoms. The doctor may refer you to a mental health specialist.

Social phobia is generally treated with psychotherapy, medication, or both.

Psychotherapy: A type of psychotherapy called cognitive behavior therapy is especially useful for treating social phobia. It teaches a person different ways of thinking, behaving, and reacting to situations that help him or her feel less anxious and fearful. It can also help people learn and practice social skills.

Medication: Doctors also may prescribe medication to help treat social phobia. The most commonly prescribed medications for social phobia are anti-anxiety medications and anti-depressants. Anti-anxiety medications are powerful and there are different types. Many types begin working right away, but they generally should not be taken for long periods.

Antidepressants are used to treat depression, but they are also helpful for social phobia. They are probably more commonly prescribed for social phobia than anti-anxiety medications. Antidepressants may take several weeks to start working. Some may cause side effects such as headache, nausea, or difficulty sleeping. These side effects are usually not a problem for most people, especially if the dose starts off low and is increased slowly over time. Talk to your doctor about any side effects that you may have.

A type of antidepressant called monoamine oxidase inhibitors (MAOIs) is especially effective in treating social phobia. However, MAOIs are rarely used as a first line of treatment because when they are combined with certain foods or other medicines, dangerous side effects can occur.

It's important to know that although antidepressants can be safe and effective for many people, they may be risky for some, especially teens and young adults. A "black box"—the most serious type of warning that a prescription drug can have—has been added to the labels of antidepressant medications. These labels warn people that antidepressants may cause some people to have suicidal thoughts or make suicide attempts.

Anyone taking antidepressants should be monitored closely, especially when they first start treatment with medications.

Another type of medication called beta-blockers can help control some of the physical symptoms of social phobia such as excessive sweating, shaking, or a racing heart. They are most commonly prescribed when the symptoms of social phobia occur in specific situations, such as "stage fright."

Some people do better with cognitive behavior therapy, while others do better with medication. Still others do best with a combination of the two. Talk with your doctor about the best treatment for you.

Chapter 13

Post-Traumatic Stress Disorder

Understanding Post-Traumatic Stress Disorder (PTSD)

PTSD is an anxiety disorder that some people get after seeing or living through a dangerous event.

When in danger, it's natural to feel afraid. This fear triggers many split-second changes in the body to prepare to defend against the danger or to avoid it. This "fight-or-flight" response is a healthy reaction meant to protect a person from harm. But in PTSD, this reaction is changed or damaged. People who have PTSD may feel stressed or frightened even when they're no longer in danger.

Anyone can get PTSD at any age. This includes war veterans and survivors of physical and sexual assault, abuse, accidents, disasters, and many other serious events.

Not everyone with PTSD has been through a dangerous event. Some people get PTSD after a friend or family member experiences danger or is harmed. The sudden, unexpected death of a loved one can also cause PTSD.

Symptoms Of PTSD

PTSD can cause many symptoms. These symptoms can be grouped into three categories: re-experiencing symptoms, avoidance symptoms, and hyperarousal symptoms.

About This Chapter: Excerpted from "Post-Traumatic Stress Disorder (PTSD)," National Institute of Mental Health (www.nimh.nih.gov), December 2012.

Re-Experiencing Symptoms

Re-experiencing symptoms may cause problems in a person's everyday routine. They can start from the person's own thoughts and feelings. Words, objects, or situations that are reminders of the event can also trigger re-experiencing. Re-experiencing symptoms can include flashbacks (reliving the trauma over and over, including physical symptoms like a racing heart or sweating), bad dreams, and/or frightening thoughts.

Avoidance Symptoms

Things that remind a person of the traumatic event can trigger avoidance symptoms. These symptoms may cause a person to change his or her personal routine. For example, after a bad car accident, a person who usually drives may avoid driving or riding in a car. Avoidance symptoms can include staying away from places, events, or objects that are reminders of the experience. Other symptoms include:

- Feeling emotionally numb,
- Feeling strong guilt, depression, or worry,
- Losing interest in activities that were enjoyable in the past
- Having trouble remembering the dangerous event

Hyperarousal Symptoms

Hyperarousal symptoms are usually constant, instead of being triggered by things that remind one of the traumatic event. They can make the person feel stressed and angry. These symptoms may make it hard to do daily tasks, such as sleeping, eating, or concentrating. Hyperarousal symptoms can include being easily startled, feeling tense or "on edge," having difficulty sleeping, and/or having angry outbursts.

It's natural to have some of these symptoms after a dangerous event. Sometimes people have very serious symptoms that go away after a few weeks. This is called acute stress disorder, or ASD. When the symptoms last more than a few weeks and become an ongoing problem, they might be PTSD. Some people with PTSD don't show any symptoms for weeks or months.

Teens React Differently To PTSD Than Adults

Teens usually show symptoms like those seen in adults. They may also develop disruptive, disrespectful, or destructive behaviors, feel guilty for not preventing injury or deaths, or have thoughts of revenge.

PTSD Detection

A doctor who has experience helping people with mental illnesses, such as a psychiatrist or psychologist, can diagnose PTSD. The diagnosis is made after the doctor talks with the person who has symptoms of PTSD.

To be diagnosed with PTSD, a person must have all of the following for at least one month:

- At least one re-experiencing symptom
- At least three avoidance symptoms
- At least two hyperarousal symptoms
- Symptoms that make it hard to go about daily life, go to school or work, be with friends, and take care of important tasks

PTSD Risk Factors

It is important to remember that not everyone who lives through a dangerous event gets PTSD. In fact, most will not get the disorder.

Many factors play a part in whether a person will get PTSD. Some of these are risk factors that make a person more likely to get PTSD. Other factors, called resilience factors, can help reduce the risk of the disorder. Some of these risk and resilience factors are present before the trauma and others become important during and after a traumatic event.

Risk factors for PTSD include:

- Living through dangerous events and traumas
- Having a history of mental illness
- Getting hurt
- Seeing people hurt or killed
- Feeling horror, helplessness, or extreme fear
- Having little or no social support after the event
- Dealing with extra stress after the event, such as loss of a loved one, pain and injury, or loss of a job or home

Resilience factors that may reduce the risk of PTSD include:

- Seeking out support from other people, such as friends and family
- Finding a support group after a traumatic event

- Feeling good about one's own actions in the face of danger

- Having a coping strategy, or a way of getting through the bad event and learning from it

- Being able to act and respond effectively despite feeling fear

Researchers are studying the importance of various risk and resilience factors. With more study, it may be possible someday to predict who is likely to get PTSD and prevent it.

Treating PTSD

The main treatments for people with PTSD are psychotherapy ("talk" therapy), medications, or both. Everyone is different, so a treatment that works for one person may not work for another. It is important for anyone with PTSD to be treated by a mental health care provider who is experienced with PTSD. Some people with PTSD need to try different treatments to find what works for their symptoms.

If someone with PTSD is going through an ongoing trauma, such as being in an abusive relationship, both of the problems need to be treated. Other ongoing problems can include panic disorder, depression, substance abuse, and feeling suicidal.

Psychotherapy

Psychotherapy is "talk" therapy. It involves talking with a mental health professional to treat a mental illness. Psychotherapy can occur one-on-one or in a group. Talk therapy treatment for PTSD usually lasts six to 12 weeks, but can take more time. Research shows that support from family and friends can be an important part of therapy.

Many types of psychotherapy can help people with PTSD. Some types target the symptoms of PTSD directly. Other therapies focus on social, family, or job-related problems. The doctor or therapist may combine different therapies depending on each person's needs.

One helpful therapy is called cognitive behavioral therapy, or CBT. There are several parts to CBT, including:

- **Exposure Therapy:** This therapy helps people face and control their fear. It exposes them to the trauma they experienced in a safe way. It uses mental imagery, writing, or visits to the place where the event happened. The therapist uses these tools to help people with PTSD cope with their feelings.

- **Cognitive Restructuring:** This therapy helps people make sense of the bad memories. Sometimes people remember the event differently than how it happened. They may feel guilt or shame about what is not their fault. The therapist helps people with PTSD look at what happened in a realistic way.

- **Stress Inoculation Training:** This therapy tries to reduce PTSD symptoms by teaching a person how to reduce anxiety. Like cognitive restructuring, this treatment helps people look at their memories in a healthy way.

Other types of treatment can also help people with PTSD. People with PTSD should talk about all treatment options with their therapist.

How can talk therapies help people overcome PTSD?

Talk therapies teach people helpful ways to react to frightening events that trigger their PTSD symptoms. Based on this general goal, different types of therapy may:

- Teach about trauma and its effects
- Use relaxation and anger control skills
- Provide tips for better sleep, diet, and exercise habits
- Help people identify and deal with guilt, shame, and other feelings about the event
- Focus on changing how people react to their PTSD symptoms (For example, therapy helps people visit places and people that are reminders of the trauma.)

Source: NIMH, December 2012.

Medications

The U.S. Food and Drug Administration (FDA) has approved two medications for treating adults with PTSD, sertraline (Zoloft) and paroxetine (Paxil). Both of these medications are antidepressants, which are also used to treat depression. They may help control PTSD symptoms such as sadness, worry, anger, and feeling numb inside. Taking these medications may make it easier to go through psychotherapy.

Sometimes people taking these medications have side effects. The effects can be annoying, but they usually go away. However, medications affect everyone differently. Any side effects or unusual reactions should be reported to a doctor immediately. The most common side effects of antidepressants like sertraline and paroxetine are:

- Headache, which usually goes away within a few days
- Nausea (feeling sick to your stomach), which usually goes away within a few days

- Sleeplessness or drowsiness, which may occur during the first few weeks but then goes away (Sometimes the medication dose needs to be reduced or the time of day it is taken needs to be adjusted to help lessen these side effects.)

- Agitation (feeling jittery)

- Sexual problems, which can affect both men and women (including reduced sex drive, and problems having and enjoying sex)

Other Medications

Doctors may also prescribe other types of medications, such as the ones listed below. There is little information on how well these work for people with PTSD.

- **Benzodiazepines:** These medications may be given to help people relax and sleep. People who take benzodiazepines may have memory problems or become dependent on the medication.

- **Antipsychotics:** These medications are usually given to people with other mental disorders, like schizophrenia. People who take antipsychotics may gain weight and have a higher chance of getting heart disease and diabetes.

- **Other Antidepressants:** Like sertraline and paroxetine, the antidepressants fluoxetine (Prozac) and citalopram (Celexa) can help people with PTSD feel less tense or sad. For people with PTSD who also have other anxiety disorders or depression, antidepressants may be useful in reducing symptoms of these co-occurring illnesses.

Food And Drug Administration (FDA) Warnings About Antidepressants

Despite the relative safety and popularity of selective serotonin reuptake inhibitors (SSRIs) and other antidepressants, some studies have suggested that they may have unintentional effects on some people, especially adolescents and young adults. In 2004, the Food and Drug Administration (FDA) conducted a thorough review of published and unpublished controlled clinical trials of antidepressants that involved nearly 4,400 children and adolescents. The review revealed that four percent of those taking antidepressants thought about or attempted suicide (although no suicides occurred), compared to two percent of those receiving placebos.

This information prompted the FDA, in 2005, to adopt a "black box" warning label on all antidepressant medications to alert the public about the potential increased risk of suicidal thinking or attempts in children and adolescents taking antidepressants. In 2007, the FDA proposed that makers of all antidepressant medications extend the warning to include young adults up through age 24. A "black box" warning is the most serious type of warning on prescription drug labeling.

The warning emphasizes that patients of all ages taking antidepressants should be closely monitored, especially during the initial weeks of treatment. Possible side effects to look for are worsening depression, suicidal thinking or behavior, or any unusual changes in behavior such as sleeplessness, agitation, or withdrawal from normal social situations. The warning adds that families and caregivers should also be told of the need for close monitoring, and should report any changes to the physician. The latest information can be found on the FDA website (www .fda.gov).

Results of a comprehensive review of pediatric trials conducted between 1988 and 2006 suggested that the benefits of antidepressant medications likely outweigh their risks to children and adolescents with major depression and anxiety disorders. The study was funded in part by the National Institute of Mental Health.

Treating Mass Trauma

Sometimes large numbers of people are affected by the same event. For example, a lot of people needed help after Hurricane Katrina in 2005 and the terrorist attacks of September 11, 2001. Most people will have some PTSD symptoms in the first few weeks after events like these. This is a normal and expected response to serious trauma, and for most people, symptoms generally lessen with time. Most people can be helped with basic support, such as getting to a safe place, seeing a doctor if injured, getting food and water, contacting loved ones or friends, and learning what is being done to help.

But some people do not get better on their own. A study of Hurricane Katrina survivors found that, over time, more people were having problems with PTSD, depression, and related mental disorders. This pattern is unlike the recovery from other natural disasters, where the number of people who have mental health problems gradually lessens. As communities try to rebuild after a mass trauma, people may experience ongoing stress from loss of jobs and schools, and trouble paying bills, finding housing, and getting health care. This delay in community recovery may in turn delay recovery from PTSD.

In the first couple weeks after a mass trauma, brief versions of cognitive behavioral therapy (CBT) may be helpful to some people who are having severe distress. Sometimes other treatments are used, but their effectiveness is not known. For example, there is growing interest in an approach called psychological first aid. The goal of this approach is to make people feel safe and secure, connect people to health care and other resources, and reduce stress reactions. There are guides for carrying out the treatment, but experts do not know yet if it helps prevent or treat PTSD.

In single-session psychological debriefing, another type of mass trauma treatment, survivors talk about the event and express their feelings one-on-one or in a group. Studies show that it is not likely to reduce distress or the risk for PTSD, and may actually increase distress and risk.

Mass Trauma Affects Health Care Providers

Hospitals, health care systems, and health care providers are also affected by a mass trauma. The number of people who need immediate physical and psychological help may be too much for health systems to handle. Some patients may not find help when they need it because hospitals do not have enough staff or supplies. In some cases, health care providers themselves may be struggling to recover as well.

Scientists at the National Institute of Mental Health (NIMH) are working on this problem. For example, researchers are testing how to give CBT and other treatments using the phone and the Internet. In one study, people with PTSD met with a therapist to learn about the disorder, made a list of things that trigger their symptoms, and learned basic ways to reduce stress. After this meeting, the participants could visit a website with more information about PTSD. Participants could keep a log of their symptoms and practice coping skills. Overall, the researchers found the Internet-based treatment helped reduce symptoms of PTSD and depression. These effects lasted after treatment ended.

Researchers will carry out more studies to find out if other such approaches to therapy can be helpful after mass trauma.

PTSD Research

Researchers have learned a lot in the last decade about fear, stress, and PTSD. Scientists are also learning about how people form memories. This is important because creating very powerful fear-related memories seems to be a major part of PTSD. Researchers are also exploring how people can create "safety" memories to replace the bad memories that form after a trauma. NIMH's goal in supporting this research is to improve treatment and find ways to prevent the disorder.

PTSD research also includes the following examples:

- Using powerful new research methods, such as brain imaging and the study of genes, to find out more about what leads to PTSD (when it happens and who is most at risk)

- Trying to understand why some people get PTSD and others do not (Knowing this can help healthcare professionals predict who might get PTSD and provide early treatment.)

- Focusing on ways to examine pre-trauma, trauma, and post-trauma risk and resilience factors all at once

- Looking for treatments that reduce the impact traumatic memories have on our emotions

- Improving the way people are screened for PTSD, given early treatment, and tracked after a mass trauma

- Developing new approaches in self-testing and screening to help people know when it's time to call a doctor.

- Testing ways to help family doctors detect and treat PTSD or refer people with PTSD to mental health specialists

Helping A Friend Or Relative Who Has PTSD?

If you know someone who has PTSD, it affects you too. The first and most important thing you can do to help a friend or relative is to help him or her get the right diagnosis and treatment. You may need to make an appointment for your friend or relative and go with him or her to see the doctor. Encourage him or her to stay in treatment, or to seek different treatment if his or her symptoms don't get better after six to eight weeks.

To help a friend or relative, you can offer emotional support, understanding, patience, and encouragement. Learn about PTSD, so you can understand what your friend or relative is experiencing, then talk to your friend or relative, and listen carefully. Listen to feelings your friend or relative expresses, and be understanding of situations that may trigger PTSD symptoms. Invite your friend or relative out for positive distractions such as walks, outings, and other activities. Finally, remind your friend or relative that, with time and treatment, he or she can get better.

Never ignore comments about your friend or relative harming him or herself, and report such comments to your friend's or relative's therapist or doctor.

Helping Yourself

It may be very hard to take that first step to help yourself. It is important to realize that although it may take some time, with treatment, you can get better.

To help yourself, talk to your doctor about treatment options. Engage in mild activity or exercise to help reduce stress. Set realistic goals for yourself. Break up large tasks into small ones, set some priorities, and do what you can as you can. Try to spend time with other people and confide in a trusted friend or relative. Tell others about things that may trigger symptoms. Expect your symptoms to improve gradually, not immediately. Finally, identify and seek out comforting situations, places, and people.

Where To Go For Help

If you are unsure where to go for help, ask your family doctor. Others who can help you, include mental health resources, mental health specialists (such as psychiatrists, psychologists, social workers, or mental health counselors) health maintenance organizations, community mental health centers, hospital psychiatry departments and outpatient clinics, mental health programs at universities or medical schools, state hospital outpatient clinics, family services, social agencies, or clergy, peer support groups, private clinics and facilities, and local medical and/or psychiatric societies.

You can also check the phone book under "mental health," "health," "social services," "hotlines," or "physicians" for phone numbers and addresses. An emergency room doctor can also provide temporary help and can tell you where and how to get further help.

If Someone Is In Crisis

If you are thinking about harming yourself, or know someone who is, tell someone who can help immediately:

- Call your doctor.

- Call 911 or go to a hospital emergency room to get immediate help or ask a friend or family member to help you do these things.

- Call the toll-free, 24-hour hotline of the National Suicide Prevention Lifeline at 1-800-273-TALK (1-800-273-8255); TTY: 1-800-799-4TTY (1-800-799-4889) to talk to a trained counselor.

- Make sure you or the suicidal person is not left alone.

Chapter 14

Obsessive-Compulsive Disorder: When Unwanted Thoughts Take Over

Do you feel the need to check and re-check things over and over? Do you have the same thoughts constantly? Do you feel a very strong need to perform certain rituals repeatedly and feel like you have no control over what you are doing? If so, you may have a type of anxiety disorder called obsessive-compulsive disorder (OCD).

What is OCD?

Everyone double checks things sometimes. For example, you might double check to make sure the stove or iron is turned off before leaving the house. But people with OCD feel the need to check things repeatedly, or have certain thoughts or perform routines and rituals over and over. The thoughts and rituals associated with OCD cause distress and get in the way of daily life.

The frequent upsetting thoughts are called obsessions. To try to control them, a person will feel an overwhelming urge to repeat certain rituals or behaviors called compulsions. People with OCD can't control these obsessions and compulsions.

For many people, OCD starts during childhood or the teen years. Most people are diagnosed by about age 19. Symptoms of OCD may come and go and be better or worse at different times.

What are the signs and symptoms of OCD?

People with OCD generally:

- Have repeated thoughts or images about many different things, such as fear of germs, dirt, or intruders; acts of violence; hurting loved ones; sexual acts; conflicts with religious beliefs; or being overly tidy

About This Chapter: Excerpted from "Obsessive-Compulsive Disorder: When Unwanted Thoughts Take Over," National Institute of Mental Health (www.nimh.nih.gov), March 2012.

- Do the same rituals over and over such as washing hands, locking and unlocking doors, counting, keeping unneeded items, or repeating the same steps again and again

- Can't control the unwanted thoughts and behaviors

- Don't get pleasure when performing the behaviors or rituals, but get brief relief from the anxiety the thoughts cause

- Spend at least one hour a day on the thoughts and rituals, which cause distress and get in the way of daily life

What causes OCD?

OCD sometimes runs in families, but no one knows for sure why some people have it, while others don't. Researchers have found that several parts of the brain are involved in fear and anxiety. By learning more about fear and anxiety in the brain, scientists may be able to

Possible Causes Of Sudden Onset OCD In Kids Broadened

Criteria for a broadened syndrome of acute-onset obsessive compulsive disorder (OCD) have been proposed by National Institutes of Health (NIH) researchers. The syndrome, pediatric acute-onset neuropsychiatric syndrome (PANS), includes children and teens that suddenly develop on-again/off-again OCD symptoms or abnormal eating behaviors, along with other psychiatric symptoms—without any known cause.

PANS expands on pediatric autoimmune neuropsychiatric disorder associated with streptococcus (PANDAS), which is limited to a subset of cases traceable to an autoimmune process triggered by a strep infection. According to scientists, parents have described children with PANS as overcome by a "ferocious" onset of obsessive thoughts, compulsive rituals, and overwhelming fears.

Differing Causes Sharing A "Common Presentation"

The PANS criteria grew out of a PANDAS workshop. It brought together a broad range of researchers, clinicians, and advocates. The participants considered all cases of acute-onset OCD, regardless of potential cause. Clinicians confirmed that boys outnumbered girls two to one—with psychiatric symptoms, always including OCD, usually beginning before eight years of age.

Although debate continues about the fine points, the field is now of one mind on the core concept of "acute and dramatic" onset of a constellation of psychiatric symptoms. There is also broad agreement on the need for a "centralized registry" that will enable the research community to analyze evidence from studies that will eventually pinpoint causes and treatments.

Since a diagnosis of PANS implies no specific cause, clinicians will have to evaluate and treat each affected youth on a case-by-case basis. The researchers propose that a patient must meet three diagnostic criteria for a diagnosis of PANS:

create better treatments. Researchers are also looking for ways in which stress and environmental factors may play a role.

How is OCD treated?

First, talk to your doctor about your symptoms. Your doctor should do an exam to make sure that another physical problem isn't causing the symptoms. The doctor may refer you to a mental health specialist.

OCD is generally treated with psychotherapy, medication, or both.

Psychotherapy: A type of psychotherapy called cognitive behavior therapy is especially useful for treating OCD. It teaches a person different ways of thinking, behaving, and reacting to situations that help him or her feel less anxious or fearful without having obsessive thoughts or acting compulsively. One type of therapy called exposure and response prevention is especially helpful in reducing compulsive behaviors in OCD.

- Abrupt, dramatic onset of OCD or anorexia
- Concurrent presence of at least two additional symptoms with similarly severe and acute onset, including: anxiety; mood swings and depression; aggression, irritability, and oppositional behaviors; developmental regression; sudden deterioration in school performance or learning abilities; sensory and motor abnormalities; and somatic signs and symptoms
- Symptoms are unexplainable by a known neurologic or medical disorder

Among the wide range of accompanying symptoms, children may appear terror stricken or suffer extreme separation anxiety, shift from laughter to tears for no apparent reason, or regress to temper tantrums, "baby talk" or bedwetting. In some cases, their handwriting and other fine motor skills worsen dramatically.

PANDAS Treatment Study Targets Errant Antibodies

Meanwhile, scientists are collaborating on a new study, testing the effectiveness of intravenous immunoglobulin (IVIG) for reducing OCD symptoms in children with PANDAS.

Previous human and animal research suggested that strep-triggered antibodies mistakenly attack specific brain circuitry, resulting in obsessional thoughts and compulsive behaviors. IVIG, a medication derived from normal antibodies, neutralizes such harmful antibodies, restoring normal immune function. It is used to treat other autoimmune illnesses and showed promise in a pilot study with PANDAS patients.

Source: Excerpted from "Possible Causes of Sudden Onset OCD in Kids Broadened," National Institutes of Mental Health (www.nimh.nih.gov), February 2013.

Medication: Doctors also may prescribe medication to help treat OCD. The most commonly prescribed medications for OCD are anti-anxiety medications and antidepressants. Anti-anxiety medications are powerful and there are different types. Many types begin working right away, but they generally should not be taken for long periods.

Antidepressants are used to treat depression, but they are also particularly helpful for OCD, probably more so than anti-anxiety medications. They may take several weeks—10 to 12 weeks for some—to start working. Some of these medications may cause side effects such as headache, nausea, or difficulty sleeping. These side effects are usually not a problem for most people, especially if the dose starts off low and is increased slowly over time. Talk to your doctor about any side effects that you may have.

It's important to know that although antidepressants can be safe and effective for many people, they may be risky for some, especially teens and young adults. A "black box"—the most serious type of warning that a prescription drug can have—has been added to the labels of antidepressant medications. These labels warn people that antidepressants may cause some people to have suicidal thoughts or make suicide attempts. Anyone taking antidepressants should be monitored closely, especially when they first start treatment with medications.

Some people with OCD do better with cognitive behavior therapy, especially exposure and response prevention. Others do better with medication. Still others do best with a combination of the two. Talk with your doctor about the best treatment for you.

What is it like having OCD?

"I couldn't do anything without rituals. They invaded every aspect of my life. Counting really bogged me down. I would wash my hair three times as opposed to once because three was a good luck number and one wasn't. It took me longer to read because I'd count the lines in a paragraph. When I set my alarm at night, I had to set it to a number that wouldn't add up to a 'bad' number."

"Getting dressed in the morning was tough, because I had a routine, and if I didn't follow the routine, I'd get anxious and would have to get dressed again. I always worried that if I didn't do something, my parents were going to die. I'd have these terrible thoughts of harming my parents. I knew that was completely irrational, but the thoughts triggered more anxiety and more senseless behavior. Because of the time I spent on rituals, I was unable to do a lot of things that were important to me."

"I knew the rituals didn't make sense, and I was deeply ashamed of them, but I couldn't seem to overcome them until I got treatment."

Chapter 15

Phobias And Fears: Symptoms, Treatment, And Self Help

Almost everyone has an irrational fear or two—of mice, for example, or your annual dental checkup. For most people, these fears are minor. But, when fears become so severe that they cause tremendous anxiety and interfere with your normal life, they're called phobias. The good news is that phobias can be managed and cured. Self-help strategies and therapy can help you overcome your fears and start living the life you want.

What Is A Phobia?

A phobia is an intense fear of something that, in reality, poses little or no actual danger. Common phobias and fears include closed-in places, heights, highway driving, flying insects, snakes, and needles. However, we can develop phobias of virtually anything. Most phobias develop in childhood, but they can also develop in adults.

If you have a phobia, you probably realize that your fear is unreasonable, yet you still can't control your feelings. Just thinking about the feared object or situation may make you anxious. And when you're actually exposed to the thing you fear, the terror is automatic and overwhelming.

The experience is so nerve wracking that you may go to great lengths to avoid it—inconveniencing yourself or even changing your lifestyle. If you have claustrophobia, for example, you might turn down a lucrative job offer if you have to ride the elevator to get to the office. If you have a fear of heights, you might drive an extra twenty miles in order to avoid a tall bridge.

About This Chapter: Reprinted from "Phobias and Fears: Symptoms, Treatment, and Self Help for Phobias and Fears," by Melinda Smith, M.A., Robert Segal, M.A., and Jeanne Segal, Ph.D. Updated August 2013 © 2013 Helpguide.org. All rights reserved. Reprinted with permission. Helpguide provides a detailed list of references and resources for this article, with links to related Helpguide topics and information from other websites. For a complete list of these resources, go to http://www.helpguide.org/mental/phobia_symptoms_types_treatment.htm.

Understanding your phobia is the first step to overcoming it. It's important to know that phobias are common. Having a phobia doesn't mean you're crazy! It also helps to know that phobias are highly treatable. You can overcome your anxiety and fear, no matter how out of control it feels.

"Normal" Fear Vs. Phobias

It is normal and even helpful to experience fear in dangerous situations. Fear is an adaptive human response. It serves a protective purpose, activating the automatic "fight-or-flight" response. With our bodies and minds alert and ready for action, we are able to respond quickly and protect ourselves.

But with phobias the threat is greatly exaggerated or nonexistent. For example, it is only natural to be afraid of a snarling Doberman, but it is irrational to be terrified of a friendly poodle on a leash, as you might be if you have a dog phobia.

Normal Fears In Children

Many childhood fears are natural and tend to develop at specific ages. For example, many young children are afraid of the dark and may need a nightlight to sleep. That doesn't mean they have a phobia. In most cases, they will grow out of this fear as they get older.

If [a] child's fear is not interfering with his or her daily life or causing him or her a great deal of distress, then there's little cause for undue concern. However, if the fear is interfering with [the] child's social activities, school performance, or sleep, [he/she] may want to see a qualified child therapist.

Table 15.1. The Difference Between Normal Fear And A Phobia

Normal Fear	Phobia
Feeling anxious when flying through turbulence or taking off during a storm	Not going to your best friend's island wedding because you'd have to fly there
Experiencing butterflies when peering down from the top of a skyscraper or climbing a tall ladder	Turning down a great job because it's on the 10th floor of the office building
Getting nervous when you see a pit bull or a Rottweiler	Steering clear of the park because you might see a dog
Feeling a little queasy when getting a shot or when your blood is being drawn	Avoiding necessary medical treatments or doctor's checkups because you're terrified of needles

Source: Helpguide © 2013.

Barbara's Fear Of Flying

Barbara is terrified of flying. Unfortunately, she has to travel a lot for work, and this traveling takes a terrible toll. For weeks before every trip, she has a knot in her stomach and a feeling of anxiety that won't go away. On the day of the flight, she wakes up feeling like she's going to throw up. Once she's on the plane, her heart pounds, she feels lightheaded, and she starts to hyperventilate. Every time it gets worse and worse.

Barbara's fear of flying has gotten so bad that she finally told her boss she can only travel to places within driving distance. Her boss was not happy about this, and Barbara's not sure what will happen at work. She's afraid she'll be demoted or lose her job altogether. But better that, she tells herself, than getting on a plane again.

Source: Helpguide © 2013.

Common Types Of Phobias And Fears

There are four general types of phobias and fears:

- **Animal Phobias:** Examples include fear of snakes, fear of spiders, fear of rodents, and fear of dogs.

- **Natural Environment Phobias:** Examples include fear of heights, fear of storms, fear of water, and fear of the dark.

- **Situational Phobias**: Fears triggered by a specific situation. Examples include fear of enclosed spaces (claustrophobia), fear of flying, fear of driving, fear of tunnels, and fear of bridges.

Which Child's Fears Are Normal?

According to the Child Anxiety Network, the following fears are extremely common and considered normal:

- **Ages 0–2 Years:** Loud noises, strangers, separation from parents, large objects
- **Ages 3–6 Years:** Imaginary things such as ghosts, monsters, the dark, sleeping alone, strange noises
- **Ages 7–16 Years:** More realistic fears such as injury, illness, school performance, death, natural disasters

Source: Helpguide © 2013.

- **Blood-Injection-Injury Phobia:** The fear of blood, fear or injury, or a fear of needles or other medical procedures.

Some phobias don't fall into one of the four common categories. Such phobias include fear of choking, fear of getting a disease such as cancer, and fear of clowns.

Social Phobia And Fear Of Public Speaking

Social phobia, also called social anxiety disorder, is fear of social situations where you may be embarrassed or judged. If you have social phobia you may be excessively self-conscious and afraid of humiliating yourself in front of others. Your anxiety over how you will look and what others will think may lead you to avoid certain social situations you'd otherwise enjoy.

Fear of public speaking, an extremely common phobia, is a type of social phobia. Other fears associated with social phobia include fear of eating or drinking in public, talking to strangers, taking exams, mingling at a party, and being called on in class.

Agoraphobia (Fear Of Open Spaces)

Agoraphobia is another phobia that doesn't fit neatly into any of the four categories. Traditionally thought to involve a fear of public places and open spaces, it is now believed that agoraphobia develops as a complication of panic attacks.

Afraid of having another panic attack, you become anxious about being in situations where escape would be difficult or embarrassing, or where help wouldn't be immediately available. For example, you are likely to avoid crowded places such as shopping malls and movie theaters. You may also avoid cars, airplanes, subways, and other forms of travel. In more severe cases, you might only feel safe at home.

Signs And Symptoms Of Phobias

The symptoms of a phobia can range from mild feelings of apprehension and anxiety to a full-blown panic attack. Typically, the closer you are to the thing you're afraid of, the greater your fear will be. Your fear will also be higher if getting away is difficult.

Physical Signs And Symptoms Of A Phobia

- Difficulty breathing
- Racing or pounding heart

- Chest pain or tightness
- Trembling or shaking
- Feeling dizzy or lightheaded
- A churning stomach
- Hot or cold flashes; tingling sensations
- Sweating

Common Phobias And Fears

- Fear of spiders
- Fear of heights
- Fear of storms
- Fear of public speaking
- Fear of germs

- Fear of snakes
- Fear or closed spaces
- Fear of needles and injections
- Fear of flying
- Fear of illness or death

Source: Helpguide© 2013.

Emotional Signs And Symptoms Of A Phobia

- Feeling of overwhelming anxiety or panic
- Feeling an intense need to escape
- Feeling "unreal" or detached from yourself
- Fear of losing control or going crazy
- Feeling like you're going to die or pass out
- Knowing that you're overreacting, but feeling powerless to control your fear

Symptoms Of Blood-Injection-Injury Phobia

The symptoms of blood-injection-injury phobia are slightly different from other phobias. When confronted with the sight of blood or a needle, you experience not only fear but disgust.

Like other phobias, you initially feel anxious as your heart speeds up. However, unlike other phobias, this acceleration is followed by a quick drop in blood pressure, which leads to nausea, dizziness, and fainting. Although a fear of fainting is common in all specific phobias, blood-injection-injury phobia is the only phobia where fainting can actually occur.

When To Seek Help For Phobias And Fears

Although phobias are common, they don't always cause considerable distress or significantly disrupt your life. For example, if you have a snake phobia, it may cause no problems in your everyday activities if you live in a city where you are not likely to run into one. On the other hand, if you have a severe phobia of crowded spaces, living in a big city would pose a problem.

If your phobia doesn't really impact your life that much, it's probably nothing to be concerned about. But if avoidance of the object, activity, or situation that triggers your phobia interferes with your normal functioning or keeps you from doing things you would otherwise enjoy, it's time to seek help.

Consider treatment for your phobia if:

- It causes intense and disabling fear, anxiety, and panic
- You recognize that your fear is excessive and unreasonable
- You avoid certain situations and places because of your phobia
- Your avoidance interferes with your normal routine or causes significant distress
- You've had the phobia for at least six months

Self-Help Or Therapy For Phobias: Which Treatment Is Best?

When it comes to treating phobias, self-help strategies and therapy can both be effective. What's best for you depends on a number of factors, including the severity of your phobia, your insurance coverage, and the amount of support you need.

As a general rule, self-help is always worth a try. The more you can do for yourself, the more in control you'll feel—which goes a long way when it comes to phobias and fears. However, if your phobia is so severe that it triggers panic attacks or uncontrollable anxiety, you may want to get additional support.

The good news is that therapy for phobias has a great track record. Not only does it work extremely well, but you tend to see results very quickly—sometimes in as a little as 1–4 sessions.

However, support doesn't have to come in the guise of a professional therapist. Just having someone to hold your hand or stand by your side as you face your fears can be extraordinarily helpful.

Phobia Treatment Tip 1: Face Your Fears, One Step At A Time

It's only natural to want to avoid the thing or situation you fear. But when it comes to conquering phobias, facing your fears is the key. While avoidance may make you feel better in the short-term, it prevents you from learning that your phobia may not be as frightening or overwhelming as you think. You never get the chance to learn how to cope with your fears and experience control over the situation. As a result, the phobia becomes increasingly scarier and more daunting in your mind.

Exposure: Gradually And Repeatedly Facing Your Fears

The most effective way to overcome a phobia is by gradually and repeatedly exposing yourself to what you fear in a safe and controlled way. During this exposure process, you'll learn to ride out the anxiety and fear until it inevitably passes.

Through repeated experiences facing your fear, you'll begin to realize that the worst isn't going to happen; You're not going to die or "lose it." With each exposure, you'll feel more confident and in control. The phobia begins to lose its power.

Successfully facing your fears takes planning, practice, and patience. The following tips will help you get the most out of the exposure process.

Climbing Up The "Fear Ladder"

If you've tried exposure in the past and it didn't work, you may have started with something too scary or overwhelming. It's important to begin with a situation that you can handle, and work your way up from there, building your confidence and coping skills as you move up the "fear ladder."

- **Make a list.** Make a list of the frightening situations related to your phobia. If you're afraid of flying, your list (in addition to the obvious, such as taking a flight or getting through takeoff) might include booking your ticket, packing your suitcase, driving to the airport, watching planes take off and land, going through security, boarding the plane, and listening to the flight attendant present the safety instructions.

- **Build your fear ladder.** Arrange the items on your list from the least scary to the most scary. The first step should make you slightly anxious, but not so frightened that you're too intimidated to try it. When creating the ladder, it can be helpful to think about your end goal (for example, to be able to be near dogs without panicking) and then break down the steps needed to reach that goal.

- **Work your way up the ladder.** Start with the first step (in this example, looking at pictures of dogs) and don't move on until you start to feel more comfortable doing it. If at all possible, stay in the situation long enough for your anxiety to decrease. The longer you expose yourself to the thing you're afraid of, the more you'll get used to it and the less anxious you'll feel when you face it the next time. If the situation itself is short (for example, crossing a bridge), do it over and over again until your anxiety starts to lessen. Once you've done a step on several separate occasions without feeling too much anxiety, you can move on to the next step. If a step is too hard, break it down into smaller steps or go slower.

- **Practice.** It's important to practice regularly. The more often you practice, the quicker your progress will be. However, don't rush. Go at a pace that you can manage without feeling overwhelmed. And remember: you will feel uncomfortable and anxious as you face your fears, but the feelings are only temporary. If you stick with it, the anxiety will fade. Your fears won't hurt you.

If You Start To Feel Overwhelmed...

While it's natural to feel scared or anxious as you face your phobia, you should never feel overwhelmed by these feelings. If you start to feel overwhelmed, immediately back off. You may need to spend more time learning to control feelings of anxiety (see the relaxation techniques), or you may feel more comfortable working with a therapist.

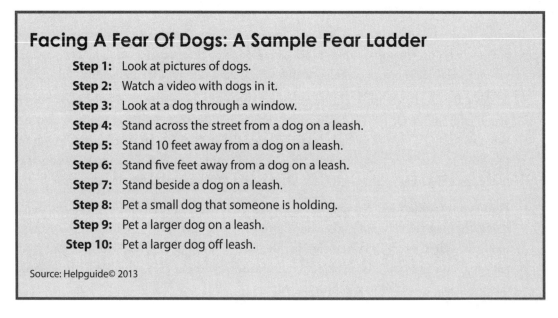

Facing A Fear Of Dogs: A Sample Fear Ladder

Step 1: Look at pictures of dogs.

Step 2: Watch a video with dogs in it.

Step 3: Look at a dog through a window.

Step 4: Stand across the street from a dog on a leash.

Step 5: Stand 10 feet away from a dog on a leash.

Step 6: Stand five feet away from a dog on a leash.

Step 7: Stand beside a dog on a leash.

Step 8: Pet a small dog that someone is holding.

Step 9: Pet a larger dog on a leash.

Step 10: Pet a larger dog off leash.

Source: Helpguide© 2013

Phobia Treatment Tip 2: Learn Relaxation Techniques

As you'll recall, when you're afraid or anxious, you experience a variety of uncomfortable physical symptoms, such as a racing heart and a suffocating feeling. These physical sensations can be frightening themselves—and a large part of what makes your phobia so distressing. However, by learning and practicing relaxation techniques, you can become more confident in your ability to tolerate these uncomfortable sensations and calm yourself down quickly.

Relaxation techniques such as deep breathing, meditation, and muscle relaxation are powerful antidotes to anxiety, panic, and fear. With regular practice, they can improve your ability to control the physical symptoms of anxiety, which will make facing your phobia less intimidating. Relaxation techniques will also help you cope more effectively with other sources of stress and anxiety in your life.

A Simple Deep Breathing Relaxation Exercise

When you're anxious, you tend to take quick, shallow breaths (also known as hyperventilating), which actually adds to the physical feelings of anxiety. By breathing deeply from the abdomen, you can reverse these physical sensations. You can't be upset when you're breathing slowly, deeply, and quietly. Within a few short minutes of deep breathing, you'll feel less tense, short of breath, and anxious.

- **Sit or stand comfortably** with your back straight. Put one hand on your chest and the other on your stomach.

- **Take a slow breath in** through your nose, counting to four. The hand on your stomach should rise. The hand on your chest should move very little.

- **Hold your breath** for a count of seven.

- **Exhale through your mouth** to a count of eight, pushing out as much air as you can while contracting your abdominal muscles. The hand on your stomach should move in as you exhale, but your other hand should move very little.

- **Inhale again**, repeating the cycle until you feel relaxed and centered.

Try practicing this deep breathing technique for five minutes, twice day. You don't need to feel anxious to practice. In fact, it's best to practice when you're feeling calm until you're familiar and comfortable with the exercise. Once you're comfortable with this deep breathing technique, you can start to use it when you're facing your phobia or in other stressful situations.

Evaluating Negative Thoughts

Once you've identified your negative thoughts, evaluate them. Use the following example to get started.

Negative thought: "The elevator will break down and I'll get trapped and suffocate."

Is there any evidence that contradicts this thought?

- "I see many people using the elevator and it has never broken down."
- "I cannot remember ever hearing of anyone dying from suffocation in an elevator."
- "I have never actually been in an elevator that has broken down."
- "There are air vents in an elevator which will stop the air running out."

Could you do anything to resolve this situation if it does occur?

- "I guess I could press the alarm button or use the telephone to call for assistance."

Are you making a thinking error?

- "Yes. I'm fortune telling, as I have no evidence to suggest that the elevator will break down."

What would you say to a friend who has this fear?

- "I would probably say that the chances of it happening are very slim as you don't see or hear about it very often."

Source [of information included in the Helpguide document cited at the beginning of this chapter]: Mood Juice.

Phobia Treatment Tip 3: Challenge Negative Thoughts

Learning to challenge unhelpful thoughts is an important step in overcoming your phobia. When you have a phobia, you tend to overestimate how bad it will be if you're exposed to the situation you fear. At the same time, you underestimate your ability to cope.

The anxious thoughts that trigger and fuel phobias are usually negative and unrealistic. It can help to put these thoughts to the test. Begin by writing down any negative thoughts you have when confronted with your phobia. Many times, these thoughts fall into the following categories:

- **Fortune Telling:** For example, "This bridge is going to collapse;" "I'll make a fool of myself for sure;" "I will definitely lose it when the elevator doors close."

- **Overgeneralization:** "I fainted once while getting a shot. I'll never be able to get a shot again without passing out;" "That pit bull lunged at me. All dogs are dangerous."

- **Catastrophizing:** "The captain said we're going through turbulence. The plane is going to crash!" "The person next to me coughed. Maybe it's the swine flu. I'm going to get very sick!"

It's also helpful to come up with some positive coping statements that you can tell yourself when facing your phobia. For example:

- "I've felt this way before and nothing terrible happened. It may be unpleasant, but it won't harm me."

- "If the worst happens and I have a panic attack while I'm driving, I'll simply pull over and wait for it to pass."

- "I've flown many times and the plane has never crashed. In fact, I don't know anyone who's ever been in a plane crash. Statistically, flying is very safe."

Chapter 16

Panic Disorder: When Fear Overwhelms

Do you sometimes have sudden attacks of fear that last for several minutes? Do you feel like you are having a heart attack or can't breathe? Do these attacks occur at unpredictable times causing you to worry about the possibility of having another one at any time? If so, you may have a type of anxiety disorder called panic disorder.

What is panic disorder?

People with panic disorder have sudden and repeated attacks of fear that last for several minutes. Sometimes symptoms may last longer. These are called panic attacks. Panic attacks are characterized by a fear of disaster or of losing control even when there is no real danger. A person may also have a strong physical reaction during a panic attack. It may feel like having a heart attack. Panic attacks can occur at any time, and many people with panic disorder worry about and dread the possibility of having another attack.

A person with panic disorder may become discouraged and feel ashamed because he or she cannot carry out normal routines like going to the grocery store or driving. Having panic disorder can also interfere with school or work.

Panic disorder often begins in the late teens or early adulthood. More women than men have panic disorder. But not everyone who experiences panic attacks will develop panic disorder.

What are the signs and symptoms of panic disorder?

People with panic disorder may have:

About This Chapter: Excerpted from "Panic Disorder: When Fear Overwhelms," National Institute of Mental Health (www.nimh.nih.gov), January 2013.

- Sudden and repeated attacks of fear

- A feeling of being out of control during a panic attack

- An intense worry about when the next attack will happen

- A fear or avoidance of places where panic attacks have occurred in the past

- Physical symptoms during an attack, such as a pounding or racing heart, sweating, breathing problems, weakness or dizziness, feeling hot or a cold chill, tingly or numb hands, chest pain, or stomach pain

What causes panic disorder?

Panic disorder sometimes runs in families, but no one knows for sure why some people have it, while others don't. Researchers have found that several parts of the brain are involved in fear and anxiety. By learning more about fear and anxiety in the brain, scientists may be able to create better treatments. Researchers are also looking for ways in which stress and environmental factors may play a role.

How is panic disorder treated?

First, talk to your doctor about your symptoms. Your doctor should do an exam to make sure that another physical problem isn't causing the symptoms. The doctor may refer you to a mental health specialist.

Panic disorder is generally treated with psychotherapy, medication, or both.

Psychotherapy: A type of psychotherapy called cognitive behavior therapy is especially useful for treating panic disorder. It teaches a person different ways of thinking, behaving, and reacting to situations that help him or her feel less anxious and fearful.

Medication: Doctors also may prescribe medication to help treat panic disorder. The most commonly prescribed medications for panic disorder are anti-anxiety medications and anti-depressants. Anti-anxiety medications are powerful and there are different types. Many types begin working right away, but they generally should not be taken for long periods.

Antidepressants are used to treat depression, but they also are helpful for panic disorder. They may take several weeks to start working. Some of these medications may cause side effects such as headache, nausea, or difficulty sleeping. These side effects are usually not a problem for most people, especially if the dose starts off low and is increased slowly over time. Talk to your doctor about any side effects that you may have.

What is it like to have panic disorder?

"One day, without any warning or reason, I felt terrified. I was so afraid, I thought I was going to die. My heart was pounding and my head was spinning. I would get these feelings every couple of weeks. I thought I was losing my mind."

"The more attacks I had, the more afraid I got. I was always living in fear. I didn't know when I might have another attack. I became so afraid that I didn't want to leave my house."

"My friend saw how afraid I was and told me to call my doctor for help. My doctor told me I was physically healthy but that I have panic disorder. My doctor gave me medicine that helps me feel less afraid. I've also been working with a counselor learning ways to cope with my fear. I had to work hard, but after a few months of medicine and therapy, I'm starting to feel like myself again."

Source: NIMH, January 2013.

It's important to know that although antidepressants can be safe and effective for many people, they may be risky for some, especially teens and young adults. A "black box"—the most serious type of warning that a prescription drug can have—has been added to the labels of antidepressant medications. These labels warn people that antidepressants may cause some people to have suicidal thoughts or make suicide attempts. Anyone taking antidepressants should be monitored closely, especially when they first start treatment with medications.

Another type of medication called beta-blockers can help control some of the physical symptoms of panic disorder such as excessive sweating, a pounding heart, or dizziness. Although beta blockers are not commonly prescribed, they may be helpful in certain situations that bring on a panic attack.

Some people do better with cognitive behavior therapy, while others do better with medication. Still others do best with a combination of the two. Talk with your doctor about the best treatment for you.

Part Three
Personality And Psychotic Disorders

Chapter 17

Antisocial Disorders

Antisocial personality disorder is a mental health condition in which a person has a long-term pattern of manipulating, exploiting, or violating the rights of others. This behavior is often criminal.

Causes

Cause of antisocial personality disorder is unknown. Genetic factors and environmental factors, such as child abuse, are believed to contribute to the development of this condition. People with an antisocial or alcoholic parent are at increased risk. Far more men than women are affected. The condition is common among people who are in prison.

Fire-setting and cruelty to animals during childhood are linked to the development of antisocial personality.

Some doctors believe that psychopathic personality (psychopathy) is the same disorder. Others believe that psychopathic personality is a similar but more severe disorder.

Symptoms

A person with antisocial personality disorder may: be able to act witty and charming; be good at flattery and manipulating other people's emotions; break the law repeatedly; disregard the safety of self and others; have problems with substance abuse; lie, steal, and fight often; not show guilt or remorse; and/or often be angry or arrogant.

About This Chapter: Excerpted from "Antisocial Personality Disorder," © 2013 A.D.A.M., Inc. Reprinted with permission.

Exams And Tests

Antisocial personality disorder is diagnosed based on a psychological evaluation that assesses the history and severity of symptoms. To be diagnosed with antisocial personality disorder, a person must have had conduct disorder during childhood.

Treatment

Antisocial personality disorder is one of the most difficult personality disorders to treat. People with this condition rarely seek treatment on their own. They may only start therapy when required to by a court.

Behavioral treatments, such as those that reward appropriate behavior and have negative consequences for illegal behavior, may hold the most promise. Certain forms of talk therapy are also being explored.

Persons with antisocial personality who have other disorders, such as a mood or substance disorder, are often treated for those problems as well.

Outlook (Prognosis)

Symptoms tend to peak during the late teenage years and early 20s. They sometimes improve on their own by a person's 40s.

Possible Complications

Complications can include imprisonment, drug abuse, violence, and suicide.

When To Contact A Medical Professional

See your health care provider or a mental health professional if you or someone you know has symptoms of antisocial personality disorder.

Alternative Names

- Sociopathic personality
- Sociopathy
- Personality disorder (antisocial)

Chapter 18

Borderline Personality Disorder

What is borderline personality disorder?

Borderline personality disorder is a serious mental illness marked by unstable moods, behavior, and relationships. In 1980, the *Diagnostic and Statistical Manual for Mental Disorders, Third Edition* (*DSM-III*) listed borderline personality disorder as a diagnosable illness for the first time. Most psychiatrists and other mental health professionals use the DSM to diagnose mental illnesses.

Because some people with severe borderline personality disorder have brief psychotic episodes, experts originally thought of this illness as atypical, or borderline, versions of other mental disorders. While mental health experts now generally agree that the name "borderline personality disorder" is misleading, a more accurate term does not exist yet.

Most people who have borderline personality disorder suffer from:

- Problems with regulating emotions and thoughts
- Impulsive and reckless behavior
- Unstable relationships with other people

People with this disorder also have high rates of co-occurring disorders, such as depression, anxiety disorders, substance abuse, and eating disorders, along with self-harm, suicidal behaviors, and completed suicides.

According to data from a subsample of participants in a national survey on mental disorders, about 1.6 percent of adults in the United States have borderline personality disorder in a given year.

About This Chapter: Excerpted from "Borderline Personality Disorder," National Institute of Mental Health (www .nimh.nih.gov), March 2012.

Borderline personality disorder is often viewed as difficult to treat. However, recent research shows that borderline personality disorder can be treated effectively, and that many people with this illness improve over time.

What are the symptoms of borderline personality disorder?

According to the *Diagnostic and Statistical Manual for Mental Disorders, Fourth Edition, Text Revision* (*DSM-IV-TR*), to be diagnosed with borderline personality disorder, a person must show an enduring pattern of behavior that includes at least five of the following symptoms:

- Extreme reactions (including panic, depression, rage, or frantic actions) to abandonment, whether real or perceived

- A pattern of intense and stormy relationships with family, friends, and loved ones, often veering from extreme closeness and love (idealization) to extreme dislike or anger (devaluation)

- Distorted and unstable self-image or sense of self, which can result in sudden changes in feelings, opinions, values, or plans and goals for the future (such as school or career choices)

- Impulsive and often dangerous behaviors, such as spending sprees, unsafe sex, substance abuse, reckless driving, and binge eating

- Recurring suicidal behaviors or threats or self-harming behavior, such as cutting

- Intense and highly changeable moods, with each episode lasting from a few hours to a few days

- Chronic feelings of emptiness and/or boredom

- Inappropriate, intense anger or problems controlling anger

- Having stress-related paranoid thoughts or severe dissociative symptoms, such as feeling cut off from oneself, observing oneself from outside the body, or losing touch with reality

Seemingly mundane events may trigger symptoms. For example, people with borderline personality disorder may feel angry and distressed over minor separations—such as vacations, business trips, or sudden changes of plans—from people to whom they feel close. Studies show that people with this disorder may see anger in an emotionally neutral face and have a stronger reaction to words with negative meanings than people who do not have the disorder.

Suicide And Self-Harm

Self-injurious behavior includes suicide and suicide attempts, as well as self-harming behaviors. As many as 80 percent of people with borderline personality disorder have suicidal behaviors, and about 4–9 percent commit suicide.

Suicide is one of the most tragic outcomes of any mental illness. Some treatments can help reduce suicidal behaviors in people with borderline personality disorder. For example, one study showed that dialectical behavior therapy (DBT) reduced suicide attempts in women by half compared with other types of psychotherapy, or talk therapy. DBT also reduced use of emergency room and inpatient services and retained more participants in therapy, compared to other approaches to treatment. For more information about DBT, see the section, "How is borderline personality disorder treated?"

Unlike suicide attempts, self-harming behaviors do not stem from a desire to die. However, some self-harming behaviors may be life threatening. Self-harming behaviors linked with borderline personality disorder include cutting, burning, hitting, head banging, hair pulling, and other harmful acts. People with borderline personality disorder may self-harm to help regulate their emotions, to punish themselves, or to express their pain. They do not always see these behaviors as harmful.

Source: NIMH, March 2012.

When does borderline personality disorder start?

Borderline personality disorder usually begins during adolescence or early adulthood. Some studies suggest that early symptoms of the illness may occur during childhood.

Some people with borderline personality disorder experience severe symptoms and require intensive, often inpatient, care. Others may use some outpatient treatments but never need hospitalization or emergency care. Some people who develop this disorder may improve without any treatment.

What illnesses often co-exist with borderline personality disorder?

Borderline personality disorder often occurs with other illnesses. These co-occurring disorders can make it harder to diagnose and treat borderline personality disorder, especially if symptoms of other illnesses overlap with the symptoms of borderline personality disorder.

Women with borderline personality disorder are more likely to have co-occurring disorders such as major depression, anxiety disorders, or eating disorders. In men, borderline personality disorder is more likely to co-occur with disorders such as substance abuse or antisocial personality disorder.

According to the National Comorbidity Survey Replication funded by the National Institute of Mental Health (NIMH)—the largest national study to date of mental disorders in U.S. adults—about 85 percent of people with borderline personality disorder also meet the diagnostic criteria for another mental illness.

Other illnesses that often occur with borderline personality disorder include diabetes, high blood pressure, chronic back pain, arthritis, and fibromyalgia. These conditions are associated with obesity, which is a common side effect of the medications prescribed to treat borderline personality disorder and other mental disorders. For more information, see the section, "How is borderline personality disorder treated?"

What are the risk factors for borderline personality disorder?

Research on the possible causes and risk factors for borderline personality disorder is still at a very early stage. However, scientists generally agree that genetic and environmental factors are likely to be involved.

Studies on twins with borderline personality disorder suggest that the illness is strongly inherited. Another study shows that a person can inherit his or her temperament and specific personality traits, particularly impulsiveness and aggression. Scientists are studying genes that help regulate emotions and impulse control for possible links to the disorder.

Social or cultural factors may increase the risk for borderline personality disorder. For example, being part of a community or culture in which unstable family relationships are common may increase a person's risk for the disorder. Impulsiveness, poor judgment in lifestyle choices, and other consequences of borderline personality disorder may lead individuals to risky situations. Adults with borderline personality disorder are considerably more likely to be the victim of violence, including rape and other crimes.

How is borderline personality disorder diagnosed?

Unfortunately, borderline personality disorder is often underdiagnosed or misdiagnosed.

A mental health professional experienced in diagnosing and treating mental disorders—such as a psychiatrist, psychologist, clinical social worker, or psychiatric nurse—can detect borderline personality disorder based on a thorough interview and a discussion about symptoms. A careful and thorough medical exam can help rule out other possible causes of symptoms.

The mental health professional may ask about symptoms and personal and family medical histories, including any history of mental illnesses. This information can help the mental health professional decide on the best treatment. In some cases, co-occurring mental illnesses may have symptoms that overlap with borderline personality disorder, making it difficult to distinguish borderline personality disorder from other mental illnesses. For example, a person may describe feelings of depression but may not bring other symptoms to the mental health professional's attention.

No single test can diagnose borderline personality disorder. Scientists funded by NIMH are looking for ways to improve diagnosis of this disorder. One study found that adults with borderline personality disorder showed excessive emotional reactions when looking at words with unpleasant meanings, compared with healthy people. People with more severe borderline personality disorder showed a more intense emotional response than people who had less severe borderline personality disorder.

What studies are being done to improve the diagnosis of borderline personality disorder?

Recent neuroimaging studies show differences in brain structure and function between people with borderline personality disorder and people who do not have this illness. Some research suggests that brain areas involved in emotional responses become overactive in people with borderline personality disorder when they perform tasks that they perceive as negative. People with the disorder also show less activity in areas of the brain that help control emotions and aggressive impulses and allow people to understand the context of a situation. These findings may help explain the unstable and sometimes explosive moods characteristic of borderline personality disorder.

Another study showed that, when looking at emotionally negative pictures, people with borderline personality disorder used different areas of the brain than people without the disorder. Those with the illness tended to use brain areas related to reflexive actions and alertness, which may explain the tendency to act impulsively on emotional cues.

These findings could inform efforts to develop more specific tests to diagnose borderline personality disorder.

How is borderline personality disorder treated?

Borderline personality disorder can be treated with psychotherapy, or "talk" therapy. In some cases, a mental health professional may also recommend medications to treat specific symptoms. When a person is under more than one professional's care, it is essential for the professionals to coordinate with one another on the treatment plan.

The following treatments are just some of the options that may be available to a person with borderline personality disorder. However, the research on treatments is still in very early stages.

More studies are needed to determine the effectiveness of these treatments, who may benefit the most, and how best to deliver treatments.

Psychotherapy: Psychotherapy is usually the first treatment for people with borderline personality disorder. Current research suggests psychotherapy can relieve some symptoms, but further studies are needed to better understand how well psychotherapy works.

It is important that people in therapy get along with and trust their therapist. The very nature of borderline personality disorder can make it difficult for people with this disorder to maintain this type of bond with their therapist.

Types of psychotherapy used to treat borderline personality disorder include the following:

- **Cognitive Behavioral Therapy (CBT):** CBT can help people with borderline personality disorder identify and change core beliefs and/or behaviors that underlie inaccurate perceptions of themselves and others and problems interacting with others. CBT may help reduce a range of mood and anxiety symptoms and reduce the number of suicidal or self-harming behaviors.

- **Dialectical Behavior Therapy (DBT):** This type of therapy focuses on the concept of mindfulness, or being aware of and attentive to the current situation. DBT teaches skills to control intense emotions, reduces self-destructive behaviors, and improves relationships. This therapy differs from CBT in that it seeks a balance between changing and accepting beliefs and behaviors.

- **Schema-Focused Therapy:** This type of therapy combines elements of CBT with other forms of psychotherapy that focus on reframing schemas, or the ways people view themselves. This approach is based on the idea that borderline personality disorder stems from a dysfunctional self-image—possibly brought on by negative childhood experiences—that affects how people react to their environment, interact with others, and cope with problems or stress.

Therapy can be provided one-on-one between the therapist and the patient or in a group setting. Therapist-led group sessions may help teach people with borderline personality disorder how to interact with others and how to express themselves effectively.

One type of group therapy, Systems Training for Emotional Predictability and Problem Solving (STEPPS), is designed as a relatively brief treatment consisting of 20 two-hour sessions led by an experienced social worker. Scientists funded by NIMH reported that STEPPS, when used with other types of treatment (medications or individual psychotherapy), can help reduce symptoms and problem behaviors of borderline personality disorder, relieve symptoms of depression, and improve quality of life. The effectiveness of this type of therapy has not been extensively studied.

Families of people with borderline personality disorder may also benefit from therapy. The challenges of dealing with an ill relative on a daily basis can be very stressful, and family members may unknowingly act in ways that worsen their relative's symptoms.

Some therapies, such as DBT-family skills training (DBT-FST), include family members in treatment sessions. These types of programs help families develop skills to better understand and support a relative with borderline personality disorder. Other therapies, such as Family Connections, focus on the needs of family members. More research is needed to determine the effectiveness of family therapy in borderline personality disorder. Studies with other mental disorders suggest that including family members can help in a person's treatment.

Other types of therapy not listed in this chapter may be helpful for some people with borderline personality disorder. Therapists often adapt psychotherapy to better meet a person's needs. Therapists may switch from one type of therapy to another, mix techniques from different therapies, or use a combination therapy.

Some symptoms of borderline personality disorder may come and go, but the core symptoms of highly changeable moods, intense anger, and impulsiveness tend to be more persistent. People whose symptoms improve may continue to face issues related to co-occurring disorders, such as depression or post-traumatic stress disorder. However, encouraging research suggests that relapse, or the recurrence of full-blown symptoms after remission, is rare. In one study, six percent of people with borderline personality disorder had a relapse after remission.

Medications: No medications have been approved by the U.S. Food and Drug Administration to treat borderline personality disorder. Only a few studies show that medications are necessary or effective for people with this illness. However, many people with borderline personality disorder are treated with medications in addition to psychotherapy. While medications do not cure borderline personality disorder, some medications may be helpful in managing specific symptoms. For some people, medications can help reduce symptoms such as anxiety, depression, or aggression. Often, people are treated with several medications at the same time, but there is little evidence that this practice is necessary or effective.

Medications can cause different side effects in different people. People who have borderline personality disorder should talk with their prescribing doctor about what to expect from a particular medication.

Omega-3 Fatty Acids: One study done on 30 women with borderline personality disorder showed that omega-3 fatty acids may help reduce symptoms of aggression and depression. The treatment seemed to be as well tolerated as commonly prescribed mood stabilizers and had few side effects. Fewer women who took omega-3 fatty acids dropped out of the study, compared to women who took a placebo (sugar pill).

With proper treatment, many people experience fewer or less severe symptoms. However, many factors affect the amount of time it takes for symptoms to improve, so it is important for people with borderline personality disorder to be patient and to receive appropriate support during treatment.

How can I help a friend or relative who has borderline personality disorder?

If you know someone who has borderline personality disorder, it affects you too. The first and most important thing you can do is help your friend or relative get the right diagnosis and treatment. You may need to make an appointment and go with your friend or relative to see the doctor. Encourage him or her to stay in treatment or to seek different treatment if symptoms do not appear to improve with the current treatment.

To help a friend or relative you can:

- Offer emotional support, understanding, patience, and encouragement—change can be difficult and frightening to people with borderline personality disorder, but it is possible for them to get better over time.

- Learn about mental disorders, including borderline personality disorder, so you can understand what your friend or relative is experiencing.

- With permission from your friend or relative, talk with his or her therapist to learn about therapies that may involve family members, such as DBT-FST.

Never ignore comments about someone's intent or plan to harm himself or herself or someone else. Report such comments to the person's therapist or doctor. In urgent or potentially life-threatening situations, you may need to call the police.

How can I help myself if I have borderline personality disorder?

Taking that first step to help yourself may be hard. It is important to realize that, although it may take some time, you can get better with treatment.

To help yourself:

- Talk to your doctor about treatment options and stick with treatment.

- Try to maintain a stable schedule of meals and sleep times.

- Engage in mild activity or exercise to help reduce stress.

- Set realistic goals for yourself.

- Break up large tasks into small ones, set some priorities, and do what you can, as you can.

- Try to spend time with other people and confide in a trusted friend or family member.

- Tell others about events or situations that may trigger symptoms.

- Expect your symptoms to improve gradually, not immediately.

- Identify and seek out comforting situations, places, and people.

- Continue to educate yourself about this disorder.

Where can I go for help?

If you are unsure where to go for help, ask your family doctor. Other people who can help are:

- Mental health professionals, such as psychiatrists, psychologists, social workers, or mental health counselors

- Health maintenance organizations

- Community mental health centers

- Hospital psychiatry departments and outpatient clinics

- Mental health programs at universities or medical schools

- State hospital outpatient clinics

- Family services, social agencies, or clergy

- Peer support groups

- Private clinics and facilities

- Local medical and psychiatric societies

You can also check the phone book under "mental health," "health," "social services," "hotlines," or "physicians" for phone numbers and addresses. An emergency room doctor can provide temporary help and can tell you where and how to get further help.

What if I or someone I know is in crisis?

If you are thinking about harming yourself, or know someone who is:

- Call your doctor.

- Call 911 or go to a hospital emergency room to get immediate help or ask a friend or family member to help you do these things.

- Call the toll-free, 24-hour hotline of the National Suicide Prevention Lifeline at 1-800-273-TALK (1-800-273-8255) or TTY: 1-800-799-4TTY (1-800-799-4889) to talk to a trained counselor.

- If you are in a crisis, make sure you are not left alone.

- If someone else is in a crisis, make sure he or she is not left alone.

Chapter 19

Histrionic Personality Disorder

Histrionic personality disorder is a mental health condition in which people act in a very emotional and dramatic way that draws attention to themselves.

Causes

Cause of histrionic personality disorder is unknown. Genes and early childhood events may be responsible. It is diagnosed more often in women than in men. Doctors believe that more men may have the disorder than are diagnosed.

Histrionic personality disorder usually begins by late teens or early 20s.

Symptoms

People with this disorder are usually able to function at a high level and can be successful socially and at work.

Symptoms include:

- Acting or looking overly seductive
- Being easily influenced by other people
- Being overly concerned with their looks
- Being overly dramatic and emotional
- Being overly sensitive to criticism or disapproval
- Believing that relationships are more intimate than they actually are

About This Chapter: Excerpted from "Histrionic Personality Disorder," © 2013 A.D.A.M., Inc. Reprinted with permission.

- Blaming failure or disappointment on others
- Constantly seeking reassurance or approval
- Having a low tolerance for frustration or delayed gratification
- Needing to be the center of attention (self-centeredness)
- Quickly changing emotions, which may seem shallow to others

Exams And Tests

Histrionic personality disorder is diagnosed based on a psychological evaluation that assesses the history and severity of the symptoms.

The health care provider can diagnose histrionic personality disorder by looking at the person's: Behavior; History; Overall appearance; Psychological evaluation.

Treatment

People with this condition often seek treatment when they experience depression or anxiety from failed romantic relationships or other conflicts with people. Medicine may help the symptoms. Talk therapy is the best treatment for the condition itself.

Outlook (Prognosis)

Histrionic personality disorder can improve with talk therapy and sometimes medicines. Left untreated, it can cause problems in people's personal lives and prevent them doing their best at work.

Possible Complications

Histrionic personality disorder may affect a person's social or romantic relationships. The person may be unable to cope with losses or failures. The person may change jobs often because of boredom and not being able to deal with frustration. A person with this disorder craves new things and excitement, which leads to risky situations. All of these factors may lead to a higher chance of depression.

When To Contact A Medical Professional

See your health care provider or mental health professional if you or someone you know has symptoms of histrionic personality disorder.

Chapter 20

Factitious Disorders

What is factitious disorder?

Mental illness describes abnormal cognitive or emotional patterns related to how a person thinks, feels, acts, and/or relates to others and his or her surroundings. Factitious disorder is a mental disorder in which a person acts as if he or she has a physical or mental illness when, in fact, he or she has consciously created their symptoms. The name "factitious" comes from the Latin word for "artificial."

People with factitious disorder deliberately create or exaggerate symptoms of an illness in several ways. They may lie about or mimic symptoms, hurt themselves to bring on symptoms, or alter diagnostic tests (such as contaminating a urine sample). Those with factitious disorders have an inner need to be seen as ill or injured, but not to achieve a concrete benefit, such as a financial gain. Individuals with factitious disorder are even willing to undergo painful or risky tests and operations in order to obtain the sympathy and special attention given to people who are truly ill. Factitious disorder is considered a mental illness because it is associated with severe emotional difficulties.

Many people with factitious disorder may also suffer from other mental disorders, particularly personality disorders. People with personality disorders have long-standing patterns of thinking and acting that differ from what society considers usual or normal. People with personality disorders generally also have poor coping skills and problems forming healthy relationships.

About This Chapter: Excerpted from "An Overview of Factitious Disorders," © 2013 The Cleveland Clinic Foundation, 9500 Euclid Avenue, Cleveland, OH 44195. All rights reserved. Reprinted with permission. Additional information is available from the Cleveland Clinic Health Information Center, 216-444-3771, toll-free 800-223-2273 extension 43771, or at http://my.clevelandclinic.org/health.

Factitious disorder is similar to somatic symptom disorder, another mental disorder that involves the presence of symptoms that are not due to actual physical illnesses. The main difference between the two groups of disorders is that people with somatic symptom disorder do not intentionally fake symptoms or mislead others about their symptoms. Similarly, the behavior of people with factitious disorder is not malingering, a term that refers to faking illness for financial gain (such as to collect insurance money), food or shelter, or to avoid criminal prosecution or other responsibilities. Malingering is potentially criminal behavior and not a mental illness.

What are the symptoms of factitious disorder?

Possible warning signs of factitious disorder include the following:

- Dramatic but inconsistent medical history

Types Of Factitious Disorder

In *The Diagnostic and Statistical Manual of Mental Disorders, Fifth Edition* (*DSM-5*), which is the standard reference book for recognized mental illnesses in the United States, factitious disorder falls under the section of Somatic Symptom and Related Disorders. The *DSM-5* categorizes factitious disorder into two types: factitious disorder imposed on self and factious disorder imposed on another. "Falsification of physical or psychological signs or symptoms" or a combination of those occurs in factitious disorder, but it may also include inducing an injury such as making a skin cut to produce blood to mix with urine. There are no obvious rewards like money or time off of work to explain why the individual is deceiving others. To make the diagnosis it is necessary to rule out delusions or other evidence of psychosis. Factitious disorder can occur as a single episode or be a recurrent pattern.

One example of factitious disorder is to mimic behavior that is typical of a mental illness, such as schizophrenia. The person may appear confused, make absurd statements, and report hallucinations (the experience of sensing things that are not there; for example, hearing voices).

Another example is deceptively laying claim to having symptoms related to a physical illness, such as chest pain, stomach problems, or fever. In the past this was referred to as Munchausen syndrome, named for Baron von Munchausen, an 18th century German officer who was known for embellishing the stories of his life and experiences.

Factitious disorder imposed on another was formerly called factitious disorder by proxy or Munchausen syndrome by proxy. Individuals with this disorder produce or fabricate symptoms of illness in another under their care: children, elderly adults, disabled persons, or pets. It most often occurs in mothers, although it can occur in fathers, who intentionally harm their children in order to receive attention. The diagnosis is not given to the victim, but rather to the perpetrator.

Source: The Cleveland Clinic © 2013.

- Unclear symptoms that are not controllable, become more severe, or change once treatment has begun

- Predictable relapses following improvement in the condition

- Extensive knowledge of hospitals and/or medical terminology, as well as the textbook descriptions of illness

- Presence of many surgical scars

- Appearance of new or additional symptoms following negative test results

- Presence of symptoms only when the patient is alone or not being observed

- Willingness or eagerness to have medical tests, operations, or other procedures

- History of seeking treatment at many hospitals, clinics, and doctors' offices, possibly even in different cities

- Reluctance by the patient to allow health care professionals to meet with or talk to family members, friends, and prior health care providers

What causes factitious disorder?

The exact cause of factitious disorder is not known, but researchers believe both biological and psychological factors play a role in the development of this disorder. Some theories suggest that a history of abuse or neglect as a child, or a history of frequent illnesses in themselves or family that required hospitalization, may be factors in the development of the disorder.

How common is factitious disorder?

There are no reliable statistics regarding the number of people in the United States who suffer from factitious disorder. Obtaining accurate statistics is difficult because dishonesty is common with this disorder. In addition, people with factitious disorders tend to seek treatment at many different health care facilities, resulting in statistics that are misleading. It is estimated that about one percent of those admitted to hospitals are believed to have factitious disorder.

How is factitious disorder diagnosed?

Due to the dishonesty involved, diagnosing factitious disorder is very difficult. In addition, doctors must rule out any possible physical and mental illnesses, and often use a variety of diagnostic tests and procedures before considering a diagnosis of factitious disorder.

If the health care provider finds no physical reason for the symptoms, he or she may refer the person to a psychiatrist or psychologist (mental health professionals who are specially trained to diagnose and treat mental illnesses). Psychiatrists and psychologists use thorough history, physical, laboratory tests, imagery, and psychological testing to evaluate a person for physical and mental conditions. The doctor bases his or her diagnosis on the exclusion of actual physical or mental illness, and his or her observation of the patient's attitude and behavior. For example, delusional disorder and various forms of psychosis are not examples of factitious disorder.

Questions to be answered include:

- Do the patient's reported symptoms make sense in the context of all test results and assessments?

- Do we have collateral information from other sources that confirm the patient's information? (If the patient does not allow this, this is a helpful clue.)

- Is the patient more willing to take the risk for more procedures and tests than you would expect?

- Are treatments working in a predictable way?

The doctor then determines if the patient's symptoms point to factitious disorder as outlined in *DSM-5*.

How is factitious disorder treated?

The first goal of treatment is to modify the person's behavior and reduce his or her misuse or overuse of medical resources. In the case of factitious disorder imposed on another, the main goal is to ensure the safety and protection of any real or potential victims. Once the initial goal is met, treatment aims to resolve any underlying psychological issues that may be causing the person's behavior or help them find solutions to housing or other social needs.

The primary treatment for factitious disorder is psychotherapy (a type of counseling). Treatment likely will focus on changing the thinking and behavior of the individual with the disorder (cognitive behavioral therapy). Family therapy also may be helpful in teaching family members not to reward or reinforce the behavior of the person with the disorder.

There are no medications to actually treat factitious disorder. Medication may be used, however, to treat any related disorder, such as depression or anxiety. The use of medications must be carefully monitored in people with factitious disorder due to the risk that the drugs may never be picked up from the pharmacy or may be used in a harmful way.

What are the complications of factitious disorder?

People with factitious disorder are at risk for health problems associated with hurting themselves by causing symptoms. In addition, they may suffer health problems related to multiple tests, procedures, and treatments, and are at high risk for substance abuse and suicide attempts. A complication of factitious disorder imposed on another is the abuse and potential death of the victims.

What is the prognosis (outlook) for people with factitious disorder?

Some people with factitious disorder suffer one or two brief episodes of symptoms. In most cases, however, factitious disorder is a chronic, or long-term, condition that can be very difficult to treat. Additionally, many people with factitious disorder deny they are faking symptoms and will not seek or follow treatment.

Can factitious disorder be prevented?

There is no known way to prevent factitious disorder. However, it may be helpful to start treatment in people as soon as they begin to have symptoms.

Chapter 21

Delusional Disorder

Delusional Disorder Symptoms

Delusional disorder is characterized by the presence of non-bizarre delusions which have persisted for at least one month. Non-bizarre delusions typically are beliefs of something occurring in a person's life which is not out of the realm of possibility. For example, the person may believe their significant other is cheating on them, that someone close to them is about to die, a friend is really a government agent, etc. All of these situations could be true or possible, but the person suffering from this disorder knows them not to be (for example, through fact-checking, third-person confirmation, etc.).

People who have this disorder generally don't experience a marked impairment in their daily functioning in a social, occupational, or other important setting. Outward behavior is not noticeably bizarre or objectively characterized as out-of-the-ordinary.

The delusions cannot be better accounted for by another disorder, such as schizophrenia, which is also characterized by delusions (which are bizarre). The delusions also cannot be better accounted for by a mood disorder, if the mood disturbances have been relatively brief.

Specific Diagnostic Criteria

- Non-bizarre delusions (that is, involving situations that occur in real life, such as being followed, poisoned, infected, loved at a distance, or deceived by spouse or lover, or having a disease) of at least one month's duration

- Criterion A for schizophrenia has never been met. **Note:** Tactile and olfactory hallucinations may be present in delusional disorder if they are related to the delusional theme. Criterion A of schizophrenia requires two (or more) of the following, each present for a significant portion of time during a one-month period (or less, if successfully treated):
  - Delusions
  - Hallucinations
  - Disorganized speech (for example, frequent derailment or incoherence)
  - Grossly disorganized or catatonic behavior
  - Negative symptoms (that is, affective flattening [loss or lack of emotional expressiveness], alogia [inability to speak], or avolition [lack of motivation])

  Note: Criteria A of Schizophrenia requires only one symptom if delusions are bizarre or hallucinations consist of a voice keeping up a running commentary on the person's behavior or thoughts, or two or more voices conversing with each other.

- Apart from the impact of the delusion(s) or its ramifications, functioning is not markedly impaired and behavior is not obviously odd or bizarre.

- If mood episodes have occurred concurrently with delusions, their total duration has been brief relative to the duration of the delusional periods.

- The disturbance is not due to the direct physiological effects of a substance (for example, a drug of abuse; a medication) or a general medical condition.

Specify Type

The following types are assigned based on the predominant delusional theme:

- **Erotomanic Type:** Delusions that another person, usually of higher status, is in love with the individual

- **Grandiose Type:** Delusions of inflated worth, power, knowledge, identity, or special relationship to a deity or famous person

- **Jealous Type:** Delusions that the individual's sexual partner is unfaithful

- **Persecutory Type:** Delusions that the person (or someone to whom the person is close) is being malevolently treated in some way

- **Somatic Type:** Delusions that the person has some physical defect or general medical condition
- **Mixed Type:** Delusions characteristic of more than one of the above types but no one theme predominates
- **Unspecified Type**

Delusional Disorder Treatment

Psychotherapy

Psychotherapy is usually the most effective help in person suffering from delusional disorder. The overriding important factor in this therapy is the quality of the patient/therapist relationship. Trust is a key issue, as is unconditional support. If the client believes that the therapist really does think he or she is "crazy," the therapy can terminate abruptly. Early in the therapy, it is vital not to directly challenge the delusion system or beliefs and instead to concentrate on realistic and concrete problems and goals within the person's life.

Once a firm, supportive therapeutic relationship has been established, the therapist can begin reinforcing positive gains and behaviors the individual makes in his or her life, such as in educational or occupational gains. It is important to reinforce these life events (such as getting a job), because it reinforces in the patient a sense of self-confidence and self-reliance.

Only when the client has begun to feel more secure in their social or occupational world can more productive work be accomplished in therapy. This involves the gradual but gentle challenging of the client's delusional beliefs, starting with the smallest and least important items. Occasionally making these types of gentle challenges throughout therapy will give the clinician a greater understanding of how far along the individual has come. If the patient refuses to give up his or her delusion beliefs, even the smallest ones, then therapy is likely to be very long term. Even if the client is willing, therapy is likely to take a fair amount of time, from at least six months to a year.

Clinicians should always be very direct and honest, especially with people who suffer from delusion disorder. Professionals should be even more careful than usual not to impinge on the client's privacy or confidentiality, and to say plainly what they mean in therapy sessions. Subtlety and sarcasm may be easily misinterpreted by the patient. Therapy approaches which focus on insight or self-knowledge may not be as beneficial as those stressing social skills training and other behaviorally and solution-oriented therapies.

Medications

Suggesting the use of medication for use in this disorder, while possibly indicated to help temporarily relieve the delusions, is usually difficult. The client may be suspicious of any professional suggesting the use of a medication and therefore this treatment approach (and successful maintenance of the individual on the medication) is problematic.

Anti-psychotic medication is the preferred medication used, though, although it is only marginally effective. There are few studies done which confirm the use of any specific medications for this disorder.

Hospitalization should be avoided at all costs, since this will usually go to reinforce the individual's distorted cognitive schema. Partial hospitalization and/or day treatment programs are preferred to help manage the individual under close supervision on a daily basis.

Phillip W. Long, MD writes that "other treatments have been tried (electroconvulsive therapy, insulin shock therapy, and psychosurgery), but these approaches are not recommended."

Self-Help

There are not any self-help support groups or communities that we are aware of that would be conducive to someone suffering from this disorder. Such approaches would likely not be very effective because a person with this disorder is likely to be mistrustful and suspicious of others and their motivations, making group help and dynamics unlikely and possibly harmful.

Chapter 22

Dissociative Disorders

What is dissociation?

A number of people with mental illnesses experience dissociation: a disturbance of thinking, awareness, identity, consciousness or memory. Dissociation is more severe than just ordinary forgetfulness and is also not associated with any underlying cause of memory deficits or altered consciousness (for example, neurological illnesses; substance or alcohol abuse). Some people have dissociative events that last only moments where as others experience extended periods of dissociation.

Some people will experience having limited ability to regulate their bodily functions and may feel like they are "going crazy" or are "out of my body" during dissociative events. Other people may lose control of their emotions or actions during a dissociative event and can do things that are otherwise quite uncharacteristic. Some people will have limited memory of the dissociative event and may feel surprised or disoriented when it ends. Many people may later recall what happened during their dissociation, but others may not be able to remember significant parts of what occurred, sometimes for even for a time before they dissociated.

There is an association between traumatic events and the process of dissociation. It may be that dissociation is a way the mind/brain contends with overwhelming stimuli. There is much more to be learned about the process of dissociation and the best strategies to address it. Dissociation can be part of a symptom of an existing mental illness. For example, many people who have experienced a traumatic event, such as physical or sexual abuse, may have some aspect of

About This Chapter: Information in this chapter is reprinted from, "Dissociative Disorders Fact Sheet," November 2012, © NAMI, the National Alliance on Mental Illness, www.nami.org.

dissociation during the event itself and will be unable to recall details regarding their victimization. Dissociation can be a symptom associated with posttraumatic stress disorder (PTSD) and with certain anxiety disorders, including panic disorder and obsessive-compulsive disorder.

What are dissociative disorders?

Dissociative disorders are a controversial sub-group of mental illnesses. The most dramatic condition in this area is called dissociative identity disorder, formerly called multiple personality disorder. The media has a history of sensational portrayals of dissociative [disorders] and of persons who have pretended to have dissociative illnesses in order to avoid criminal charges. Researchers, clinicians, and the public alike find the topic compelling and challenging to understand.

There is controversy over whether or not dissociative disorders are over diagnosed or improperly diagnosed by certain mental health professionals. This is an ongoing debate that is unlikely to be resolved soon.

In rare cases, some individuals have severe symptoms of dissociation in the absence of another primary mental or medical illness. In these situations, the *Diagnostic and Statistical Manual of Mental Disorders, 4th Edition, Text Revision* (*DSM-IV-TR*) lists criteria by which dissociative disorders may be diagnosed. Dissociative disorders as defined by the DSM-IV-TR include:

- **Dissociative Amnesia:** [This amnesia is] characterized by severe impairment in remembering important information about one's self. This is perhaps the most common of the dissociative disorders and—like all other dissociative illnesses—is associated with traumatic events. This amnesia can be limited to specific details or events but can also encompass entire aspects of a person's life.

- **Dissociative Fugue:** [This amnesia is characterized by] a massive disorientation of self that leads to confusion about one's personal identity and potentially the assumption of a new identity.

- **Depersonalization Disorder:** [A disorder] marked by recurrent feelings of detachment or distance from one's own experiences and can be associated with the experience that the world is unreal. While many people experience these sensations at one point in their lives, an individual with depersonalization disorder has this experience so frequently or severely that it interrupts his or her functioning.

- **Dissociative Identify Disorder (DID):** Previously called multiple personality disorder, DID is the most famous and controversial of the dissociative disorders. This is characterized by having multiple "alters" (personal identities) that control an individual's behavior and actions at different times.

What are some available treatments?

In patients where dissociation is thought to be a symptom of another mental illness (for example, borderline personality disorder or PTSD), treatment of the primary cause is of upmost importance. This can involve psychotherapy and psychiatric medications when appropriate. It is important to note that there is no clear consensus on the treatment of dissociative symptoms themselves with medications for it is unclear whether or not psychiatric drugs can help to decrease symptoms of dissociation and depersonalization.

Psychotherapy is generally helpful for people who experience dissociative episodes. Different cognitive behavioral therapy (CBT) and dialectical behavioral therapy (DBT) techniques have been specifically developed by mental health professionals to decrease symptom frequency and improve coping strategies for the experience of dissociation. As with any mental illness, the caring support of loved ones cannot be underestimated, particularly for individuals with a traumatic past.

Chapter 23

Psychosis

Psychosis is a loss of contact with reality that usually includes false beliefs about what is taking place or who one is (delusions), and seeing (or hearing) things that aren't there (hallucinations).

Causes

A number of medical problems can cause psychosis, including: alcohol and certain illegal drugs, both during use and during withdrawal; brain diseases, such as Parkinson disease, Huntington disease, and certain chromosomal disorders; brain tumors or cysts; dementia (including Alzheimer disease); HIV and other infections that affect the brain; some prescription drugs, such as steroids and stimulants; some types of epilepsy; and stroke.

Psychosis (or psychotic symptoms) may also be found in: most people with schizophrenia; some people with bipolar disorder (manic-depressive) or severe depression; and some personality disorders.

Symptoms

Psychotic symptoms may include: disorganized thought and speech; false beliefs that are not based in reality (delusions), especially unfounded fear or suspicion; hearing, seeing, or feeling things that are not there (hallucinations); and/or thoughts that "jump" between unrelated topics (disordered thinking).

Exams And Tests

Psychiatric evaluation and testing are used to diagnose the cause of the psychosis. Laboratory testing and brain scans may not be needed, but sometimes can help pinpoint the diagnosis. Tests may include: blood tests for abnormal electrolyte and hormone levels; blood tests for syphilis and other infections; drug screens; and magnetic resonance imaging (MRI) of the brain.

Treatment

Treatment depends on the cause of the psychosis. Care in a hospital is often needed to ensure the patient's safety.

Antipsychotic drugs, which reduce hallucinations and delusions and improve thinking and behavior are helpful, whether the cause is a medical or psychiatric disorder.

Outlook (Prognosis)

How well a person does depends on the cause of the psychosis. If the cause can be corrected, the outlook is often good, and treatment with antipsychotic medication may be brief.

Some chronic conditions, such as schizophrenia, may need life-long treatment with antipsychotic medications to control symptoms.

Possible Complications

Psychosis can prevent people from functioning normally and caring for themselves. If the condition is left untreated, people can sometimes harm themselves or others.

When To Contact A Medical Professional

Call your health care provider or mental health professional if you or a member of your family is losing contact with reality. If there is any concern about safety, immediately take the person to the nearest emergency room to be seen by a doctor.

Prevention

Prevention depends on the cause. For example, avoiding alcohol abuse prevents alcohol-induced psychosis.

Chapter 24

Schizophrenia And Schizoaffective Disorder

Schizophrenia: An Overview

Schizophrenia is a chronic, severe, and disabling brain disorder that has affected people throughout history. About one percent of Americans have this illness.

People with the disorder may hear voices other people don't hear. They may believe other people are reading their minds, controlling their thoughts, or plotting to harm them. This can terrify people with the illness and make them withdrawn or extremely agitated.

People with schizophrenia may not make sense when they talk. They may sit for hours without moving or talking. Sometimes people with schizophrenia seem perfectly fine until they talk about what they are really thinking.

Families and society are affected by schizophrenia too. Many people with schizophrenia have difficulty holding a job or caring for themselves, so they rely on others for help.

Treatment helps relieve many symptoms of schizophrenia, but most people who have the disorder cope with symptoms throughout their lives. However, many people with schizophrenia can lead rewarding and meaningful lives in their communities. Researchers are developing more effective medications and using new research tools to understand the causes of schizophrenia. In the years to come, this work may help prevent and better treat the illness.

About This Chapter: Excerpted from "Schizophrenia," National Institute of Mental Health (www.nimh.nih.gov), March 2012.

Symptoms Of Schizophrenia

The symptoms of schizophrenia fall into three broad categories: positive symptoms, negative symptoms, and cognitive symptoms.

Positive Symptoms

Positive symptoms are psychotic behaviors not seen in healthy people. People with positive symptoms often "lose touch" with reality. These symptoms can come and go. Sometimes they are severe and at other times hardly noticeable, depending on whether the individual is receiving treatment. They include the following:

Hallucinations: Hallucinations are things a person sees, hears, smells, or feels that no one else can see, hear, smell, or feel. "Voices" are the most common type of hallucination in schizophrenia. Many people with the disorder hear voices. The voices may talk to the person about his or her behavior, order the person to do things, or warn the person of danger. Sometimes the voices talk to each other. People with schizophrenia may hear voices for a long time before family and friends notice the problem.

Other types of hallucinations include seeing people or objects that are not there, smelling odors that no one else detects, and feeling things like invisible fingers touching their bodies when no one is near.

Delusions: Delusions are false beliefs that are not part of the person's culture and do not change. The person believes delusions even after other people prove that the beliefs are not true or logical. People with schizophrenia can have delusions that seem bizarre, such as believing that neighbors can control their behavior with magnetic waves. They may also believe that people on television are directing special messages to them, or that radio stations are broadcasting their thoughts aloud to others. Sometimes they believe they are someone else, such as a famous historical figure. They may have paranoid delusions and believe that others are trying to harm them, such as by cheating, harassing, poisoning, spying on, or plotting against them or the people they care about. These beliefs are called "delusions of persecution."

Thought Disorders: Thought disorders are unusual or dysfunctional ways of thinking. One form of thought disorder is called "disorganized thinking." This is when a person has trouble organizing his or her thoughts or connecting them logically. They may talk in a garbled way that is hard to understand. Another form is called "thought blocking." This is when a person stops speaking abruptly in the middle of a thought. When asked why he or she stopped talking, the person may say that it felt as if the thought had been taken out of his or her head. Finally, a person with a thought disorder might make up meaningless words, or "neologisms."

Movement Disorders: Movement disorders may appear as agitated body movements. A person with a movement disorder may repeat certain motions over and over. In the other extreme, a person may become catatonic. Catatonia is a state in which a person does not move and does not respond to others. Catatonia is rare today, but it was more common when treatment for schizophrenia was not available.

Negative Symptoms

Negative symptoms are associated with disruptions to normal emotions and behaviors. These symptoms are harder to recognize as part of the disorder and can be mistaken for depression or other conditions. These symptoms include the following:

- "Flat affect" (a person's face does not move or he or she talks in a dull or monotonous voice)

- Lack of pleasure in everyday life

- Lack of ability to begin and sustain planned activities

- Speaking little, even when forced to interact

People with negative symptoms need help with everyday tasks. They often neglect basic personal hygiene. This may make them seem lazy or unwilling to help themselves, but the problems are symptoms caused by the schizophrenia.

Cognitive Symptoms

Cognitive symptoms are subtle. Like negative symptoms, cognitive symptoms may be difficult to recognize as part of the disorder. Often, they are detected only when other tests are performed. Cognitive symptoms include the following:

- Poor "executive functioning" (the ability to understand information and use it to make decisions)

- Trouble focusing or paying attention

- Problems with "working memory" (the ability to use information immediately after learning it)

Cognitive symptoms often make it hard to lead a normal life and earn a living. They can cause great emotional distress.

What is schizoaffective disorder?

Schizoaffective disorder is a serious mental illness that affects about one in 100 people. Schizoaffective disorder, as a diagnostic entity, has features that resemble both schizophrenia and also serious mood (affective) symptoms. Many of the strategies used to treat both schizophrenia and affective conditions can be employed for this condition. These include antipsychotic and mood stabilizing medications, family involvement, psychosocial strategies, self-care peer support, psychotherapy, and integrated care for co-occurring substance abuse (when appropriate).

A person who has schizoaffective disorder will experience delusions, hallucinations, other symptoms that are characteristic of schizophrenia, and significant disturbances in their mood (for example, affective symptoms). According to the *Diagnostic and Statistical Manual of Mental Disorders, 4th Edition, Text Revision (DSM-IV-TR)*, people who experience more than two weeks of psychotic symptoms in the absence of severe mood disturbances—and then have symptoms of either depression or bipolar disorder—may have schizoaffective disorder. Schizoaffective disorder is thought to be between the bipolar and schizophrenia diagnoses as it has features of both.

Depressive symptoms associated with schizoaffective disorder can include—but are not limited to—hopelessness, helplessness, guilt, worthlessness, disrupted appetite, disturbed sleep, inability to concentrate, and depressed mood (with or without suicidal thoughts). Manic symptoms associated with schizoaffective disorder can include increased energy, decreased sleep (or decreased need for sleep), distractibility, fast ("pressured") speech, and increased impulsive behaviors (for example, sexual activities, drug and alcohol abuse, or gambling).

While it is a hot topic of debate within the mental health field, most experts believe that schizoaffective disorder is a type of chronic mental illness that has psychotic symptoms at the core and with depressive and manic symptoms as a secondary—but equally debilitating—component. Because it consists of a wide range of symptoms, some people may be inappropriately diagnosed with schizoaffective disorder. This is problematic because it can lead to unnecessary treatments, specifically medication treatment, with antipsychotics, when they are not otherwise indicated.

People who have depression or mania as their primary mental illness may experience symptoms of psychosis (including disorganized speech, disorganized behavior, delusions, or hallucinations) during severe episodes of their mood disorder but will not have these symptoms if their mood disorder is well treated. Sometimes people with other mental illnesses including borderline personality disorder may also be incorrectly diagnosed with schizoaffective disorder. This further underscores how important it is to have regular and complete mental health assessments from one's doctors, preferably over time so that patterns of what is happening and what works can be fully understood together.

Source: "Schizoaffective Disorder Fact Sheet," November 2012, © NAMI, the National Alliance on Mental Illness, www.nami.org.

Identifying Schizophrenia

Schizophrenia affects men and women equally. It occurs at similar rates in all ethnic groups around the world. Symptoms such as hallucinations and delusions usually start between ages 16 and 30. Men tend to experience symptoms a little earlier than women. Most of the time, people do not get schizophrenia after age 45. Schizophrenia rarely occurs in children, but awareness of childhood-onset schizophrenia is increasing.

It can be difficult to diagnose schizophrenia in teens. This is because the first signs can include a change of friends, a drop in grades, sleep problems, and irritability—behaviors that are common among teens. A combination of factors can predict schizophrenia in up to 80 percent of youth who are at high risk of developing the illness. These factors include isolating oneself and withdrawing from others, an increase in unusual thoughts and suspicions, and a family history of psychosis. In young people who develop the disease, this stage of the disorder is called the "prodromal" period.

Schizophrenia And Violence

People with schizophrenia are not usually violent. In fact, most violent crimes are not committed by people with schizophrenia. However, some symptoms are associated with violence, such as delusions of persecution. Substance abuse may also increase the chance a person will become violent. If a person with schizophrenia becomes violent, the violence is usually directed at family members and tends to take place at home.

The risk of violence among people with schizophrenia is small. But people with the illness attempt suicide much more often than others. About 10 percent (especially young adult males) die by suicide. It is hard to predict which people with schizophrenia are prone to suicide. If you know someone who talks about or attempts suicide, help him or her find professional help right away.

Schizophrenia And Substance Abuse

Some people who abuse drugs show symptoms similar to those of schizophrenia. Therefore, people with schizophrenia may be mistaken for people who are affected by drugs. Most researchers do not believe that substance abuse causes schizophrenia. However, people who have schizophrenia are much more likely to have a substance or alcohol abuse problem than the general population.

Substance abuse can make treatment for schizophrenia less effective. Some drugs, like marijuana and stimulants such as amphetamines or cocaine, may make symptoms worse.

In fact, research has found increasing evidence of a link between marijuana and schizophrenia symptoms. In addition, people who abuse drugs are less likely to follow their treatment plan.

Schizophrenia And Smoking

Addiction to nicotine is the most common form of substance abuse in people with schizophrenia. They are addicted to nicotine at three times the rate of the general population (75–90 percent versus 25–30 percent).

The relationship between smoking and schizophrenia is complex. People with schizophrenia seem to be driven to smoke, and researchers are exploring whether there is a biological basis for this need. In addition to its known health hazards, several studies have found that smoking may make antipsychotic drugs less effective.

Quitting smoking may be very difficult for people with schizophrenia because nicotine withdrawal may cause their psychotic symptoms to get worse for a while. Quitting strategies that include nicotine replacement methods may be easier for patients to handle. Doctors who treat people with schizophrenia should watch their patients' response to antipsychotic medication carefully if the patient decides to start or stop smoking.

Causes Of Schizophrenia

Experts think schizophrenia is caused by several factors.

Genes And Environment

Scientists have long known that schizophrenia runs in families. The illness occurs in one percent of the general population, but it occurs in 10 percent of people who have a first-degree relative with the disorder, such as a parent, brother, or sister. People who have second-degree relatives (aunts, uncles, grandparents, or cousins) with the disease also develop schizophrenia more often than the general population. The risk is highest for an identical twin of a person with schizophrenia. He or she has a 40–65 percent chance of developing the disorder.

We inherit our genes from both parents. Scientists believe several genes are associated with an increased risk of schizophrenia, but that no gene causes the disease by itself. In fact, recent research has found that people with schizophrenia tend to have higher rates of rare genetic mutations. These genetic differences involve hundreds of different genes and probably disrupt brain development.

Other recent studies suggest that schizophrenia may result in part when a certain gene that is key to making important brain chemicals malfunctions. This problem may affect the part of the brain involved in developing higher functioning skills. Research into this gene is ongoing, so it is not yet possible to use the genetic information to predict who will develop the disease.

Despite this, tests that scan a person's genes can be bought without a prescription or a health professional's advice. Ads for the tests suggest that with a saliva sample, a company can determine if a client is at risk for developing specific diseases, including schizophrenia. However, scientists don't yet know all of the gene variations that contribute to schizophrenia. Those that are known raise the risk only by very small amounts. Therefore, these "genome scans" are unlikely to provide a complete picture of a person's risk for developing a mental disorder like schizophrenia.

In addition, it probably takes more than genes to cause the disorder. Scientists think interactions between genes and the environment are necessary for schizophrenia to develop. Many environmental factors may be involved, such as exposure to viruses or malnutrition before birth, problems during birth, and other not yet known psychosocial factors.

Different Brain Chemistry And Structure

Scientists think that an imbalance in the complex, interrelated chemical reactions of the brain involving the neurotransmitters dopamine and glutamate, and possibly others, plays a role in schizophrenia. Neurotransmitters are substances that allow brain cells to communicate with each other. Scientists are learning more about brain chemistry and its link to schizophrenia.

Also, in small ways the brains of people with schizophrenia look different than those of healthy people. For example, fluid-filled cavities at the center of the brain, called ventricles, are larger in some people with schizophrenia. The brains of people with the illness also tend to have less gray matter, and some areas of the brain may have less or more activity.

Studies of brain tissue after death also have revealed differences in the brains of people with schizophrenia. Scientists found small changes in the distribution or characteristics of brain cells that likely occurred before birth. Some experts think problems during brain development before birth may lead to faulty connections. The problem may not show up in a person until puberty. The brain undergoes major changes during puberty, and these changes could trigger psychotic symptoms. Scientists have learned a lot about schizophrenia, but more research is needed to help explain how it develops.

Treating Schizophrenia

Because the causes of schizophrenia are still unknown, treatments focus on eliminating the symptoms of the disease. Treatments include antipsychotic medications and various psychosocial treatments.

Antipsychotic Medications

Antipsychotic medications have been available since the mid-1950s. The older types are called conventional or "typical" antipsychotics. Some of the more commonly used typical medications include chlorpromazine (Thorazine), haloperidol (Haldol), perphenazine (Etrafon, Trilafon), and fluphenazine (Prolixin).

In the 1990s, new antipsychotic medications were developed. These new medications are called second generation, or "atypical" antipsychotics.

One of these medications, clozapine (Clozaril) is an effective medication that treats psychotic symptoms, hallucinations, and breaks with reality. But clozapine can sometimes cause a serious problem called agranulocytosis, which is a loss of the white blood cells that help a person fight infection. People who take clozapine must get their white blood cell counts checked every week or two. This problem and the cost of blood tests make treatment with clozapine difficult for many people. But clozapine is potentially helpful for people who do not respond to other antipsychotic medications.

Other atypical antipsychotics were also developed. None cause agranulocytosis. Examples include risperidone (Risperdal), olanzapine (Zyprexa), quetiapine (Seroquel), ziprasidone (Geodon), aripiprazole (Abilify), and paliperidone (Invega).

When a doctor says it is okay to stop taking a medication, it should be gradually tapered off, never stopped suddenly.

Side Effects: Some people have side effects when they start taking these medications. Most side effects go away after a few days and often can be managed successfully. People who are taking antipsychotics should not drive until they adjust to their new medication. Side effects of many antipsychotics include:

- Drowsiness
- Dizziness when changing positions
- Blurred vision
- Rapid heartbeat

- Sensitivity to the sun
- Skin rashes
- Menstrual problems for women

Atypical antipsychotic medications can cause major weight gain and changes in a person's metabolism. This may increase a person's risk of getting diabetes and high cholesterol. A person's weight, glucose levels, and lipid levels should be monitored regularly by a doctor while taking an atypical antipsychotic medication.

Typical antipsychotic medications can cause side effects related to physical movement, such as:

- Rigidity
- Persistent muscle spasms
- Tremors
- Restlessness

Long term use of typical antipsychotic medications may lead to a condition called tardive dyskinesia (TD). TD causes muscle movements a person can't control. The movements commonly happen around the mouth. TD can range from mild to severe, and in some people the problem cannot be cured. Sometimes people with TD recover partially or fully after they stop taking the medication.

TD happens to fewer people who take the atypical antipsychotics, but some people may still get TD. People who think that they might have TD should check with their doctor before stopping their medication.

Administration: Antipsychotics are usually in pill or liquid form. Some anti-psychotics are shots that are given once or twice a month.

Symptoms of schizophrenia, such as feeling agitated and having hallucinations, usually go away within days. Symptoms like delusions usually go away within a few weeks. After about six weeks, many people will see a lot of improvement.

However, people respond in different ways to antipsychotic medications, and no one can tell beforehand how a person will respond. Sometimes a person needs to try several medications before finding the right one. Doctors and patients can work together to find the best medication or medication combination, as well as the right dose.

Some people may have a relapse—their symptoms come back or get worse. Usually, relapses happen when people stop taking their medication, or when they only take it sometimes.

Some people stop taking the medication because they feel better or they may feel they don't need it anymore. But no one should stop taking an antipsychotic medication without talking to his or her doctor. When a doctor says it is okay to stop taking a medication, it should be gradually tapered off, never stopped suddenly.

Interactions With Other Medications: Antipsychotics can produce unpleasant or dangerous side effects when taken with certain medications. For this reason, all doctors treating a patient need to be aware of all the medications that person is taking. Doctors need to know about prescription and over-the-counter medicine, vitamins, minerals, and herbal supplements. People also need to discuss any alcohol or other drug use with their doctor.

To find out more about how antipsychotics work, the National Institute of Mental Health (NIMH) funded a study called CATIE (Clinical Antipsychotic Trials of Intervention Effectiveness). This study compared the effectiveness and side effects of five antipsychotics used to treat people with schizophrenia. In general, the study found that the older typical antipsychotic perphenazine (Trilafon) worked as well as the newer, atypical medications. But because people respond differently to different medications, it is important that treatments be designed carefully for each person.

Psychosocial Treatments

Psychosocial treatments can help people with schizophrenia who are already stabilized on antipsychotic medication. Psychosocial treatments help these patients deal with the everyday challenges of the illness, such as difficulty with communication, self-care, work, and forming and keeping relationships. Learning and using coping mechanisms to address these problems allow people with schizophrenia to socialize and attend school and work.

Patients who receive regular psychosocial treatment also are more likely to keep taking their medication, and they are less likely to have relapses or be hospitalized. A therapist can help patients better understand and adjust to living with schizophrenia. The therapist can provide education about the disorder, common symptoms or problems patients may experience, and the importance of staying on medications.

Illness Management Skills: People with schizophrenia can take an active role in managing their own illness. Once patients learn basic facts about schizophrenia and its treatment, they can make informed decisions about their care. If they know how to watch for the early warning signs of relapse and make a plan to respond, patients can learn to prevent relapses. Patients can also use coping skills to deal with persistent symptoms.

Integrated Treatment For Co-Occurring Substance Abuse: Substance abuse is the most common co-occurring disorder in people with schizophrenia. But ordinary substance abuse treatment programs usually do not address this population's special needs. When schizophrenia treatment programs and drug treatment programs are used together, patients get better results.

Rehabilitation: Rehabilitation emphasizes social and vocational training to help people with schizophrenia function better in their communities. Because schizophrenia usually develops in people during the critical career-forming years of life (ages 18–35), and because the disease makes normal thinking and functioning difficult, most patients do not receive training in the skills needed for a job.

Rehabilitation programs can include job counseling and training, money management counseling, help in learning to use public transportation, and opportunities to practice communication skills. Rehabilitation programs work well when they include both job training and specific therapy designed to improve cognitive or thinking skills. Programs like this help patients hold jobs, remember important details, and improve their functioning.

Family Education: People with schizophrenia are often discharged from the hospital into the care of their families. So it is important that family members know as much as possible about the disease. With the help of a therapist, family members can learn coping strategies and problem-solving skills. In this way the family can help make sure their loved one sticks with treatment and stays on his or her medication. Families should learn where to find outpatient and family services.

Cognitive Behavioral Therapy: Cognitive behavioral therapy (CBT) is a type of psychotherapy that focuses on thinking and behavior. CBT helps patients with symptoms that do not go away even when they take medication. The therapist teaches people with schizophrenia how to test the reality of their thoughts and perceptions, how to "not listen" to their voices, and how to manage their symptoms overall. CBT can help reduce the severity of symptoms and reduce the risk of relapse.

Self-Help Groups: Self-help groups for people with schizophrenia and their families are becoming more common. Professional therapists usually are not involved, but group members support and comfort each other. People in self-help groups know that others are facing the same problems, which can help everyone feel less isolated. The networking that takes place in self-help groups can also prompt families to work together to advocate for research and more hospital and community treatment programs. Also, groups may be able to draw public attention to the discrimination many people with mental illnesses face.

Once patients learn basic facts about schizophrenia and its treatment, they can make informed decisions about their care.

Helping A Person With Schizophrenia

People with schizophrenia can get help from professional case managers and caregivers at residential or day programs. However, family members usually are a patient's primary caregivers.

People with schizophrenia often resist treatment. They may not think they need help because they believe their delusions or hallucinations are real. In these cases, family and friends may need to take action to keep their loved one safe. Laws vary from state to state, and it can be difficult to force a person with a mental disorder into treatment or hospitalization. But when a person becomes dangerous to himself or herself, or to others, family members or friends may have to call the police to take their loved one to the hospital.

Hospital Treatment

In the emergency room, a mental health professional will assess the patient and determine whether a voluntary or involuntary admission is needed. For a person to be admitted involuntarily, the law states that the professional must witness psychotic behavior and hear the person voice delusional thoughts. Family and friends can provide needed information to help a mental health professional make a decision.

After Leaving The Hospital

Family and friends can help their loved ones get treatment and take their medication once they go home. If patients stop taking their medication or stop going to follow-up appointments, their symptoms likely will return. Sometimes symptoms become severe for people who stop their medication and treatment. This is dangerous, since they may become unable to care for themselves. Some people end up on the street or in jail, where they rarely receive the kind of help they need.

Family and friends can also help patients set realistic goals and learn to function in the world. Each step toward these goals should be small and taken one at a time. The patient will need support during this time. When people with a mental illness are pressured and criticized, they usually do not get well. Often, their symptoms may get worse. Telling them when they are doing something right is the best way to help them move forward.

It can be difficult to know how to respond to someone with schizophrenia who makes strange or clearly false statements. Remember that these beliefs or hallucinations seem very real to the person. It is not helpful to say they are wrong or imaginary. But going along with the delusions is not helpful, either. Instead, calmly say that you see things differently. Tell them that you acknowledge that everyone has the right to see things his or her own way. In addition, it is important to understand that schizophrenia is a biological illness. Being respectful, supportive, and kind without tolerating dangerous or inappropriate behavior is the best way to approach people with this disorder.

People with schizophrenia can get help from professional case managers and caregivers at residential or day programs.

The Outlook For The Future

The outlook for people with schizophrenia continues to improve. Although there is no cure, treatments that work well are available. Many people with schizophrenia improve enough to lead independent, satisfying lives.

Continued research and understanding in genetics, neuroscience, and behavioral science will help scientists and health professionals understand the causes of the disorder and how it may be predicted and prevented. This work will help experts develop better treatments to help people with schizophrenia achieve their full potential. Families and individuals who are living with schizophrenia are encouraged to participate in clinical research.

Part Four
Behavioral, Impulse Control, And Addiction Disorders

Chapter 25

Eating Disorders

Eating Disorders: An Overview

An eating disorder is an illness that causes serious disturbances to your everyday diet, such as eating extremely small amounts of food or severely overeating. A person with an eating disorder may have started out just eating smaller or larger amounts of food, but at some point, the urge to eat less or more spiraled out of control. Severe distress or concern about body weight or shape may also characterize an eating disorder.

Eating disorders frequently appear during the teen years or young adulthood but may also develop during childhood or later in life. Common eating disorders include anorexia nervosa, bulimia nervosa, and binge eating disorder.

Eating disorders affect both men and women. It is unknown how many adults and children suffer with other serious, significant eating disorders, including one category of eating disorders called eating disorders not otherwise specified (EDNOS). EDNOS includes eating disorders that do not meet the criteria for anorexia or bulimia nervosa. Binge eating disorder is a type of eating disorder called EDNOS. EDNOS is the most common diagnosis among people who seek treatment.

Eating disorders are real, treatable medical illnesses. They frequently coexist with other illnesses such as depression, substance abuse, or anxiety disorders. Other symptoms can become life-threatening if a person does not receive treatment. People with anorexia nervosa are 18 times more likely to die early compared with people of similar age in the general population.

About This Chapter: Excerpts from "Eating Disorders," National Institute of Mental Health (www.nimh.nih.gov), January 2013.

Body Image

Have you ever thought that there was something wrong with the way you look? Do you think that you are too short or too tall, too heavy or too skinny?

If you have had thoughts like these, you are not alone. These feelings about how you look are called body image. Body image and self-esteem are tied together since body image can affect how you feel about your whole self. When you put yourself down about how you look, it can lead to negative feelings about yourself in general. Poor self-esteem can also lead to eating disorders that can put your health in danger.

If you start to have negative thoughts about your body and the way you look, think about all of the traits that make you special and unique. Look at your whole self—body and mind—in a positive way and write down what you see. Or before you go to bed at night, name three things you did that day that made you happy. By focusing on the positive aspects of your life you can feel more positive about yourself. Don't forget to give yourself compliments too.

Remember, during adolescence, your body is going through many changes that are happening at a fast pace. These changes might make you feel unsure of yourself at times, or stressed. They might make you worry about your size and wanting to fit in with the rest of the crowd.

During puberty, not only will you get taller, you will also see other changes in your body such as wider hips, bottoms, and thighs. Because your body is starting to produce new hormones (like estrogen), your weight may change and your body, which has both muscle and fat, will also start to have more fat compared to muscle than it did before. Changes in estrogen levels can also cause mood swings—especially around your period.

Try not to worry. Each woman changes at her own pace and all of these new changes are normal. While you are experiencing these changes keep your self-confidence up. How? By taking good care of yourself, eating healthy foods, and getting regular exercise.

Source: Excerpted from "Your Feelings: Body Image," Girls Health, Office on Women's Health, U.S. Department of Health and Human Resources (www.girlshealth.gov), July 2013.

Different Types Of Eating Disorders

Anorexia Nervosa

Many people with anorexia nervosa see themselves as overweight, even when they are clearly underweight. Eating, food, and weight control become obsessions. People with anorexia nervosa typically weigh themselves repeatedly, portion food carefully, and eat very small quantities of only certain foods. Some people with anorexia nervosa may also engage in binge eating followed by extreme dieting, excessive exercise, self-induced vomiting, and/or misuse of laxatives, diuretics, or enemas.

Some who have anorexia nervosa recover with treatment after only one episode. Others get well but have relapses. Still others have a more chronic, or long-lasting, form of anorexia nervosa, in which their health declines as they battle the illness.

Bulimia Nervosa

Bulimia nervosa is characterized by recurrent and frequent episodes of eating unusually large amounts of food and feeling a lack of control over these episodes. This binge eating is followed by behavior that compensates for the overeating such as forced vomiting, excessive use of laxatives or diuretics, fasting, excessive exercise, or a combination of these behaviors.

Unlike anorexia nervosa, people with bulimia nervosa usually maintain what is considered a healthy or normal weight, while some are slightly overweight. But like people with anorexia nervosa, they often fear gaining weight, want desperately to lose weight, and are intensely unhappy with their body size and shape. Usually, bulimic behavior is done secretly because it is often accompanied by feelings of disgust or shame. The binge eating and purging cycle happens anywhere from several times a week to many times a day.

Binge Eating Disorder

With binge eating disorder, a person loses control over his or her eating. Unlike bulimia nervosa, periods of binge eating are not followed by purging, excessive exercise, or fasting. As a result, people with binge eating disorder often are over-weight or obese. People with binge eating disorder who are obese are at higher risk for developing cardiovascular disease and high blood pressure. They also experience guilt, shame, and distress about their binge eating, which can lead to more binge eating.

Treating Eating Disorders

Adequate nutrition, reducing excessive exercise, and stopping purging behaviors are the foundations of treatment. Specific forms of psychotherapy, or talk therapy, and medication are effective for many eating disorders. However, in more chronic cases, specific treatments have not yet been identified. Treatment plans often are tailored to individual needs and may include individual, group, and/or family psychotherapy; medical care and monitoring; nutritional counseling; and/or medications. Some patients may also need to be hospitalized to treat problems caused by mal-nutrition or to ensure they eat enough if they are very underweight.

Treating Anorexia Nervosa

Treating anorexia nervosa involves three components:

- Restoring the person to a healthy weight

- Treating the psychological issues related to the eating disorder

- Reducing or eliminating behaviors or thoughts that lead to insufficient eating and preventing relapse

Some research suggests that the use of medications, such as antidepressants, antipsychotics, or mood stabilizers, may be modestly effective in treating patients with anorexia nervosa. These medications may help resolve mood and anxiety symptoms that often occur along with anorexia nervosa. It is not clear whether antidepressants can prevent some weight-restored

---

About Eating Disorders

Eating disorders are serious medical problems. Anorexia nervosa, bulimia nervosa, and binge eating disorder are all types of eating disorders. Eating disorders frequently develop during adolescence or early adulthood, but can occur during childhood or later in adulthood. Females are more likely than males to develop an eating disorder.

Eating disorders are more than just a problem with food. Food is used to feel in control of other feelings that may seem overwhelming. For example, starving is a way for people with anorexia to feel more in control of their lives and to ease tension, anger, and anxiety. Purging and other behaviors to prevent weight gain are ways for people with bulimia to feel more in control of their lives and to ease stress and anxiety.

Although there is no single known cause of eating disorders, several things may contribute to the development of these disorders:

- **Culture:** In the United States, extreme thinness is a social and cultural ideal, and women partially define themselves by how physically attractive they are.

- **Personal Characteristics:** Feelings of helplessness, worthlessness, and poor self-image often accompany eating disorders.

- **Other Emotional Disorders:** Other mental health problems, like depression or anxiety, occur along with eating disorders.

- **Stressful Events Or Life Changes:** Things like starting a new school or job or being teased and traumatic events like rape can lead to the onset of eating disorders.

- **Biology:** Studies are being done to look at genes, hormones, and chemicals in the brain that may have an effect on the development of, and recovery from, eating disorders.

patients with anorexia nervosa from relapsing. Although research is still ongoing, no medication yet has shown to be effective in helping someone gain weight to reach a normal level.

Different forms of psychotherapy, including individual, group, and family-based, can help address the psychological reasons for the illness. In a therapy called the Maudsley approach, parents of adolescents with anorexia nervosa assume responsibility for feeding their child. This approach appears to be very effective in helping people gain weight and improve eating habits and moods. Shown to be effective in case studies and clinical trials, the Maudsley approach is discussed in some guidelines and studies for treating eating disorders in younger, non-chronic patients.

Other research has found that a combined approach of medical attention and supportive psychotherapy designed specifically for anorexia nervosa patients is more effective than psychotherapy alone. The effectiveness of a treatment depends on the person involved and his or her situation. Unfortunately, no specific psychotherapy appears to be consistently effective for

---

- **Families:** Parents' attitudes about appearance and diet can affect their kids' attitudes. Also, if your mother or sister has bulimia, you are more likely to have it.

Over-Exercising

Too much of a good thing can be very bad for you. Just like eating disorders, societal pressures to be thin can also push women to exercise too much. Over-exercise is when someone engages in strenuous physical activity to the point that is unsafe and unhealthy. In fact, some studies indicate that young women who are compelled to exercise at excessive levels are at risk for developing eating disorders.

Eating disorders and over-exercising go hand-in-hand—they both can be a result of an unhealthy obsession with your body. The most dangerous aspect of over-exercising is the ease with which it can go unrecognized. The condition can be easily hidden by an emphasis on fitness or a desire to be healthy. Like bulimia and anorexia, in which persons deny themselves adequate nutrition by restrictive eating behaviors, over-exercising is a controlled behavior that denies the body the energy and nutrition needed to maintain a healthy weight.

According to the *American Journal of Sports Medicine*, a host of physical consequences can result from over-exercising—pulled muscles, stress fractures, knee trauma, shin splints, strained hamstrings, and ripped tendons.

Remember, fitness should be done within limits and integrated into your lifestyle, done in moderation like everything else in life. If exercising is getting in the way of your daily activities or relationships, you may need to slow down.

Source: Excerpted from "Body Image: Eating Disorders," Office on Women's Health, U.S. Department of Health and Human Services (www.womenshealth.gov), September 2010.

treating adults with anorexia nervosa. However, research into new treatment and prevention approaches is showing some promise. One study suggests that an online intervention program may prevent some at-risk women from developing an eating disorder. Also, specialized treatment of anorexia nervosa may help reduce the risk of death.

Treating Bulimia Nervosa

As with anorexia nervosa, treatment for bulimia nervosa often involves a combination of options and depends upon the needs of the individual. To reduce or eliminate binge eating and purging behaviors, a patient may undergo nutritional counseling and psychotherapy, especially cognitive behavioral therapy (CBT), or be prescribed medication. CBT helps a person focus on his or her current problems and how to solve them. The therapist helps the patient learn how to identify distorted or unhelpful thinking patterns, recognize, and change inaccurate beliefs, relate to others in more positive ways, and change behaviors accordingly.

CBT that is tailored to treat bulimia nervosa is effective in changing binge eating and purging behaviors and eating attitudes. Therapy may be individual or group-based.

Some antidepressants, such as fluoxetine (Prozac), which is the only medication approved by the U.S. Food and Drug Administration (FDA) for treating bulimia nervosa, may help patients who also have depression or anxiety. Fluoxetine also appears to help reduce binge eating and purging behaviors, reduce the chance of relapse, and improve eating attitudes.

Treating Binge Eating Disorder

Treatment options for binge eating disorder are similar to those used to treat bulimia nervosa. Psychotherapy, especially CBT that is tailored to the individual, has been shown to be effective. Again, this type of therapy can be offered in an individual or group environment.

FDA Warnings On Antidepressants

Antidepressants are safe and popular, but some studies have suggested that they may have unintentional effects on some people, especially in adolescents and young adults. The FDA warning says that patients of all ages taking antidepressants should be watched closely, especially during the first few weeks of treatment. Possible side effects to look for are depression that gets worse, suicidal thinking or behavior, or any unusual changes in behavior such as trouble sleeping, agitation, or withdrawal from normal social situations. Families and caregivers should report any changes to the doctor.

Source: NIMH, January 2013.

Fluoxetine and other antidepressants may reduce binge eating episodes and help lessen depression in some patients.

Males Are Also Affected

Like females who have eating disorders, males also have a distorted sense of body image. For some, their symptoms are similar to those seen in females. Others may have muscle dysmorphia, a type of disorder that is characterized by an extreme concern with becoming more muscular. Unlike girls with eating disorders, who mostly want to lose weight, some boys with muscle dysmorphia see themselves as smaller than they really are and want to gain weight or bulk up. Men and boys are more likely to use steroids or other dangerous drugs to increase muscle mass.

Although males with eating disorders exhibit the same signs and symptoms as females, they are less likely to be diagnosed with what is often considered a female disorder. More research is needed to understand the unique features of these disorders among males.

Research Regarding Eating Disorders

Researchers are finding that eating disorders are caused by a complex interaction of genetic, biological, behavioral, psychological, and social factors. But many questions still need answers. Researchers are using the latest in technology and science to better understand eating disorders.

One approach involves the study of human genes. Researchers are studying various combinations of genes to determine if any DNA variations are linked to the risk of developing eating disorders.

Neuroimaging studies are also providing a better understanding of eating disorders and possible treatments. One study showed different patterns of brain activity between women with bulimia nervosa and healthy women. Using functional magnetic resonance imaging (fMRI), researchers were able to see the differences in brain activity while the women performed a task that involved self-regulation (a task that requires overcoming an automatic or impulsive response).

Psychotherapy interventions are also being studied. One such study of adolescents found that more adolescents with bulimia nervosa recovered after receiving Maudsley model family-based treatment than those receiving supportive psychotherapy, that did not specifically address the eating disorder.

Researchers are studying questions about behavior, genetics, and brain function to better understand risk factors, identify biological markers, and develop specific psychotherapies and medications that can target areas in the brain that control eating behavior. Neuroimaging and genetic studies may provide clues for how each person may respond to specific treatments for these medical illnesses.

Chapter 26

Anorexia Nervosa

What is anorexia nervosa?

A person with anorexia nervosa (an-uh-RECK-see-uh nur-VOH-suh), often called anorexia, has an intense fear of gaining weight. Someone with anorexia thinks about food a lot and limits the food she or he eats, even though she or he is too thin. Anorexia is more than just a problem with food. It's a way of using food or starving oneself to feel more in control of life and to ease tension, anger, and anxiety. Most people with anorexia are female. An anorexic:

- Has a low body weight for her or his height
- Resists keeping a normal body weight
- Has an intense fear of gaining weight
- Thinks she or he is fat even when very thin
- Misses three menstrual periods in a row (for girls/women who have started having their periods)

Who becomes anorexic?

While anorexia mostly affects girls and women (85–95 percent of anorexics are female), it can also affect boys and men. It was once thought that women of color were shielded from eating disorders by their cultures, which tend to be more accepting of different body sizes. It is not known for sure whether African American, Latina, Asian/Pacific Islander, and American Indian and Alaska Native people develop eating disorders because American culture values

About This Chapter: Excerpted from "Anorexia Nervosa Fact Sheet," Office on Women's Health, U.S. Department of Health and Human Services (www.womenshealth.gov), July 2012.

thin people. People with different cultural backgrounds may develop eating disorders because it's hard to adapt to a new culture (a theory called "culture clash"). The stress of trying to live in two different cultures may cause some minorities to develop their eating disorders.

What causes anorexia?

There is no single known cause of anorexia. Eating disorders are real, treatable medical illnesses with causes in both the body and the mind. Some of these things may play a part:

- **Culture:** Women in the U.S. are under constant pressure to fit a certain ideal of beauty. Seeing images of flawless, thin females everywhere makes it hard for women to feel good about their bodies. More and more, women are also feeling pressure to have a perfect body.

- **Families:** If you have a mother or sister with anorexia, you are more likely to develop the disorder. Parents who think looks are important, diet themselves, or criticize their children's bodies are more likely to have a child with anorexia.

- **Life Changes Or Stressful Events:** Traumatic events (like rape) as well as stressful things (like starting a new job), can lead to the onset of anorexia.

- **Personality Traits:** Someone with anorexia may not like her or himself, hate the way she or he looks, or feel hopeless. She or he often sets hard-to-reach goals for her or himself and tries to be perfect in every way.

- **Biology:** Genes, hormones, and chemicals in the brain may be factors in developing anorexia.

What are signs of anorexia?

Someone with anorexia may look very thin. She or he may use extreme measures to lose weight by:

- Making her or himself throw up

- Taking pills to urinate or have a bowel movement

- Taking diet pills

- Not eating or eating very little

- Exercising a lot, even in bad weather or when hurt or tired

- Weighing food and counting calories

- Eating very small amounts of only certain foods

- Moving food around the plate instead of eating it

Someone with anorexia may also have a distorted body image, shown by thinking she or he is fat, wearing baggy clothes, weighing her or himself many times a day, and fearing weight gain.

Anorexia can also cause someone to not act like her or himself. She or he may talk about weight and food all the time, not eat in front of others, be moody or sad, or not want to go out with friends. People with anorexia may also have other psychiatric and physical illnesses, including:

- Depression
- Anxiety
- Obsessive behavior
- Substance abuse
- Issues with the heart and/or brain
- Problems with physical development

What happens to your body with anorexia?

With anorexia, your body doesn't get the energy from foods that it needs, so it slows down. Figure 26.1 shows how anorexia affects your health.

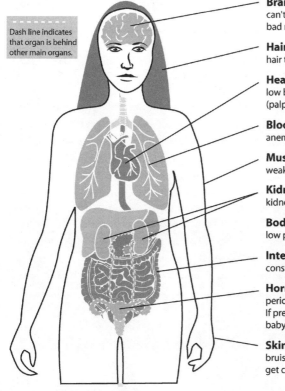

Dash line indicates that organ is behind other main organs.

Brain and Nerves
can't think right, fear of gaining weight, sad, moody, irritable, bad memory, fainting, changes in brain chemistry

Hair
hair thins and gets brittle

Heart
low blood pressure, slow heart rate, fluttering of the heart (palpitations), heart failure

Blood
anemia and other blood problems

Muscles, Joints, and Bones
weak muscles, swollen joints, fractures, osteoporosis

Kidneys
kidney stones, kidney failure

Body Fluids
low potassium, magnesium, and sodium

Intestines
constipation, bloating

Hormones
periods stop, problems growing, trouble getting pregnant. If pregnant, higher risk for miscarriage, having a C-section, baby with low birthweight, and post partum depression.

Skin
bruise easily, dry skin, growth of fine hair all over body, get cold easily, yellow skin, nails get brittle

Figure 26.1. Anorexia affects your whole body. Without enough energy from food, body functions are altered.

Can someone with anorexia get better?

Yes. Someone with anorexia can get better. A health care team of doctors, nutritionists, and therapists will help the patient get better. They will:

- Help bring the person back to a normal weight

- Treat any psychological issues related to anorexia

- Help the person get rid of any actions or thoughts that cause the eating disorder

These three steps will prevent "relapse." (Relapse means to get sick again, after feeling well for a while.)

Some research suggests that the use of medicines—such as antidepressants, antipsychotics, or mood stabilizers—may sometimes work for anorexic patients. It is thought that these medicines help the mood and anxiety symptoms that often co-exist with anorexia. Other recent studies, however, suggest that antidepressants may not stop some patients with anorexia from relapsing. Also, no medicine has shown to work one hundred percent of the time during

---

What should I do if I think someone I know has anorexia?

If someone you know is showing signs of anorexia, you may be able to help.

- **Set a time to talk.** Set aside a time to talk privately with your friend. Make sure you talk in a quiet place where you won't be distracted.

- **Share your concerns.** Be honest. Tell your friend about your worries about her or his not eating or over exercising. Tell your friend you are concerned and that you think these things may be a sign of a problem that needs professional help.

- **Ask your friend to talk to a professional.** Your friend can talk to a counselor or doctor who knows about eating issues. Offer to help your friend find a counselor or doctor and make an appointment, and offer to go with her or him to the appointment.

- **Avoid conflicts.** If your friend won't admit that she or he has a problem, don't push. Be sure to tell your friend you are always there to listen if she or he wants to talk.

- **Don't place shame, blame, or guilt.** Don't tell your friend, "You just need to eat." Instead, say things like, "I'm concerned about you because you won't eat breakfast or lunch." Or, "It makes me afraid to hear you throwing up."

- **Don't give simple solutions.** Don't say, "If you'd just stop, then things would be fine!"

- **Assure your friend.** Let your friend know that you will always be there no matter what.

Source: These tips, excerpted from the document by the Office on Women's Health which was cited at the beginning of this chapter, were adapted from "What Should I Say? Tips for Talking to a Friend Who May Be Struggling with an Eating Disorder," from the National Eating Disorders Association.

the important first step of restoring a patient to healthy weight. So, it is not clear if and how medications can help anorexic patients get better, but research is still happening.

Some forms of psychotherapy can help make the psychological reasons for anorexia better. Psychotherapy is sometimes known as "talk therapy." It uses different ways of communicating to change a patient's thoughts or behavior. This kind of therapy can be useful for treating eating disorders in young patients who have not had anorexia for a long time.

Individual counseling can help someone with anorexia. If the patient is young, counseling may involve the whole family. Support groups may also be a part of treatment. In support groups, patients, and families meet and share what they've been through.

Some researchers point out that prescribing medicines and using psychotherapy designed just for anorexic patients works better at treating anorexia than just psychotherapy alone. Whether or not a treatment works, though, depends on the person involved and his or her situation. Unfortunately, no one kind of psychotherapy always works for treating adults with anorexia.

What is outpatient care for anorexia treatment and how is it different from inpatient care?

With outpatient care, the patient receives treatment through visits with members of their health care team. Often this means going to a doctor's office. Outpatients usually live at home.

Some patients may need "partial hospitalization." This means that the person goes to the hospital during the day for treatment, but sleeps at home at night.

Sometimes, the patient goes to a hospital and stays there for treatment. This is called inpatient care. After leaving the hospital, the patient continues to get help from her health care team and becomes an outpatient.

Can women who had anorexia in the past still get pregnant?

It depends. When a woman has "active anorexia," meaning she currently has anorexia, she does not get her period and usually does not ovulate. This makes it hard to get pregnant. Women who have recovered from anorexia and are at a healthy weight have a better chance of getting pregnant.

Can anorexia hurt a baby when the mother is pregnant?

Yes. Women who have anorexia while they are pregnant are more likely to lose the baby. If a woman with anorexia doesn't lose the baby, she is more likely to have the baby early, deliver by C-section, deliver a baby with a lower birth weight, and have depression after the baby is born.

Chapter 27

Bulimia Nervosa

What is bulimia?

Bulimia nervosa (buh-LEE-me-ah nur-VOH-suh), often called bulimia, is a type of eating disorder. A person with bulimia eats a lot of food in a short amount of time (binging) and then tries to prevent weight gain by getting rid of the food (purging). Purging might be done by making yourself throw up or taking laxatives (pills or liquids that speed up the movement of food through your body and lead to a bowel movement).

A person with bulimia feels he or she cannot control the amount of food eaten. Also, bulimics might exercise a lot, eat very little or not at all, or take pills to pass urine often to prevent weight gain.

Unlike anorexia, people with bulimia can fall within the normal range for their age and weight. But like people with anorexia, bulimics:

- Fear gaining weight
- Want desperately to lose weight
- Are very unhappy with their body size and shape

Who becomes bulimic?

Many people think that eating disorders affect only young, upper-class white females. It is true that most bulimics are women (around 85–90 percent). But bulimia affects people from all walks of life, including males, women of color, and even older women. It is not known for sure

About This Chapter: Excerpted from "Bulimia Nervosa Fact Sheet," Office on Women's Health, U.S. Department of Health and Human Services (www.womenshealth.gov), July 2012.

whether African American, Latina, Asian/Pacific Islander, and American Indian and Alaska Native people develop eating disorders because American culture values thin people. People with different cultural backgrounds may develop eating disorders because it's hard to adapt to a new culture (a theory called "culture clash"). The stress of trying to live in two different cultures may cause some minorities to develop their eating disorders.

What causes bulimia?

Bulimia is more than just a problem with food. A binge can be triggered by dieting, stress, or uncomfortable emotions, such as anger or sadness. Purging and other actions to prevent weight gain are ways for people with bulimia to feel more in control of their lives and ease stress and anxiety. There is no single known cause of bulimia, but there are some factors that may play a part.

- **Culture:** Women in the U.S. are under constant pressure to fit a certain ideal of beauty. Seeing images of flawless, thin females everywhere makes it hard for women to feel good about their bodies.

- **Families:** If you have a mother or sister with bulimia, you are more likely to also have bulimia. Parents who think looks are important, diet themselves, or criticize their children's bodies are more likely to have a child with bulimia.

- **Life Changes Or Stressful Events:** Traumatic events (like rape), as well as stressful things (like starting a new job), can lead to bulimia.

- **Personality Traits:** A person with bulimia may not like herself, hate the way she looks, or feel hopeless. She may be very moody, have problems expressing anger, or have a hard time controlling impulsive behaviors.

- **Biology:** Genes, hormones, and chemicals in the brain may be factors in developing bulimia.

What are signs of bulimia?

A person with bulimia may be thin, overweight, or have a normal weight. Also, bulimic behavior, such as throwing up, is often done in private because the person with bulimia feels shame or disgust. This makes it hard to know if someone has bulimia. But there are warning signs to look out for. Someone with bulimia may use extreme measures to lose weight by:

- Using diet pills, or taking pills to urinate or have a bowel movement

- Going to the bathroom all the time after eating (to throw up)

- Exercising a lot, even in bad weather or when hurt or tired

Someone with bulimia may show signs of throwing up, such as:

- Swollen cheeks or jaw area
- Calluses or scrapes on the knuckles (if using fingers to induce vomiting)
- Teeth that look clear
- Broken blood vessels in the eyes

People with bulimia often have other mental health conditions, including:

- Depression
- Anxiety
- Substance abuse problems

Someone with bulimia may also have a distorted body image, shown by thinking she or he is fat, hating her or his body, and fearing weight gain.

Bulimia can also cause someone to not act like her or himself. She or he may be moody or sad, or may not want to go out with friends.

What happens to someone who has bulimia?

Bulimia can be very harmful to the body. Look at Figure 27.1 to find out how bulimia affects your health.

Can someone with bulimia get better?

Yes. Someone with bulimia can get better. A health care team of doctors, nutritionists, and therapists will help the patient recover. They will help the person learn healthy eating patterns and cope with their thoughts and feelings. Treatment for bulimia uses a combination of options. Whether or not the treatment works depends on the patient.

To stop a person from binging and purging, a doctor may recommend the patient:

- Receive nutritional advice and psychotherapy, especially cognitive behavioral therapy (CBT)
- Be prescribed medicine

CBT is a form of psychotherapy that focuses on the important role of thinking in how we feel and what we do. CBT that has been tailored to treat bulimia has shown to be effective in changing binging and purging behavior, and eating attitudes. Therapy for a person with bulimia may be one-on-one with a therapist or group-based.

Some antidepressants, such as fluoxetine (Prozac), which is the only medication approved by the U.S. Food and Drug Administration (FDA) for treating bulimia, may help patients who also have depression and/or anxiety. It also appears to help reduce binge-eating and purging behavior, reduces the chance of relapse, and improves eating attitudes. ("Relapse" means to get sick again, after feeling well for a while.)

Can women who had bulimia in the past still get pregnant?

Active bulimia can cause a woman to miss her period sometimes. Or, she may never get her period. If this happens, she usually does not ovulate. This makes it hard to get pregnant. Women who have recovered from bulimia have a better chance of getting pregnant once their monthly cycle is normal.

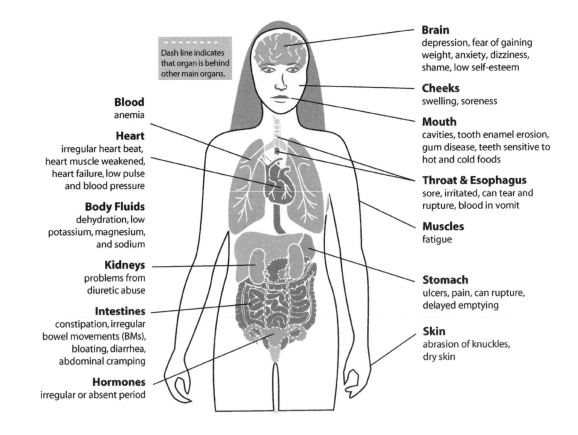

Figure 27.1. How bulimia affects your whole body. Bulimia can be very harmful to the body.

Jen's Story

It was ten years ago when I became bulimic. I had always worried about my weight and how I looked. I thought I looked fat, no matter what the scale showed or anyone said. But I had never made myself throw up—not until after college. I felt stressed out after graduating from college. I was very overwhelmed with my new job and turned to food to feel more in control of my life. Sometimes, I'd eat a lot of food and throw it up. Other times, I'd throw up a normal meal. At the time, it seemed like the only way I could cope with my stress. Luckily, I got help from a doctor, after a friend talked to me about the problem. It took a lot of work, but I am better now.

Source: Office on Women's Health, U.S. Department of Health and Human Services (www.womenshealth.gov), July 2012.

How does bulimia affect pregnancy?

If a woman with active bulimia gets pregnant, these problems may result:

- Miscarriage

- High blood pressure in the mother

- Baby isn't born alive

- Baby tries to come out with feet or bottom first

- Birth by C-section

- Baby is born early

- Low birth weight

- Birth defects, such as blindness or mental retardation

- Problems breastfeeding

- Depression in the mother after the baby is born

- Diabetes in the mother during pregnancy

If a woman takes laxatives or diuretics during pregnancy, her baby could be harmed. These things take away nutrients and fluids from a woman before they are able to feed and nourish the baby. It is possible they may lead to birth defects as well, particularly if they are used regularly.

Chapter 28

Binge Eating Disorder

What is binge eating disorder?

People with binge eating disorder often eat an unusually large amount of food and feel out of control during the binges. Unlike bulimia or anorexia, binge eaters do not throw up their food, exercise a lot, or eat only small amounts of only certain foods. Because of this, binge eaters are often overweight or obese. People with binge eating disorder also may:

- Eat more quickly than usual during binge episodes

- Eat until they are uncomfortably full

- Eat when they are not hungry

- Eat alone because of embarrassment

- Feel disgusted, depressed, or guilty after overeating

About two percent of all adults in the United States (as many as four million Americans) have binge eating disorder. Binge eating disorder affects women slightly more often than men.

What causes binge eating disorder?

Researchers are unsure of the causes and nature of binge eating and other eating disorders. Eating disorders likely involve abnormal activity in several different areas of the brain. Researchers are looking at the following factors that may affect binge eating:

About This Chapter: Excerpted from "Binge Eating Disorder Fact Sheet," Office on Women's Health, U.S. Department of Health and Human Services (www.womenshealth.gov), July 2012.

- **Depression:** As many as half of all people with binge eating disorder are depressed or have been depressed in the past.

- **Dieting:** Some people binge after skipping meals, not eating enough food each day, or avoiding certain kinds of food.

- **Coping Skills:** Studies suggest that people with binge eating may have trouble handling some of their emotions. Many people who are binge eaters say that being angry, sad, bored, worried, or stressed can cause them to binge eat.

- **Biology:** Researchers are looking into how brain chemicals and metabolism (the way the body uses calories) affect binge eating disorder. Research also suggests that genes may be involved in binge eating, since the disorder often occurs in several members of the same family. Neuroimaging, or pictures of the brain, may also lead to a better understanding of binge eating disorder.

Certain behaviors and emotional problems are more common in people with binge eating disorder. These include abusing alcohol, acting quickly without thinking (impulsive behavior), not feeling in charge of themselves, and not feeling a part of their communities.

What are the health consequences of binge eating disorder?

People with binge eating disorder are usually very upset by their binge eating and may become depressed. Research has shown that people with binge eating disorder report more health problems, stress, trouble sleeping, and suicidal thoughts than people without an eating disorder. People with binge eating disorder often feel badly about themselves and may miss work, school, or social activities to binge eat.

People with binge eating disorder may gain weight. Weight gain can lead to obesity, and obesity raises the risk for these health problems:

- Type 2 diabetes
- High blood pressure
- High cholesterol
- Gallbladder disease
- Heart disease
- Certain types of cancer

Obese people with binge eating disorder often have other mental health conditions, including:

- Anxiety

- Depression

- Personality disorders

Can someone with binge eating disorder get better?

Yes. Someone with binge eating disorder can get better.

People with binge eating disorder should get help from a health care professional, such as a psychiatrist, psychologist, or clinical social worker. As with bulimia, there are different ways to treat binge eating disorder that may be helpful for some people, including:

- Nutritional advice and psychotherapy, especially cognitive behavioral therapy (CBT)

- Drug therapy, such as antidepressants like fluoxetine (Prozac) or appetite suppressants prescribed by a doctor

CBT is a form of psychotherapy that focuses on the important role of thinking in how we feel and what we do. Therapy for a person with binge eating disorder may be one-on-one with a therapist or group-based.

Chapter 29

Body Dysmorphic Disorder

Focusing On Appearance

Most of us spend time in front of the mirror checking our appearance. Some people spend more time than others, but taking care of our bodies and being interested in our appearance is natural.

How we feel about our appearance is part of our body image and self-image. Many people have some kind of dissatisfaction with their bodies. This can be especially true during the teen years when our bodies and appearance go through lots of changes.

Although many people feel dissatisfied with some aspect of their appearance, these concerns usually don't constantly occupy their thoughts or cause them to feel tormented. But for some people, concerns about appearance become quite extreme and upsetting.

Some people become so focused on imagined or minor imperfections in their looks that they can't seem to stop checking or obsessing about their appearance. Being constantly preoccupied and upset about body imperfections or appearance flaws is called body dysmorphic disorder.

What Is Body Dysmorphic Disorder?

Body dysmorphic disorder (BDD) is a condition that involves obsessions, which are distressing thoughts that repeatedly intrude into a person's awareness. With BDD, the distressing thoughts are about perceived appearance flaws.

About This Chapter: "Body Dysmorphic Disorder," May 2013, reprinted with permission from www.kidshealth .org. This information was provided by KidsHealth®, one of the largest resources online for medically reviewed health information written for parents, kids, and teens. For more articles like this, visit www.KidsHealth.org, or www.TeensHealth.org. Copyright © 1995–2013 The Nemours Foundation. All rights reserved.

People with BDD might focus on what they think is a facial flaw, but they can also worry about other body parts, such as short legs, breast size, or body shape. Just as people with eating disorders obsess about their weight, those with BDD become obsessed over an aspect of their appearance. They may worry their hair is thin, their face is scarred, their eyes aren't exactly the same size, their nose is too big, or their lips are too thin.

BDD has been called "imagined ugliness" because the appearance issues the person is obsessing about usually are so small that others don't even notice them. Or, if others do notice them, they consider them minor. But for someone with BDD, the concerns feel very real, because the obsessive thoughts distort and magnify any tiny imperfection.

Because of the distorted body image caused by BDD, a person might believe that he or she is too horribly ugly or disfigured to be seen.

When Your Body Image Doesn't Measure Up

Do you like what you see when you look in the mirror? If your answer is "No," you're not alone. For many of us, there's a growing gap between how our bodies look and how we'd like them to look.

Americans have generally gotten wider and flabbier over the past few decades, as obesity rates continue to climb. But at the same time, the media bombard us with images of people who seem impossibly thin or muscular. The gap between reality and expectations can leave many people feeling inadequate.

It's normal to look in the mirror occasionally and wish for a firmer body or more glamorous hair. But some people find they can't stop thinking about body flaws they believe they have. They may avoid going out with friends or even stop going to work because they feel ashamed of their skin, hair, weight or other features.

"They say they look ugly, flawed or deformed, but in reality they look fine," says Dr. Katharine A. Phillips, a psychiatrist at Brown University. "The physical flaws they perceive are things we can't see at all, or they're really quite minimal."

Having a negative body image like this isn't just an attitude problem. It can take a toll on your mental and physical health. If excessive thoughts about your body cause great distress or interfere with your daily life, you may have a body image disorder, also known as body dysmorphic disorder (BDD).

Source: Excerpted from "How You See Yourself: When Body Image Doesn't Measure Up," National Institutes of Health (www.nih.gov), July 2009.

Behaviors That Are Part Of BDD

Besides obsessions, BDD also involves compulsions and avoidance behaviors.

A compulsion is something a person does to try to relieve the tension caused by the obsessive thoughts. For example, someone with obsessive thoughts that her nose is horribly ugly might check her appearance in the mirror, apply makeup, or ask someone many times a day whether her nose looks ugly. These types of checking, fixing, and asking are compulsions.

Somebody with obsessions usually feels a strong or irresistible urge to do compulsions because they can provide temporary relief from the terrible distress. The compulsions seem like the only way to escape bad feelings caused by bad thoughts. Compulsive actions often are repeated many times a day, taking up lots of time and energy.

Avoidance behaviors are also a part of BDD. A person might stay home or cover up to avoid being seen by others. Avoidance behaviors also include things like not participating in class or socializing, or avoiding mirrors.

With BDD, a pattern of obsessive thoughts, compulsive actions, and avoidance sets in. Even though the checking, fixing, asking, and avoiding seem to relieve terrible feelings, the relief is just temporary. In reality, the more someone performs compulsions or avoids things, the stronger the pattern of obsessions, compulsions, and avoidance becomes.

After a while, it takes more and more compulsions to relieve the distress caused by the bad thoughts. A person with BDD doesn't want to be preoccupied with these thoughts and behaviors, but with BDD it can seem impossible to break the pattern.

What Causes BDD?

Although the exact cause of BDD is still unclear, experts believe it is related to problems with serotonin, one of the brain's chemical neurotransmitters. Poor regulation of serotonin also plays a role in obsessive compulsive disorder (OCD) and other anxiety disorders, as well as depression.

Some people may be more prone to problems with serotonin balance, including those with family members who have problems with anxiety or depression. This may help explain why some people develop BDD but others don't.

Cultural messages can also play a role in BDD by reinforcing somebody's concerns about appearance. Critical messages or unkind teasing about appearance as someone is growing up may also contribute to a person's sensitivity to BDD. But while cultural messages, criticism, and teasing might harm someone's body image, these things alone usually do not result in BDD.

It's hard to know exactly how common BDD is because most people with BDD are unwilling to talk about their concerns or seek help. But compared with those who feel somewhat dissatisfied with their appearance, very few people have true BDD. BDD usually begins in the teen years, and if it's not treated, can continue into adulthood.

Facts About Body Dysmorphic Disorder (BDD)

- BDD is a psychiatric condition that affects about 1–2 percent of the population. It occurs slightly more often in women than in men. On average, these patients report that they think about their perceived appearance flaws for about 3–8 hours a day.

- Because of their imagined flaws, many people with BDD avoid going out in public or shun friends and family. About three-quarters have had major depression, and about one in four attempt suicide.

- People with BDD might focus on any part of the body. The most common concern is with some aspect of the skin (such as perceived acne or scarring), which occurs in about three-fourths of patients with BDD. Many patients are fixated on their hair or nose. Some worry about their weight, thighs, teeth or face. More than one-third seek cosmetic surgery, although it rarely fixes the appearance problem they believe they have.

- BDD can be difficult to diagnose, because affected people look normal and are often too ashamed to talk about their concerns with appearance. Clues include frequent mirror-checking, excessive grooming, skin picking or covering up disliked body parts.

- A number of studies suggest that medications known as serotonin-reuptake inhibitors, which are used to treat depression and certain other disorders, can be effective for BDD. A type of therapy known as cognitive-behavioral therapy also seems promising.

If you don't have a body image disorder, improving your attitude about your body might just be a matter of accepting that healthy bodies come in many shapes and sizes. We all want to look good, but you should never sacrifice your health to try to achieve a "perfect" body.

For A Healthy Body Image

You can improve your attitude about your body by making healthy lifestyle choices.

- Eat wholesome foods to promote healthy skin and hair, as well as strong bones.

- Exercise regularly to improve your health and boost your self-esteem and energy.

- Move and enjoy your body. Go walking, swimming, biking and dancing.

- Get plenty of rest to help manage stress and reduce anxiety.

Source: Excerpted from "How You See Yourself: When Body Image Doesn't Measure Up," National Institutes of Health (www.nih.gov), July 2009.

How BDD Can Affect A Person's Life

Sometimes people with BDD feel ashamed and keep their concerns secret. They may think that others will consider them vain or superficial.

Other people might become annoyed or irritated with somebody's obsessions and compulsions about appearance. They don't understand BDD or what the person is going through. As a result, those with BDD may feel misunderstood, unfairly judged, or alone. Because they avoid contact with others, they may have few friends or activities to enjoy.

It's extremely upsetting to be tormented by thoughts about appearance imperfections. These thoughts intrude into a person's awareness throughout the day and are hard to ignore. People with mild to moderate symptoms of BDD usually spend a great deal of time grooming themselves in the morning. Throughout the day, they may frequently check their appearance in mirrors or windows. In addition, they may repeatedly seek reassurance from people around them that they look OK.

Although people with mild BDD usually continue to go to school, the obsessions can interfere with their daily lives. For example, someone might measure or examine the "flawed" body part repeatedly or spend large sums of money and time on makeup to cover the problem.

Some people with BDD hide from others, and avoid going places because of fear of being seen. Spending so much time and energy on appearance concerns robs a person of pleasure and happiness, and of opportunities for fun and socializing.

People with severe symptoms may drop out of school, quit their jobs, or refuse to leave their homes. Many people with BDD also develop depression. Those with the most severe BDD might even consider or attempt suicide.

Many people with BDD seek the help of a dermatologist or cosmetic surgeon to try to correct appearance flaws. But dermatology treatments or plastic surgery don't change the BDD. Those who find cosmetic surgeons willing to perform surgery are often not satisfied with the results. They may find that even though their appearance has changes, the obsessive thinking is still present, and they begin to focus on some other imperfection.

Getting Help For BDD

If you or someone you know has BDD, the first step is recognizing what might be causing the distress. Many times, people with BDD are so focused on their appearance that they believe the answer lies in correcting how they look, not with their thoughts.

Men And Boys Can Also Feel They Can't Measure Up

Much attention has been paid to how culture and the media can damage women's feelings about their own bodies. But studies suggest that men and boys can also feel they can't measure up to the broad-shouldered, narrow-waisted, muscular men they see in ads, cartoons, TV shows, movies and even action figures.

"There's a climate in American society that rewards muscularity and equates it with masculinity," says Dr. Harrison Pope, a psychiatrist at Harvard Medical School.

Pope and his colleagues have found a wide gap between what men think of their own bodies and what they believe women prefer. In one study, researchers asked men in the U.S. and Europe to select a body size and shape on a computer that they felt matched their own bodies. Then they selected a body that they thought women would find most attractive. On average, the men expected that women would prefer bodies with about 20 pounds more muscle than the men actually had.

But when the scientists asked women which body shapes they liked most, "the women chose perfectly ordinary male bodies, without any extra muscle," Pope says. "The men seemed to have a very distorted view of what women wanted."

A skewed view of how muscular you are may signal a type of BDD called muscle dysmorphia. It's sometimes found among bodybuilders. People with the disorder become obsessed with being more muscular. "They might look in a mirror and think that they look small and wimpy, even if they are actually large and muscular," Pope says. Their poor body image puts them at risk for illegal use of anabolic steroids and other drugs to gain muscle mass.

"Steroids are extremely effective at building muscle, and they aren't as negatively perceived as other drugs of abuse," Pope says. "They can give you bulging upper-body muscles that you could never achieve with even the most dedicated exercise and weight-training."

But these drug-induced muscles come at a high price. Steroid abuse can lead to serious, sometimes irreversible health problems. It can damage the liver and cause high blood pressure, high cholesterol and skin problems. Growing evidence suggests that steroids can also damage heart muscle. Males may develop breast tissue, and their testicles may shrink. Steroid abuse can also alter certain brain chemicals and affect mood and behavior.

"One surprising effect is that when men take anabolic steroids and gradually become more muscular, they sometimes become more fixated on their body size and even more dissatisfied," Pope says. "Steroids don't always relieve body image problems."

Source: Excerpted from "How You See Yourself: When Body Image Doesn't Measure Up," National Institutes of Health (www.nih.gov), July 2009.

The real problem with BDD lies in the obsessions and compulsions, which distort body image, making someone feel ugly. Because people with BDD believe what they're perceiving is true and accurate, sometimes the most challenging part of overcoming the disorder is being open to new ideas about what might help.

BDD can be treated by an experienced mental health professional. Usually, the treatment involves a type of talk therapy called cognitive behavioral therapy. This approach helps to correct the pattern that's causing the body image distortion and the extreme distress.

In cognitive behavioral therapy, a therapist helps a person to examine and change faulty beliefs, resist compulsive behaviors, and face stressful situations that trigger appearance concerns. Sometimes doctors prescribe medication along with the talk therapy.

Treatment for BDD takes time, hard work, and patience. It helps if a person has the support of a friend or loved one. If someone with BDD is also dealing with depression, anxiety, feeling isolated or alone, or other life situations, the therapy can address those issues, too.

Body dysmorphic disorder, like other obsessions, can interfere with a person's life, robbing it of pleasure and draining energy. An experienced psychologist or psychiatrist who is knowledgeable about BDD can help break the grip of the disorder so that a person can fully enjoy life.

Chapter 30

Compulsive Exercise Disorder

Rachel and her cheerleading team practice three to five times a week. Rachel feels a lot of pressure to keep her weight down—as head cheerleader, she wants to set an example to the team. So, she adds extra daily workouts to her regimen. But lately, she's been feeling worn out, and she has a hard time just making it through a regular team practice.

You may think you can't get too much of a good thing, but in the case of exercise, a healthy activity can sometimes turn into an unhealthy compulsion. Rachel is a good example of how an overemphasis on physical fitness or weight control can become unhealthy. Read on to find out more about compulsive exercise and its effects.

Too Much Of A Good Thing?

We all know the benefits of exercise, and it seems that everywhere we turn, we hear that we should exercise more. The right kind of exercise does many great things for your body and soul: It can strengthen your heart and muscles, lower your body fat, and reduce your risk of many diseases.

Many teens who play sports have higher self-esteem than their less active pals, and exercise can even help keep the blues at bay because of the endorphin rush it can cause. Endorphins are chemicals that naturally relieve pain and lift mood. These chemicals are released in your body during and after a workout and they go a long way in helping to control stress.

About This Chapter: "Compulsive Exercise," October 2010, reprinted with permission from www.kidshealth .org. This information was provided by KidsHealth®, one of the largest resources online for medically reviewed health information written for parents, kids, and teens. For more articles like this, visit www.KidsHealth.org, or www.TeensHealth.org. Copyright © 1995–2013 The Nemours Foundation. All rights reserved.

So how can something with so many benefits have the potential to cause harm?

Why Do People Overexercise?

Lots of people start working out because it's fun or it makes them feel good, but exercise can become a compulsive habit when it is done for the wrong reasons.

Some people start exercising with weight loss as their main goal. Although exercise is part of a safe and healthy way to control weight, many people may have unrealistic expectations. We are bombarded with images from advertisers of the ideal body: young and thin for women; strong and muscular for men. To try to reach these unreasonable ideals, people may turn to diets, and for some, this may develop into eating disorders such as anorexia and bulimia. And some people who grow frustrated with the results from diets alone may overexercise to speed up weight loss.

Some athletes may also think that repeated exercise will help them to win an important game. Like Rachel, they add extra workouts to those regularly scheduled with their teams without consulting their coaches or trainers. The pressure to succeed may also lead these people to exercise more than is healthy. The body needs activity but it also needs rest. Over exercising can lead to injuries like fractures and muscle strains.

Are You A Healthy Exerciser?

Fitness experts recommend that teens do at least 60 minutes of moderate to vigorous physical activity every day. Most young people exercise much less than this recommended amount (which can be a problem for different reasons), but some—such as athletes—do more.

Experts say that repeatedly exercising beyond the requirements for good health is an indicator of compulsive behavior. Some people need more than the average amount of exercise, of course—such as athletes in training for a big event. But several workouts a day, every day, when a person is not in training is a sign that the person is probably overdoing it.

People who are exercise dependent also go to extremes to fit activity into their lives. If you put workouts ahead of friends, homework, and other responsibilities, you may be developing a dependence on exercise.

Signs Of Compulsive Exercise

If you are concerned about your own exercise habits or a friend's, ask yourself the following questions. Do you:

- Force yourself to exercise, even if you don't feel well?

- Prefer to exercise rather than being with friends?

- Become very upset if you miss a workout?

- Base the amount you exercise on how much you eat?

- Have trouble sitting still because you think you're not burning calories?

- Worry that you'll gain weight if you skip exercising for a day?

If the answer to any of these questions is yes, you or your friend may have a problem. What should you do?

How To Get Help

The first thing you should do if you suspect that you are a compulsive exerciser is get help. Talk to your parents, doctor, a teacher or counselor, a coach, or another trusted adult. Compulsive exercise, especially when it is combined with an eating disorder, can cause serious and permanent health problems, and in extreme cases, death.

Because compulsive exercise is closely related to eating disorders, help can be found at community agencies specifically set up to deal with anorexia, bulimia, and other eating problems. Your school's health or physical education department may also have support programs and nutrition advice available. Ask your teacher, coach, or counselor to recommend local organizations that may be able to help.

You should also schedule a checkup with a doctor. Because our bodies go through so many important developments during the teen years, guys and girls who have compulsive exercise problems need to see a doctor to make sure they are developing normally. This is especially true if the person also has an eating disorder. Girls who overexercise and restrict their eating may stop having periods and develop osteoporosis (weakening of the bones), a condition called female athlete triad. Medical help is necessary to resolve the physical problems associated with over exercising before they cause long-term damage to the body.

Make A Positive Change

Girls and guys who exercise compulsively may have a distorted body image and low self-esteem. They may see themselves as overweight or out of shape even when they are actually a healthy weight.

Compulsive exercisers need to get professional help for the reasons described above. But there are also some things that you can do to help you take charge again:

- Work on changing your daily self-talk. When you look in the mirror, make sure you find at least one good thing to say about yourself. Be more aware of your positive attributes.

- When you exercise, focus on the positive, mood-boosting qualities.

- Give yourself a break. Listen to your body and give yourself a day of rest after a hard workout.

- Control your weight by exercising and eating moderate portions of healthy foods. Don't try to change your body into an unrealistically lean shape. Talk with your doctor, dietitian, coach, athletic trainer, or other adult about what a healthy body weight is for you and how to develop healthy eating and exercise habits.

Exercise and sports are supposed to be fun and keep you healthy. Working out in moderation will do both.

Chapter 31

Impulse Control Disorders

As humans, the ability to control our impulses—or urges—helps distinguish us from other species and marks our psychological maturity. Most of us take our ability to think before we act for granted. But this isn't easy for people who have problems controlling their impulses.

What are impulse control disorders?

People with an impulse control disorder can't resist the urge to do something harmful to themselves or others. Impulse control disorders include addictions to alcohol or drugs, eating disorders, compulsive gambling, paraphilias [socially prohibited] sexual fantasies and behaviors involving non-human objects, suffering, humiliation or children, compulsive hair pulling, stealing, fire setting, and intermittent explosive attacks of rage.

Some of these disorders, such as intermittent explosive disorder, kleptomania, pyromania, compulsive gambling, and trichotillomania [a compulsion to pull out one's own hair] are similar in terms of when they begin and how they progress. Usually, a person feels increasing tension or arousal before committing the act that characterizes the disorder. During the act, the person probably will feel pleasure, gratification or relief. Afterward, the person may blame himself or feel regret or guilt.

People with these disorders may or may not plan the acts, but the acts generally fulfill their immediate, conscious wishes. Most people, however, find their disorders highly distressing and feel a loss of control over their lives.

About This Chapter: "What Are Impulse Control Disorders?" © 2013 Psych Central (www.psychcentral.com). All rights reserved. Reprinted with permission.

How are they different from similar disorders?

While other disorders may involve difficulty controlling impulses, that is not their primary feature. For example, while people with attention-deficit hyperactivity disorder (ADHD) or in a manic state of bipolar might have difficulty controlling their impulses, it is not their main problem.

Some health professionals consider impulse control disorders subgroups of other conditions, such as anxiety disorders or obsessive-compulsive disorders. Some medications for treating depression and anxiety also have been successful in treating impulse disorders, particularly antidepressants known as serotonin reuptake inhibitors. This suggests the neurotransmitter serotonin plays a role in these disorders.

What causes impulse control disorders?

Scientists don't know what causes these disorders. But many things probably play a role, including physical or biological, psychological or emotional, and cultural or societal factors. Scientists do suspect that certain brain structures—including the limbic system, linked to emotions and memory functions, and the frontal lobe, the part of the brain's cortex linked to planning functions and controlling impulses—affect the disorder.

Hormones associated with violence and aggression, such as testosterone, also could play a role in the disorders. For example, researchers have suggested that women might be predisposed to less aggressive types of impulse control disorders such as kleptomania or trichotillomania, and men might be predisposed to more violent and aggressive types such as pyromania and intermittent explosive disorder.

Research also has shown connections between certain types of seizure disorders and violent impulsive behaviors. And studies have revealed that family members of people with impulse control disorders have a higher rate of addiction and mood disorders.

Chapter 32

Adjustment Disorders

Adjustment disorder is a group of symptoms, such as stress, feeling sad or hopeless, and physical symptoms that can occur after you go through a stressful life event. The symptoms occur because you are having a hard time coping, and the reaction is stronger or greater than what would be expected for the type of event that occurred.

Causes

Many different events may trigger symptoms of an adjustment disorder. Whatever the trigger is, the event may become too much for you.

Stressors for people of any age include:

- Death of a loved one

- Divorce or problems with a relationship

- General life changes

- Illness or other health issues in yourself or a loved one

- Moving to a different home or a different city

- Unexpected catastrophes

- Worries about money

Triggers of stress in teenagers and young adults may include:

- Family problems or conflict

- School problems

- Sexuality issues

There is no way to predict which people who are affected by the same stress are likely to develop adjustment disorder. Your social skills before the event, and how you have learned to deal with stress in the past, may play roles.

Symptoms

Symptoms of adjustment disorder are often severe enough to affect work or social life. Some of the symptoms include:

- Acting defiant or showing impulsive behavior

- Acting nervous or tense

- Crying, feeling sad or hopeless, and possibly withdrawing from other people

- Skipped heartbeats and other physical complaints

- Trembling or twitching

To have adjustment disorder, you must meet the following criteria:

- The symptoms clearly come after a stressor, most often within three months.

- The symptoms are more severe than would be expected.

- There do not appear to be other disorders involved.

- The symptoms are not part of normal grieving for the death of a loved one.

On occasion, symptoms can be severe and the person may have thoughts of suicide or make a suicide attempt.

Treatment

The main goal of treatment is to relieve symptoms and help you return to a similar level of functioning as before the stressful event occurred.

Most mental health professionals recommend some type of talk therapy. This type of therapy can help you identify or change your responses to the stressors in your life.

Cognitive behavioral therapy (CBT) can help you deal with your feelings.

- First, your therapist helps you recognize the negative feelings and thoughts that occur.

- Then, your therapist teaches you how to change these into helpful thoughts and healthy actions.

Other types of therapy may include:

- Long-term therapy, where you will explore your thoughts and feelings over many months or more

- Family therapy, where you will meet with a therapist along with your family

- Self-help groups, where the support of others may help you get better

Medicines may be used, but only along with some type of talk therapy. These medicines may help if you are:

- Nervous or anxious most of the time

- Not sleeping very well

- Very sad or depressed

Outlook (Prognosis)

With the right help and support, you should get better quickly. The problem usually does not last longer than six months, unless the stressor continues to be present.

When To Contact A Medical Professional

Call for an appointment with your health care provider if you develop symptoms of adjustment disorder.

Chapter 33

Conduct, Intermittent Explosive, And Oppositional Defiant Disorders

Conduct Disorder

Conduct disorder is a disorder of childhood and adolescence that involves long-term (chronic) behavior problems, such as:

- Defiant or impulsive behavior

- Drug use

- Criminal activity

Causes

Conduct disorder has been associated with:

- Child abuse

- Drug addiction or alcoholism in the parents

- Family conflicts

- Genetic defects

- Poverty

The diagnosis is more common among boys.

About This Chapter: Information in this chapter is reprinted from "Conduct Disorder," February 2011, and "Oppositional Defiant Disorder," January 2010, © 2013 A.D.A.M., Inc. Reprinted with permission.

It is hard to know how common the disorder is, because many of the qualities needed to make the diagnosis (such as "defiance" and "rule breaking") can be hard to define. For an accurate diagnosis, the behavior must be far more extreme than simple adolescent rebellion or boyish enthusiasm.

Conduct disorder is often associated with attention-deficit disorder. Both conditions carry a risk for alcohol or other drug addiction. Conduct disorder also can be an early sign of depression or bipolar disorder.

Symptoms

Children with conduct disorder tend to be impulsive, hard to control, and not concerned about the feelings of other people. Symptoms may include:

- Breaking rules without obvious reason
- Cruel or aggressive behavior toward people or animals (for example, bullying, fighting, using dangerous weapons, forcing sexual activity, and stealing)
- Failure to attend school (truancy—beginning before age 13)
- Heavy drinking and/or heavy illicit drug use
- Intentionally setting fires
- Lying to get a favor or avoid things they have to do
- Running away
- Vandalizing or destroying property

These children often make no effort to hide their aggressive behaviors. They may have a hard time making real friends.

Exams And Tests

There is no real test for diagnosing conduct disorder. The diagnosis is made when a child or adolescent has a history of conduct disorder behaviors. A physical examination and blood tests can help rule out medical conditions that are similar to conduct disorder. Rarely, a brain scan may also help rule out other disorders.

Treatment

For treatment to be successful, the child's family needs to be closely involved. Parents can learn techniques to help manage their child's problem behavior.

In cases of abuse, the child may need to be removed from the family and placed in a less chaotic home. Treatment with medications or talk therapy may be used for depression and attention-deficit disorder, which commonly occur with conduct disorder.

Many "behavioral modification" schools, "wilderness programs," and "boot camps" are sold to parents as solutions for conduct disorder. These programs may use a form of "attack therapy" or "confrontation," which can actually be harmful. There is no research to support these techniques. Research suggests that treating children at home, along with their families, is more effective.

If you are considering an inpatient program, be sure to check it out thoroughly. Serious injuries and deaths have occurred with some programs. They are not regulated in many states.

Outlook (Prognosis)

Children who have severe or frequent symptoms tend to have the poorest outlook. Expectations are also worse for those who have other illnesses, such as mood and drug abuse disorders.

Possible Complications

Children with conduct disorder may go on to develop personality disorders as adults, particularly antisocial personality disorder. As their behaviors worsen, these individuals may also develop drug and legal problems.

Depression and bipolar disorder may develop in adolescence and early adulthood. Suicide and violence toward others are also possible complications of this disorder.

When To Contact A Medical Professional

Seek a health care provider if someone you know:

- Regularly gets into trouble
- Has mood swings
- Is being victimized
- Seems to be overly aggressive

Early treatment may help.

Prevention

The sooner the treatment for conduct disorder is started, the more likely the child will learn adaptive behaviors and prevent some of the potential complications.

Intermittent Explosive Disorder Affects Up To 16 Million Americans

A little-known mental disorder, marked by episodes of unwarranted anger, is more common than previously thought, a study funded by the National Institutes of Health's National Institute of Mental Health (NIMH) has found. Depending upon how broadly it's defined, intermittent explosive disorder (IED) affects as many as 7.3 percent of adults in their lifetimes.

People with IED may attack others and their possessions, causing bodily injury and property damage. Typically beginning in the early teens, the disorder often precedes (and may predispose for) later depression, anxiety, and substance abuse disorders. Nearly 82 percent of those with IED also had one of these other disorders, yet only 28.8 percent ever received treatment for their anger. Researchers suggest that treating anger early might prevent some co-occurring disorders from developing.

To be diagnosed with IED, an individual must have had three episodes of impulsive aggressiveness "grossly out of proportion to any precipitating psychosocial stressor," at any time in their life, according to the standard psychiatric diagnostic manual. People who had three such episodes within the space of one year were found to have a much more persistent and severe disorder, particularly if they attacked both people and property.

Evidence suggests that IED might predispose toward depression, anxiety, alcohol, and drug abuse disorders by increasing stressful life experiences, such as financial difficulties and divorce. Given its earlier age-of-onset, identifying IED early—perhaps in school-based violence prevention programs—and providing early treatment might prevent some of the associated psychopathology, propose the researchers.

Although the new prevalence estimates for IED are somewhat higher than previous studies have found, the researchers consider them conservative. For example, anger outbursts in people with bipolar disorder, which often overlaps with IED, were excluded. Previous studies have found little overlap between IED and other mental illnesses associated with impulsive violence (such as antisocial and borderline personality disorders).

Source: Excerpted from "Intermittent Explosive Disorder Affects Up To 16 Million Americans," National Institute of Mental Health (www.nimh.nih.gov), February 2013.

Oppositional Defiant Disorder

Oppositional defiant disorder is a pattern of disobedient, hostile, and defiant behavior toward authority figures.

Causes

This disorder is more common in boys than in girls. Some studies have shown that it affects 20 percent of school-age children. However, most experts believe this figure is high due to changing definitions of normal childhood behavior, and possible racial, cultural, and gender biases.

This behavior typically starts by age eight, but it may start as early as the preschool years. This disorder is thought to be caused by a combination of biological, psychological, and social factors.

Symptoms

- Actively does not follow adults' requests
- Angry and resentful of others
- Argues with adults
- Blames others for own mistakes
- Has few or no friends or has lost friends
- Is in constant trouble in school
- Loses temper
- Spiteful or seeks revenge
- Touchy or easily annoyed

To fit this diagnosis, the pattern must last for at least six months and must be more than normal childhood misbehavior. The pattern of behaviors must be different from those of other children around the same age and developmental level. The behavior must lead to significant problems in school or social activities.

Exams And Tests

Children with symptoms of this disorder should be evaluated by a psychiatrist or psychologist. In children and adolescents, the following conditions can cause similar behavior problems and should be considered as possibilities:

- Anxiety disorders

- Attention-deficit hyperactivity disorder (ADHD)

- Bipolar disorder

- Depression

- Learning disorders

- Substance abuse disorders

Treatment

The best treatment for the child is to talk with a mental health professional in individual and possibly family therapy. The parents should also learn how to manage the child's behavior. Medications may also be helpful, especially if the behaviors occur as part of another condition (such as depression, childhood psychosis, or ADHD).

Outlook (Prognosis)

Some children respond well to treatment, while others do not.

Possible Complications

In many cases, children with oppositional defiant disorder grow up to have conduct disorder as teenagers or adults. In some cases children may grow up to have antisocial personality disorder.

When To Contact A Medical Professional

Call your health care provider if you have concerns about your development or behavior.

Prevention

Rules and consequences at home should be consistent. Punishments should not be too harsh or inconsistent. Abuse and neglect increase the chances that this condition will occur.

Chapter 34

Comorbidity: Addiction And Other Mental Disorders

What is comorbidity?

The term "comorbidity" describes two or more disorders or illnesses occurring in the same person. They can occur at the same time or one after the other. Comorbidity also implies interactions between the illnesses that can worsen the course of both.

Addiction changes the brain in fundamental ways, disturbing a person's normal hierarchy of needs and desires and substituting new priorities connected with procuring and using the drug. The resulting compulsive behaviors that weaken the ability to control impulses, despite the negative consequences, are similar to hallmarks of other mental illnesses.

Many people who are addicted to drugs are also diagnosed with other mental disorders and vice versa. For example, compared with the general population, people addicted to drugs are roughly twice as likely to suffer from mood and anxiety disorders, with the reverse also true. Although drug use disorders commonly occur with other mental illnesses, this does not mean that one caused the other, even if one appeared first. In fact, establishing which came first or why can be difficult. However, research suggests the following possibilities for this common co-occurrence:

- Drug abuse may bring about symptoms of another mental illness. Increased risk of psychosis in vulnerable marijuana users suggests this possibility.

- Mental disorders can lead to drug abuse, possibly as a means of "self-medication." Patients suffering from anxiety or depression may rely on alcohol, tobacco, and other drugs to temporarily alleviate their symptoms.

About This Chapter: Reprinted from "Comorbidity: Addiction and Other Mental Disorders," National Institute on Drug Abuse (www.drugabuse.gov), March 2011.

These disorders could also be caused by shared risk factors, such as:

- **Overlapping Genetic Vulnerabilities:** Predisposing genetic factors may make a person susceptible to both addiction and other mental disorders or to having a greater risk of a second disorder once the first appears.

- **Overlapping Environmental Triggers:** Stress, trauma (such as physical or sexual abuse), and early exposure to drugs are common environmental factors that can lead to addiction and other mental illnesses.

- **Involvement Of Similar Brain Regions:** Brain systems that respond to reward and stress, for example, are affected by drugs of abuse and may show abnormalities in patients with certain mental disorders.

- **Drug Use Disorders And Other Mental Illnesses Are Developmental Disorders:** That means they often begin in the teen years or even younger—periods when the brain experiences dramatic developmental changes. Early exposure to drugs of abuse may change the brain in ways that increase the risk for mental disorders. Also, early symptoms of a mental disorder may indicate an increased risk for later drug use.

How are these comorbid conditions diagnosed and treated?

The high rate of comorbidity between drug use disorders and other mental illnesses calls for a comprehensive approach that identifies and evaluates both. Accordingly, anyone seeking help for either drug abuse/addiction or another mental disorder should be checked for both and treated accordingly.

Several behavioral therapies have shown promise for treating comorbid conditions. These approaches can be tailored to patients according to age, specific drug abused, and other factors. Some therapies have proven more effective for adolescents, while others have shown greater effectiveness for adults; some are designed for families and groups, others for individuals.

Effective medications exist for treating opioid, alcohol, and nicotine addiction and for alleviating the symptoms of many other mental disorders, yet most have not been well studied in comorbid populations. Some medications may benefit multiple problems. For example, evidence suggests that bupropion (trade names: Wellbutrin, Zyban), approved for treating depression and nicotine dependence, might also help reduce craving and use of the drug methamphetamine. More research is needed, however, to better understand how these medications work, particularly when combined in patients with comorbidities.

Part Five
Other Situations And Disorders With Mental Health Consequences

Chapter 35

Puberty And Its Relationship To Mental Health

Adolescence can be a bewildering time—for both teens and their parents. Yet it can also be a thrilling time of growth and change. Learning about teenage development and behaviors can help nurture an adolescent's strengths and help shepherd them over the rough spots.

Why does adolescence feel so complicated and intense?

It all begins with the brain. Scientists, funded by the National Institutes of Health (NIH), have been using advanced imaging tools to take a good look at how the adolescent brain functions. They've found something they didn't expect. Although the 18th birthday means legal adulthood, important regions of the brain are still under construction until about age 25. These still-developing brain areas govern judgment, decision-making, and impulse control.

The adolescent brain can be somewhat like a rider on a racehorse with no reins. "The problem is that the incentive/reward system matures earlier than the cognitive control system," explains Dr. Lisa Freund, a developmental psychologist and neuroscientist at NIH.

In other words, the brain's "that's so cool, I want it now" part develops well before the "stop and think twice" part. That's why adolescents are especially susceptible to the immediate rewards of addiction, sexual experience, risky driving, and more.

Why is adolescence so risky?

Adolescents have trouble controlling impulses and considering the possible long-term consequences of their actions. They don't seem to realize how vulnerable they are to the risks they face.

About This Chapter: Excerpted from "Risky Business: Dealing With Your Teen's Behavior," National Institutes of Health (www.nih.gov), September 2011.

Take sex. Among U.S. high school students surveyed in 2009, almost half reported that they had engaged in sexual intercourse at least once, and over 400,000 girls (ages 15–19) gave birth. Of the 19 million new sexually transmitted diseases (STDs) recorded each year, nearly half are among young people who are 15–24 years old. This age group is also the fastest-growing group of people living with human immunodeficiency virus (HIV) in the United States.

It's important to talk about sex. "Sex is a normal part of life," says Dr. Lynne Haverkos, an NIH pediatrician specializing in health risk behaviors, "but how do you prevent the STDs, pregnancy and negative emotional consequences that can happen in these relationships? Middle childhood is the time to start talking and listening." Develop your negotiation skills and learn how to recognize and handle risky situations involving sex.

Talking about sex may feel uncomfortable to some, but you don't have to go it alone. You can find helpful resources online and in community and school programs. The most effective programs for HIV/STD prevention are taught by trained instructors, are age-appropriate, focus on skill-building, and involve parents and health organizations.

You also need to talk about other behaviors such as drinking alcohol. Alcohol depresses cognitive control and increases the risk for substance abuse and sexual activity. Alcohol and drug use might also lead to situations where teens can be sexually abused.

Why do adolescents need limits?

As a teen, you may not want limits, but you still need them. Throughout late adolescence and early adulthood, you still need guidance, and having your parents set limits is important. It takes years for kids to master the art of making decisions. Adolescents are similar to preschoolers in that activation in various parts of the brain isn't yet mature and interconnected. "This makes adolescents more emotionally reactive, especially around peers," Freund says.

As the brain's complex architecture develops, teens do begin to learn from experience and adjust their behavior accordingly. They gain the ability to grasp the wider world in more complex and nuanced ways. This helps develop your sense of right and wrong, as well as objectivity, empathy, and judgment—and you may become more motivated by self-esteem and personal achievement.

Parents can help you by encouraging your strengths. Talking, listening, and channeling your ongoing interests can have a powerful positive effect on your growth.

Use technologies—such as texting or mobile phone calls—to stay in contact with your parents. Even if you can't be there physically, they should know that you're available and that you care about them.

If you have concerns and you're unwilling to talk about it, consider making a call to your doctor—ideally, an adolescent medicine specialist. Make an appointment so you can talk privately with the care provider.

Adolescence is a stage that does have risks, and some kids may be more vulnerable than others, yet there's a lot that can be done to make you feel safe and loved. Adolescence is not a disease, but a journey towards independence. It's possible for both parents and their kids to enjoy this time—and even treasure it.

Chapter 36

Child Abuse And Its Effects On Mental Health

What is child maltreatment (child abuse)?

Child maltreatment includes all types of abuse and neglect of a child under the age of 18 by a parent, caregiver, or another person in a custodial role (for example, someone in the clergy, a coach, or a teacher). There are four common types of abuse.

- **Physical abuse** is the use of intentional physical force, such as hitting, kicking, shaking, burning or other show of force against a child.

- **Sexual abuse** involves engaging a child in sexual acts. It includes fondling, rape, and exposing a child to other sexual activities.

- **Emotional abuse** refers to behaviors that harm a child's self-worth or emotional well-being. Examples include name calling, shaming, rejection, withholding love, and threatening.

- **Neglect** is the failure to meet a child's basic needs. These needs include housing, food, clothing, education, and access to medical care.

Why is child maltreatment a public health problem?

The few cases of abuse or neglect we see in the news are only a small part of the problem. Many cases are not reported to police or social services. What we do know is that:

- 1,560 children died in the United States in 2010 from abuse and neglect.

About This Chapter: Excerpted from "Understanding Child Maltreatment," National Center for Injury Prevention and Control, Division of Violence Prevention, Centers for Disease Control and Prevention (www.cdc.gov), 2012.

- 695,000 children were found to be victims of maltreatment by child protective services in 2010.

- The total lifetime economic burden resulting from new cases of fatal and nonfatal child maltreatment in the United States is approximately $124 billion.

How does child maltreatment affect health?

Child maltreatment has a negative effect on health. Abused children often suffer physical injuries including cuts, bruises, burns, and broken bones. In addition, maltreatment causes stress that can disrupt early brain development. Extreme stress can harm the development of the nervous and immune systems. As a result, children who are abused or neglected are at higher risk for health problems as adults. These problems include alcoholism, depression, drug abuse, eating disorders, obesity, high-risk sexual behaviors, smoking, suicide, and certain chronic diseases.

Depressed Teens With History Of Abuse Less Likely To Respond To Combination Treatment

Although the relationship between childhood abuse and risk for depression or other mental disorder is well-established, few studies have examined whether a history of abuse may affect response to treatment, especially among adolescents. Some studies have suggested that a history of abuse is associated with a lower response to cognitive behavioral therapy (CBT), a type of psychotherapy that emphasizes problem-solving and behavior change.

In the Treatment of Resistant Depression in Adolescents (TORDIA) study, teens whose depression had not improved after an initial course of selective serotonin reuptake inhibitor (SSRI) antidepressant treatment were randomly assigned to one of four interventions for 12 weeks, including:

- Switching to another SSRI—paroxetine (Paxil), citalopram (Celexa) or fluoxetine (Prozac)
- Switching to a different SSRI plus CBT
- Switching to venlafaxine (Effexor), a different type of antidepressant called a serotonin and norepinephrine reuptake inhibitor (SNRI)
- Switching to venlafaxine plus CBT

About 40 percent of those who completed 24 weeks of treatment achieved remission, regardless of the treatment to which they had initially been assigned. The risk for relapse remained high, however.

About 13 percent of TORDIA participants had a history of physical abuse, 17 percent had a history of sexual abuse, and five percent had a history of both. In this most recent study, researchers examined the association between having a history of physical or sexual abuse and response to combination treatment among TORDIA participants.

Who is at risk for child maltreatment?

Some factors can increase the risk for abuse or neglect. The presence of these factors does not always mean that maltreatment will occur. Children are never to blame for the harm others do to them.

- **Age:** Children under four years of age are at greatest risk for severe injury and death from abuse.

- **Family Environment:** Abuse and neglect can occur in families where there is a great deal of stress. The stress can result from a family history of violence, drug or alcohol abuse, poverty, and chronic health problems. Families that do not have nearby friends, relatives, and other social support are also at risk.

The researchers found that teens without a history of abuse had a higher response rate to combination therapy compared to medication-only therapy. Those with a history of sexual abuse responded similarly to combination and medication-only therapy. However, those with a history of physical abuse had a much lower response rate to combination therapy compared to medication-only.

Significance

The researchers were unable to identify the specific mechanism that might affect response to combination therapy among teens with a history of physical abuse. They suggest that because abuse can affect a child's brain development, abused youth may need psychotherapeutic approaches that target trauma before engaging in traditional CBT designed to treat depression. The researchers also suggest that abused youth may have a tendency to avoid unpleasant emotions, and therefore may have been averse to CBT. It is possible that therapeutic approaches that focus more on behavior and do not rely heavily on the processing of negative thoughts and emotions may be more acceptable and effective for these youth.

The researchers concluded that more research is needed into the ways in which abuse history can confer treatment resistance among teens with hard-to-treat depression, and in developing alternative treatment approaches that are more effective.

Source: Excerpted from "Depressed Teens with History of Abuse Less Likely to Respond to Combination Treatment," National Institute of Mental Health (www.nimh.nih.gov), April 2011.

- **Community:** Poverty, on-going community violence, and weak connections between neighbors are related to a higher risk for child abuse and neglect.

Note: This is a partial list of risk factors. For more information, see www.cdc.gov/violenceprevention.

How can we prevent child maltreatment?

The ultimate goal is to stop child maltreatment before it starts. Strategies that support parents and teach positive parenting skills are very important. Positive parenting skills include good communication, appropriate discipline, and responding to children's physical and emotional needs. Programs to prevent child maltreatment also improve parent-child relationships and provide parents with social support.

Chapter 37

Bullying And Youth Violence

Understanding Bullying

What is bullying?

Bullying is a form of youth violence. Although definitions of bullying vary, most agree that bullying includes:

- Attack or intimidation with the intention to cause fear, distress, or harm;

- A real or perceived imbalance of power between the bully and the victim; and

- Repeated attacks or intimidation between the same children over time.

Bullying can include aggression that is physical (hitting, tripping), verbal (name calling, teasing), or psychological/social (spreading rumors, leaving out of group).

Bullying can also occur through technology and is called electronic aggression or cyberbullying. Electronic aggression is bullying that occurs through e-mail, a chat room, instant messaging, a website, text messaging, or videos or pictures posted on websites or sent through cell phones.

A young person can be a bully, a victim, or both (bully-victim).

About This Chapter: This chapter begins with excerpts from "Understanding Bullying Fact Sheet," Centers for Disease Control and Prevention (www.cdc.gov), 2012. It continues excerpts from "Bullying and Children and Youth with Disabilities and Special Health Needs," produced by StopBullying.gov, a project of the U.S. Department of Health and Human Services, 2012.

Bullying Facts

- Bullying is unwanted, aggressive behavior among school aged children.
- Bullying involves a real or perceived power imbalance and the behavior is repeated, or has the potential to be repeated, over time.
- Both kids who are bullied and kids who bully others may have serious, lasting problems.

Source: Excerpted from "Bullying and Children and Youth With Disabilities and Special Health Needs," StopBullying. gov (www.stopbullying.gov), 2012.

Why is bullying a public health problem?

Bullying is widespread in the United States.

- In a 2011 nationwide survey, 20% of high school students reported being bullied on school property in the 12 months preceding the survey.

- An estimated 16% of high school students reported in 2011 that they were bullied electronically in the 12 months before the survey.

- During the 2009–2010 school year, 23% of public schools reported that bullying occurred among students on a daily or weekly basis. A higher percentage of middle school students reported being bullying than high school students.

How does bullying affect health?

Bullying can result in physical injury, social and emotional distress, and even death. Victimized youth are at increased risk for depression, anxiety, sleep difficulties, and poor school adjustment. Youth who bully others are at increased risk for substance use, academic problems, and violence later in adolescence and adulthood. Compared to youth who only bully, or who are only victims, bully-victims suffer the most serious consequences and are at greater risk for both mental health and behavior problems.

Who is at risk for bullying?

A number of factors can increase the risk of a youth engaging in or experiencing bullying. However, the presence of these factors does not always mean that a young person will become a bully or a victim.

Some of the factors associated with a higher likelihood of engaging in bullying behavior include:

- Impulsivity (poor self-control)

- Harsh parenting by caregivers

- Attitudes accepting of violence

Some of the factors associated with a higher likelihood of victimization include:

- Friendship difficulties

- Poor self-esteem

- Perceived by peers as different or quiet

How can we prevent bullying?

The ultimate goal is to stop bullying before it starts. Research on preventing and addressing bullying is still developing. School-based bullying prevention programs are widely implemented, but infrequently evaluated. Based on a review of the limited research on school-based bullying prevention, the following program elements are promising:

- Improving supervision of students

- Using school rules and behavior management techniques in the classroom and throughout the school to detect and address bullying by providing consequences for bullying

- Having a whole school anti-bullying policy, and enforcing that policy consistently

- Promoting cooperation among different professionals and between school staff and parents

Bullying And Children And Youth With Disabilities And Special Health Needs

Children with physical, developmental, intellectual, emotional, and sensory disabilities are more likely to be bullied than their peers. Any number of factors—physical vulnerability, social skill challenges, or intolerant environments—may increase their risk. Research suggests that some children with disabilities may bully others as well.

Kids with special health needs, such as epilepsy or food allergies, may also be at higher risk of being bullied. For kids with special health needs, bullying can include making fun of kids because of their allergies or exposing them to the things they are allergic to. In these cases, bullying is not just serious; it can mean life or death.

A small but growing amount of research shows that:

- Children with attention-deficit or hyperactivity disorder (ADHD) are more likely than other children to be bullied. They also are somewhat more likely than others to bully their peers.

- Children with autism spectrum disorder (ASD) are at increased risk of being bullied and left out by peers. In a study of 8- to 17-year-olds, researchers found that children with ASD were more than three times as likely to be bullied as their peers.

- Children with epilepsy are more likely to be bullied by peers, as are children with medical conditions that affect their appearance, such as cerebral palsy, muscular dystrophy, and spina bifida. These children frequently report being called names related to their disability.

- Children with hemiplegia (paralysis of one side of their body) are more likely than other children their age to be bullied and have fewer friends.

- Children who have diabetes and are dependent on insulin may be especially vulnerable to peer bullying.

- Children who stutter may be more likely to be bullied. In one study, 83 percent of adults who stammered as children said that they were teased or bullied; 71 percent of those who had been bullied said it happened at least once a week.

- Children with learning disabilities (LD) are at a greater risk of being bullied. At least one study also has found that children with LD may also be more likely than other children to bullying their peers.

Effects Of Bullying

Kids who are bullied are more likely to have:

- Depression and anxiety (including, increased feelings of sadness and loneliness, changes in sleep and eating patterns, and loss of interest in activities they used to enjoy; issues may persist into adulthood)

- Health complaints

- Decreased academic achievement (including, GPA and standardized test scores and school participation; are more likely to miss, skip, or drop out of school)

Bullying, Disability Harassment, And The Law

Bullying behavior can become "disability harassment," which is prohibited under Section 504 of the *Rehabilitation Act of 1973* and Title II of the *Americans with Disabilities Act of 1990*.

According to the U.S. Department of Education, disability harassment is "intimidation or abusive behavior toward a student based on disability that creates a hostile environment by interfering with or denying a student's participation in or receipt of benefits, services, or opportunities in the institution's program." Disability harassment can take different forms including verbal harassment, physical threats, or threatening written statements.

When a school learns that disability harassment may have occurred, the school must investigate the incident(s) promptly and respond appropriately. Disability harassment can occur in any location that is connected with school—classrooms, the cafeteria, hallways, the playground, athletic fields, or school buses. It also can occur during school-sponsored events.

What You Can Do

If you believe a child with special needs is being bullied:

- Be supportive of the child and encourage him or her to describe who was involved and how and where the bullying happened. Be sure to tell the child that it is not his or her fault and that nobody deserves to be bullied or harassed. Do not encourage the child to fight back. This may make the problem worse.

- Ask the child specific questions about his or her friendships. Be aware of signs of bullying, even if the child doesn't call it that. Children with disabilities do not always realize they are being bullied. They may, for example, believe that they have a new friend although this "friend" is making fun of them.

- Talk with the child's parent or teacher immediately to see whether he or she can help to resolve the problem.

- Contact the principal if the bullying or harassment is severe or the teacher doesn't fix the problem. Explain what happened in detail.

Chapter 38

Teen Dating Violence

What is dating violence?

Dating violence is a type of intimate partner violence. It occurs between two people in a close relationship. The nature of dating violence can be physical, emotional, or sexual.

- **Physical Violence:** This occurs when a partner is pinched, hit, shoved, or kicked.

- **Emotional Violence:** This means threatening a partner or harming his or her sense of self-worth. Examples include name calling, shaming, bullying, embarrassing on purpose, or keeping him/her away from friends and family.

- **Sexual Violence:** This is forcing a partner to engage in a sex act when he or she does not or cannot consent.

- **Stalking:** This refers to a pattern of harassing or threatening tactics used by a perpetrator that is both unwanted and causes fear in the victim.

Dating violence can take place in person or electronically, such as repeated texting or posting sexual pictures of a partner online. Unhealthy relationships can start early and last a lifetime. Dating violence often starts with teasing and name calling. These behaviors are often thought to be a "normal" part of a relationship. But these behaviors can lead to more serious violence like physical assault and rape.

About This Chapter: Excerpted from "Understanding Teen Dating Violence," Centers for Disease Control and Prevention (www.cdc.gov), 2012.

Why is dating violence a public health problem?

Dating violence is a serious problem in the United States. Many teens do not report it because they are afraid to tell friends and family.

- Among adult victims of rape, physical violence, and/or stalking by an intimate partner, about 22 percent of women and 15 percent of men first experienced some form of partner violence between 11 and 17 years of age.

- Approximately nine percent of high school students report being hit, slapped, or physically hurt on purpose by a boyfriend or girlfriend in the 12 months before surveyed.

How does dating violence affect health?

Dating violence can have a negative effect on health throughout life. Teens who are victims are more likely to be depressed and do poorly in school. They may engage in unhealthy behaviors, like using drugs and alcohol, and are more likely to have eating disorders. Some teens even think about or attempt suicide. Teens who are victims in high school are at higher risk for victimization during college.

Who is at risk for dating violence?

Studies show that people who harm their dating partners are more depressed and are more aggressive than peers. Other factors that increase risk for harming a dating partner include trauma symptoms, alcohol use, having a friend involved in dating violence, having problem behaviors in other areas, belief that dating violence is acceptable, exposure to harsh parenting, exposure to inconsistent discipline, and lack of parental supervision, monitoring, and warmth.

Note: These are just some risk factors. To learn more, go to www.cdc.gov/violenceprevention.

How can we prevent dating violence?

The ultimate goal is to stop dating violence before it starts. Strategies that promote healthy relationships are vital. During the preteen and teen years, young people are learning skills they need to form positive relationships with others. This is an ideal time to promote healthy relationships and prevent patterns of dating violence that can last into adulthood.

Prevention programs change the attitudes and behaviors linked with dating violence. One example is Safe Dates, a school-based program that is designed to change social norms and improve problem solving skills.

Chapter 39

Cutting And Self-Harm

What does hurting yourself mean?

Hurting yourself, sometimes called self-injury, is when a person deliberately hurts his or her own body. Some self-injuries can leave scars that won't go away, while others leave marks or bruises that eventually will go away. Some forms of self-injury include cutting yourself (such as using a razor blade, knife, or other sharp object to cut the skin); punching yourself or punching things (like a wall); burning yourself with cigarettes, matches, or candles; pulling out your hair; poking objects through body openings; and breaking your bones or bruising yourself.

Why do some teens want to hurt themselves?

Many people cut themselves because it gives them a sense of relief. Some people use cutting as a means to cope with a problem. Some teens say that when they hurt themselves, they are trying to stop feeling lonely, angry, or hopeless. Some teens who hurt themselves have low self-esteem, they may feel unloved by their family and friends, and they may have an eating disorder, an alcohol or drug problem, or may have been victims of abuse.

Teens who hurt themselves often keep their feelings "bottled up" inside and have a hard time letting their feelings show. Some teens who hurt themselves say that feeling the pain provides a sense of relief from intense feelings. Cutting can relieve the tension from bottled up sadness or anxiety. Others hurt themselves in order to "feel." Often people who hold back strong emotions can begin feeling numb, and cutting can be a way to cope with this because it causes them to feel something. Some teens also may hurt themselves because they want to fit in with others who do it.

About This Chapter: Excerpted from "Cutting and Hurting Yourself," Office on Women's Health (www.girlshealth.gov), July 2013.

If you are hurting yourself, please get help. It is possible to overcome the urge to cut. There are other ways to find relief and cope with your emotions. Please talk to your parents, your doctor, or an adult you trust, like a teacher or religious leader.

Who are the people who hurt themselves?

People who hurt themselves come from all walks of life, no matter their age, gender, race, or ethnicity. About one in 100 people hurts himself or herself on purpose. More females hurt themselves than males. Teens usually hurt themselves by cutting with sharp objects.

What are the signs of self-injury?

Signs of self-injury include cuts or scars on the arms or legs that you can see; hiding cuts or scars by wearing long-sleeved shirts or pants, even in hot weather; and making poor excuses about how the injuries happened.

Self-injury can be dangerous. Cutting can lead to infections, scars, numbness, and even hospitalization or death. People who share tools to cut themselves are at risk of getting and spreading diseases like human immunodeficiency virus (HIV) and hepatitis. Teens who continue to hurt themselves are less likely to learn how to cope with negative feelings.

Are you or a friend depressed, angry, or having a hard time coping with life?

If you are thinking about hurting yourself, please ask for help! Talk with an adult you trust, like a teacher, minister, or doctor. There is nothing wrong with asking for help. Everyone needs help sometimes. You have a right to be strong, safe, and happy!

Do you have a friend who hurts herself or himself?

Please try to get your friend to talk to a trusted adult. Your friend may need professional counseling and treatment. Help is available. Counselors can teach positive ways to cope with problems without turning to self-injury. If your friend won't talk to a trusted adult, you should tell an adult you trust about the situation.

Have you been pressured to cut yourself by others who do it?

If so, think about how much you value that friendship or relationship. Do you really want a friend who wants you to hurt yourself, cause you pain and put you in danger? Try to hang out with other friends who don't pressure you in this way.

Chapter 40

Autism Spectrum Disorder

What is autism spectrum disorder (ASD)?

Autism is a group of developmental brain disorders, collectively called autism spectrum disorder (ASD). The term "spectrum" refers to the wide range of symptoms, skills, and levels of impairment, or disability, that children with ASD can have. Some children are mildly impaired by their symptoms, but others are severely disabled.

ASD is diagnosed according to guidelines listed in the *Diagnostic and Statistical Manual of Mental Disorders, Fourth Edition, Text Revision* (*DSM-IV-TR*). The manual currently defines five disorders as ASD:

- Autistic disorder (classic autism)

- Asperger syndrome

- Pervasive developmental disorder not otherwise specified (PDD-NOS)

- Rett syndrome

- Childhood disintegrative disorder (CDD)

What are the symptoms of ASD?

Symptoms of ASD vary from one child to the next. In general, they fall into three areas: social impairment; communication difficulties; and repetitive and stereotyped behaviors.

About This Chapter: Excerpted from "A Parent's Guide to Autism Spectrum Disorder," National Institute of Mental Health (www.nimh.nih.gov), May 2012.

Children with ASD do not follow typical patterns when developing social and communication skills. Parents are usually the first to notice unusual behaviors in their child. Often, certain behaviors become more noticeable when comparing children of the same age.

In some cases, babies with ASD may seem different very early in their development. Even before their first birthday, some babies become overly focused on certain objects, rarely make eye contact, and fail to engage in typical back-and-forth play and babbling with their parents. Other children may develop normally until the second or even third year of life, but then start to lose interest in others and become silent, withdrawn, or indifferent to social signals. Loss or reversal of normal development is called regression and occurs in some children with ASD.

Social Impairment: Most children with ASD have trouble engaging in everyday social interactions. Recent research suggests that children with ASD do not respond to emotional cues in human social interactions because they may not pay attention to the social cues that others typically notice. For example, one study found that children with ASD focus on the mouth of the person speaking to them instead of on the eyes, which is where children with typical development tend to focus. A related study showed that children with ASD appear to be drawn to repetitive movements linked to a sound, such as hand-clapping during a game of pat-a-cake. More research is needed to confirm these findings, but such studies suggest that children with ASD may misread or not notice subtle social cues—a smile, a wink, or a grimace—that could help them understand social relationships and interactions. Without the ability to interpret another person's tone of voice as well as gestures, facial expressions, and other nonverbal communications, children with ASD may not properly respond.

Likewise, it can be hard for others to understand the body language of children with ASD. Their facial expressions, movements, and gestures are often vague or do not match what they are saying.

Children with ASD also may have trouble understanding another person's point of view. For example, by school age, most children understand that other people have different information, feelings, and goals than they have. Children with ASD may lack this understanding, leaving them unable to predict or understand other people's actions.

Communication Issues: According to the American Academy of Pediatrics' developmental milestones, by the first birthday, typical toddlers can say one or two words, turn when they hear their name, and point when they want a toy. When offered something they do not want, toddlers make it clear with words, gestures, or facial expressions that the answer is "no." For children with ASD, reaching such milestones may not be so straightforward. For example, some children with autism may:

- Fail or be slow to respond to their name or other verbal attempts to gain their attention

- Fail or be slow to develop gestures, such as pointing and showing things to others

- Develop language at a delayed pace

- Learn to communicate using pictures or their own sign language

- Speak only in single words or repeat certain phrases over and over, seeming unable to combine words into meaningful sentences

- Repeat words or phrases that they hear, a condition called echolalia

- Use words that seem odd, out of place, or have a special meaning known only to those familiar with the child's way of communicating

Even children with ASD who have relatively good language skills often have difficulties with the back and forth of conversations. For example, because they find it difficult to understand and react to social cues, children with Asperger syndrome often talk at length about a favorite subject, but they won't allow anyone else a chance to respond or notice when others react indifferently.

Repetitive And Stereotyped Behaviors: Children with ASD often have repetitive motions or unusual behaviors. These behaviors may be extreme and very noticeable, or they can be mild and discreet. For example, some children may repeatedly flap their arms or walk in specific patterns, while others may subtly move their fingers by their eyes in what looks to be a gesture. These repetitive actions are sometimes called "stereotypy" or "stereotyped behaviors."

Children with ASD also tend to have overly focused interests. Children with ASD may become fascinated with moving objects or parts of objects, like the wheels on a moving car. They might spend a long time lining up toys in a certain way, rather than playing with them. They may also become very upset if someone accidentally moves one of the toys. Repetitive behavior can also take the form of a persistent, intense preoccupation. For example, they might be obsessed with learning all about vacuum cleaners, train schedules, or lighthouses. Children with ASD often have great interest in numbers, symbols, or science topics.

What are some other conditions that children with ASD may have?

Sensory Problems: Many children with ASD either overreact or underreact to certain sights, sounds, smells, textures, and tastes. For example, some may:

- Dislike or show discomfort from a light touch or the feel of clothes on their skin

- Experience pain from certain sounds, like a vacuum cleaner, a ringing telephone, or a sudden storm; sometimes they will cover their ears and scream

- Have no reaction to intense cold or pain

Researchers are trying to determine if these unusual reactions are related to differences in integrating multiple types of information from the senses.

Sleep Problems: Children with ASD tend to have problems falling asleep or staying asleep, or have other sleep problems. These problems make it harder for them to pay attention, reduce their ability to function, and lead to poor behavior.

Fortunately, sleep problems can often be treated with changes in behavior, such as following a sleep schedule or creating a bedtime routine. Some children may sleep better using medications such as melatonin, which is a hormone that helps regulate the body's sleep-wake cycle.

Intellectual Disability: Many children with ASD have some degree of intellectual disability. When tested, some areas of ability may be normal, while others—especially cognitive (thinking) and language abilities—may be relatively weak. For example, a child with ASD may do well on tasks related to sight (such as putting a puzzle together) but may not do as well on language-based problem-solving tasks. Children with a form of ASD like Asperger syndrome often have average or above-average language skills and do not show delays in cognitive ability or speech.

Seizures: One in four children with ASD has seizures, often starting either in early childhood or during the teen years. Seizures, caused by abnormal electrical activity in the brain, can result in:

- A short-term loss of consciousness, or a blackout

- Convulsions, which are uncontrollable shaking of the whole body, or unusual movements

- Staring spells

Fragile X Syndrome: Fragile X syndrome is a genetic disorder and is the most common form of inherited intellectual disability, causing symptoms similar to ASD. The name refers to one part of the X chromosome that has a defective piece that appears pinched and fragile when viewed with a microscope. Fragile X syndrome results from a change, called a mutation, on a single gene. This mutation, in effect, turns off the gene. Some people may have only a small mutation and not show any symptoms, while others have a larger mutation and more severe symptoms. This disorder is inherited.

Tuberous Sclerosis: Tuberous sclerosis is a rare genetic disorder that causes noncancerous tumors to grow in the brain and other vital organs. Tuberous sclerosis occurs in one to four percent of people with ASD. A genetic mutation causes the disorder, which has also been linked to mental retardation, epilepsy, and many other physical and mental health problems. There is no cure for tuberous sclerosis, but many symptoms can be treated.

Gastrointestinal Problems: Some children with ASD report frequent gastrointestinal (GI) or digestion problems, including stomach pain, diarrhea, constipation, acid reflux, vomiting, or bloating. Food allergies may also cause problems for children with ASD. It's unclear whether children with ASD are more likely to have GI problems than typically developing children.

Co-Occurring Mental Disorders: Children with ASD can also develop mental disorders such as anxiety disorders, attention-deficit hyperactivity disorder (ADHD), or depression. Research shows that people with ASD are at higher risk for some mental disorders than people without ASD. Managing these co-occurring conditions with medications or behavioral therapy, which teaches children how to control their behavior, can reduce symptoms that appear to worsen a child's ASD symptoms. Controlling these conditions will allow children with ASD to focus more on managing the ASD.

Improving The Diagnosis, Detection, And Treatment Of ASD

ASD diagnosis is often a two-stage process. The first stage involves general developmental screening during well-child checkups with a pediatrician or an early childhood health care provider. Children who show some developmental problems are referred for additional evaluation. The second stage involves a thorough evaluation by a team of doctors and other health professionals with a wide range of specialities. At this stage, a child may be diagnosed as having autism or another developmental disorder. Children with ASD can usually be reliably diagnosed by age two, though research suggests that some screening tests can be helpful at 18 months or even younger.

Many recent research studies have focused on finding the earliest signs of ASD. These studies aim to help doctors diagnose children at a younger age so they can get needed interventions as quickly as possible.

Current studies on ASD treatment are exploring many approaches, such as:

- A computer-based training program designed to teach children with ASD how to create and respond to facial expressions appropriately
- A medication that may help improve functioning in children with Fragile X syndrome
- New social interventions that can be used in the classroom or other "everyday" settings
- An intervention parents can follow to reduce and prevent ASD-related disability in children at high risk for the disorder

How is ASD treated?

While there's no proven cure yet for ASD, treating ASD early, using school-based programs, and getting proper medical care can greatly reduce ASD symptoms and increase a child's ability to grow and learn new skills.

Early Intervention: Research has shown that intensive behavioral therapy during the toddler or preschool years can significantly improve cognitive and language skills in young children with ASD. One type of a widely accepted treatment is applied behavior analysis (ABA). The goals of ABA are to shape and reinforce new behaviors, such as learning to speak and play, and reduce undesirable ones. ABA, which can involve intensive, one-on-one child-teacher interaction for up to 40 hours a week, has inspired the development of other, similar interventions that aim to help those with ASD reach their full potential.

Medications: Some medications can help reduce symptoms that cause problems for your child in school or at home. At this time, the only medications approved by the U.S. Food and Drug Administration (FDA) to treat aspects of ASD are the antipsychotics risperidone (Risperdal) and aripiprazole (Abilify). These medications can help reduce irritability—meaning aggression, self-harming acts, or temper tantrums—in children ages five to 16 who have ASD.

Some medications that may be prescribed off-label for children with ASD include: antipsychotic medications, which may help reduce aggression and other serious behavioral problems; antidepressant medications, to treat depression, anxiety, and repetitive behaviors; and stimulant medications, to treat hyperactivity.

How common is ASD?

Studies measuring ASD prevalence—the number of children affected by ASD over a given time period—have reported varying results, depending on when and where the studies were conducted and how the studies defined ASD.

In a 2009 government survey on ASD prevalence, the Centers for Disease Control and Prevention (CDC) found that the rate of ASD was higher than in past U.S. studies. Based on health and school records of 8-year-olds in 14 communities throughout the country, the CDC survey found that around one in 110 children has ASD. Boys face about four to five times higher risk than girls.

Experts disagree about whether this shows a true increase in ASD prevalence. Since the earlier studies were completed, guidelines for diagnosis have changed. Also, many more parents and doctors now know about ASD, so parents are more likely to take their children to be diagnosed, and more doctors are able to properly diagnose ASD. These and other changes may help explain some differences in prevalence numbers. Even so, the CDC report confirms other recent studies showing that more children are being diagnosed with ASD than ever before.

What causes ASD?

Scientists don't know the exact causes of ASD, but research suggests that both genes and environment play important roles.

Genetic Factors: In identical twins who share the exact same genetic code, if one has ASD, the other twin also has ASD in nearly nine out of 10 cases. If one sibling has ASD, the other siblings have 35 times the normal risk of also developing the disorder. Researchers are starting to identify particular genes that may increase the risk for ASD.

Most people who develop ASD have no reported family history of autism, suggesting that random, rare, and possibly many gene mutations are likely to affect a person's risk. Any change to normal genetic information is called a mutation. Mutations can be inherited, but some arise for no reason. Mutations can be helpful, harmful, or have no effect.

Having increased genetic risk does not mean a child will definitely develop ASD. Many researchers are focusing on how various genes interact with each other and environmental factors to better understand how they increase the risk of this disorder.

Environmental Factors: In medicine, "environment" refers to anything outside of the body that can affect health. This includes the air we breathe, the water we drink and bathe in, the food we eat, the medicines we take, and many other things that our bodies may come in contact with. Environment also includes our surroundings in the womb, when our mother's health directly affects our growth and earliest development.

Researchers are studying many environmental factors such as family medical conditions, parental age and other demographic factors, exposure to toxins, and complications during birth or pregnancy.

As with genes, it's likely that more than one environmental factor is involved in increasing risk for ASD. And, like genes, any one of these risk factors raises the risk by only a small amount. Most people who have been exposed to environmental risk factors do not develop ASD.

Scientists are studying how certain environmental factors may affect certain genes— turning them on or off, or increasing or decreasing their normal activity. This process is called epigenetics and is providing researchers with many new ways to study how disorders like ASD develop and possibly change over time.

ASD And Vaccines: Health experts recommend that children receive a number of vaccines early in life to protect against dangerous, infectious diseases, such as measles. Since pediatricians in the United States started giving these vaccines during regular checkups, the number of children getting sick, becoming disabled, or dying from these diseases has dropped to almost zero.

Children in the United States receive several vaccines during their first two years of life, around the same age that ASD symptoms often appear or become noticeable. A minority of parents suspect that vaccines are somehow related to their child's disorder. Some may be concerned about these vaccines due to the unproven theory that ASD may be caused by thimerosal. Thimerosal is a mercury-based chemical once added to some, but not all, vaccines to help extend their shelf life. However, except for some flu vaccines, no vaccine routinely given to preschool aged children in the United States has contained thimerosal since 2001. Despite this change, the rate of children diagnosed with ASD has continued to rise.

Other parents believe their child's illness might be linked to vaccines designed to protect against more than one disease, such as the measles-mumps-rubella (MMR) vaccine, which never contained thimerosal.

Many studies have been conducted to try to determine if vaccines are a possible cause of autism. As of 2010, none of the studies has linked autism and vaccines.

How does ASD affect teens?

The teen years can be a time of stress and confusion for any growing child, including teenagers with ASD.

During the teenage years, adolescents become more aware of other people and their relationships with them. While most teenagers are concerned with acne, popularity, grades, and dates, teens with ASD may become painfully aware that they are different from their peers. For some, this awareness may encourage them to learn new behaviors and try to improve their social skills. For others, hurt feelings and problems connecting with others may lead to depression, anxiety, or other mental disorders. One way that some teens with ASD may express the tension and confusion that can occur during adolescence is through increased autistic or aggressive behavior. Teens with ASD also need support to help them understand the physical changes and sexual maturation they experience during adolescence.

Chapter 41

Attention Deficit Hyperactivity Disorder

What is attention deficit hyperactivity disorder?

Attention deficit hyperactivity disorder (ADHD) is one of the most common childhood brain disorders and can continue through adolescence and adulthood. Symptoms include difficulty staying focused and paying attention, difficulty controlling behavior, and hyperactivity (over-activity). These symptoms can make it difficult for a child with ADHD to succeed in school, get along with other children or adults, or finish tasks at home.

Brain imaging studies have revealed that, in youth with ADHD, the brain matures in a normal pattern but is delayed, on average, by about three years. The delay is most pronounced in brain regions involved in thinking, paying attention, and planning. More recent studies have found that the outermost layer of the brain, the cortex, shows delayed maturation overall, and a brain structure important for proper communications between the two halves of the brain shows an abnormal growth pattern. These delays and abnormalities may underlie the hallmark symptoms of ADHD and help to explain how the disorder may develop.

Treatments can relieve many symptoms of ADHD, but there is currently no cure for the disorder. With treatment, most people with ADHD can be successful in school and lead productive lives. Researchers are developing more effective treatments and interventions, and using new tools such as brain imaging, to better understand ADHD and to find more effective ways to treat and prevent it.

About This Chapter: Excerpted from "Attention Deficit Hyperactivity Disorder," National Institute of Mental Health (www.nimh.nih.gov), December 2012.

What are the symptoms of ADHD?

Inattention, hyperactivity, and impulsivity are the key behaviors of ADHD. It is normal for all children to be inattentive, hyperactive, or impulsive sometimes, but for children with ADHD, these behaviors are more severe and occur more often. To be diagnosed with the disorder, a child must have symptoms for six or more months and to a degree that is greater than other children of the same age.

Children who have symptoms of inattention may:

- Be easily distracted, miss details, forget things, and frequently switch from one activity to another

- Have difficulty focusing on one thing

- Become bored with a task after only a few minutes, unless they are doing something enjoyable

- Have difficulty focusing attention on organizing and completing a task or learning something new

- Have trouble completing or turning in homework assignments, often losing things (for example, pencils, toys, assignments) needed to complete tasks or activities

- Not seem to listen when spoken to

- Daydream, become easily confused, and move slowly

- Have difficulty processing information as quickly and accurately as others

- Struggle to follow instructions

Children who have symptoms of hyperactivity may:

- Fidget and squirm in their seats

- Talk nonstop

- Dash around, touching or playing with anything and everything in sight

- Have trouble sitting still during dinner, school, and story time

- Be constantly in motion

- Have difficulty doing quiet tasks or activities.

Children who have symptoms of impulsivity may:

- Be very impatient

- Blurt out inappropriate comments, show their emotions without restraint, and act without regard for consequences

- Have difficulty waiting for things they want or waiting their turns in games

- Often interrupt conversations or others' activities

What causes ADHD?

Scientists are not sure what causes ADHD, although many studies suggest that genes play a large role. Like many other illnesses, ADHD probably results from a combination of factors. In addition to genetics, researchers are looking at possible environmental factors, and are studying how brain injuries, nutrition, and the social environment might contribute to ADHD.

Genes: Inherited from our parents, genes are the "blueprints" for who we are. Results from several international studies of twins show that ADHD often runs in families. Researchers are looking at several genes that may make people more likely to develop the disorder. Knowing the genes involved may one day help researchers prevent the disorder before symptoms develop. Learning about specific genes could also lead to better treatments.

Environmental Factors: Studies suggest a potential link between cigarette smoking and alcohol use during pregnancy and ADHD in children. In addition, preschoolers who are exposed to high levels of lead, which can sometimes be found in plumbing fixtures or paint in old buildings, have a higher risk of developing ADHD.

Brain Injuries: Children who have suffered a brain injury may show some behaviors similar to those of ADHD. However, only a small percentage of children with ADHD have suffered a traumatic brain injury.

Sugar: The idea that refined sugar causes ADHD or makes symptoms worse is popular, but more research discounts this theory than supports it. In one study, researchers gave children foods containing either sugar or a sugar substitute every other day. The children who received sugar showed no different behavior or learning capabilities than those who received the sugar substitute. Another study in which children were given higher than average amounts of sugar or sugar substitutes showed similar results.

Food Additives: There is currently no research showing that artificial food coloring causes ADHD. However, a small number of children with ADHD may be sensitive to food dyes, artificial flavors, preservatives, or other food additives. They may experience fewer ADHD symptoms on a diet without additives, but such diets are often difficult to maintain.

How is ADHD diagnosed?

Children mature at different rates and have different personalities, temperaments, and energy levels. Most children get distracted, act impulsively, and struggle to concentrate at one time or another. Sometimes, these normal factors may be mistaken for ADHD. ADHD symptoms usually appear early in life, often between the ages of three and six, and because symptoms vary from person to person, the disorder can be hard to diagnose. Parents may first notice that their child loses interest in things sooner than other children, or seems constantly "unfocused" or "out of control." Often, teachers notice the symptoms first, when a child has trouble following rules, or frequently "spaces out" in the classroom or on the playground.

No single test can diagnose a child as having ADHD. Instead, a licensed health professional needs to gather information about the child, and his or her behavior and environment. A family may want to first talk with the child's pediatrician. Some pediatricians can assess the child themselves, but many will refer the family to a mental health specialist with experience in childhood brain disorders such as ADHD. The pediatrician or mental health specialist will first try to rule out other possibilities for the symptoms. For example, certain situations, events, or health conditions may cause temporary behaviors in a child that seem like ADHD.

A specialist will also check school and medical records for clues, to see if the child's home or school settings appear unusually stressful or disrupted, and gather information from the child's parents and teachers. Coaches, babysitters, and other adults who know the child well also may be consulted.

The specialist pays close attention to the child's behavior during different situations. Some situations are highly structured, some have less structure. Others would require the child to keep paying attention. Most children with ADHD are better able to control their behaviors in situations where they are getting individual attention and when they are free to focus on enjoyable activities. These types of situations are less important in the assessment. A child also may be evaluated to see how he or she acts in social situations, and may be given tests of intellectual ability and academic achievement to see if he or she has a learning disability.

Finally, after gathering all this information, if the child meets the criteria for ADHD, he or she will be diagnosed with the disorder.

How is ADHD treated?

Currently available treatments aim at reducing the symptoms of ADHD and improving functioning. Treatments include medication, various types of psychotherapy, education and training, or a combination of treatments.

Medications: Stimulants, such as methylphenidate and amphetamines, are the most common type of medication used for treating ADHD. Although it may seem counterintuitive to treat hyperactivity with a stimulant, these medications actually activate brain circuits that support attention and focused behavior, thus reducing hyperactivity. In addition, a few non-stimulant medications, such as atomoxetine, guanfacine, and clonidine, are also available. For many children, ADHD medications reduce hyperactivity and impulsivity and improve their ability to focus, work, and learn. Medications also may improve physical coordination.

However, a one-size-fits-all approach does not apply for all children with ADHD. What works for one child might not work for another. One child might have side effects with a certain medication, while another child may not. Sometimes several different medications or dosages must be tried before finding one that works for a particular child. Any child taking medications must be monitored closely and carefully by caregivers and doctors.

Psychotherapy: Different types of psychotherapy are used for ADHD. Behavioral therapy aims to help a child change his or her behavior. It might involve practical assistance, such as help organizing tasks or completing schoolwork, or working through emotionally difficult events. Behavioral therapy also teaches a child how to monitor his or her own behavior. Learning to give oneself praise or rewards for acting in a desired way, such as controlling anger or thinking before acting, is another goal of behavioral therapy. Parents and teachers also can give positive or negative feedback for certain behaviors. In addition, clear rules, chore lists, and other structured routines can help a child control his or her behavior.

What are the side effects of stimulant medications?

The most commonly reported side effects are decreased appetite, sleep problems, anxiety, and irritability. Some children also report mild stomachaches or headaches. Most side effects are minor and disappear over time or if the dosage level is lowered.

A few children develop sudden, repetitive movements or sounds called tics. Changing the medication dosage may make tics go away. Some children also may have a personality change, such as appearing "flat" or without emotion.

Do medications cure ADHD?

Current medications do not cure ADHD. Rather, they control the symptoms for as long as they are taken. Medications can help a child pay attention and complete schoolwork. It is not clear, however, whether medications can help children learn better. Adding behavioral therapy, counseling, and practical support can help children with ADHD and their families to better cope with everyday problems. NIMH-funded research has shown that medication works best when treatment is regularly monitored by the prescribing doctor and the dose is adjusted based on the child's needs.

FDA Warning On Possible Rare Side Effects

In 2007, the FDA required that all makers of ADHD medications develop Patient Medication Guides that contain information about the risks associated with the medications. The guides must alert patients that the medications may lead to possible cardiovascular (heart and blood) or psychiatric problems.

The FDA review also found a slight increased risk (about one in 1,000) for medication-related psychiatric problems, such as hearing voices, having hallucinations, becoming suspicious for no reason, or becoming manic (an overly high mood), even in patients without a history of psychiatric problems. The FDA recommends that any treatment plan for ADHD include an initial health history, including family history, and examination for existing cardiovascular and psychiatric problems.

One ADHD medication, the non-stimulant atomoxetine (Strattera), carries another warning. Studies show that children and teenagers who take atomoxetine are more likely to have suicidal thoughts than children and teenagers with ADHD who do not take it.

Source: NIMH, December 2012.

How can parents help?

Children with ADHD need guidance and understanding from their parents and teachers to reach their full potential and to succeed in school. Before a child is diagnosed, frustration, blame, and anger may have built up within a family. Parents and children may need special help to overcome bad feelings. Mental health professionals can educate parents about ADHD and how it impacts a family. They also will help the child and his or her parents develop new skills, attitudes, and ways of relating to each other.

Sometimes, the whole family may need therapy. Therapists can help family members find better ways to handle disruptive behaviors and to encourage behavior changes.

What conditions can coexist with ADHD?

Some children with ADHD also have other illnesses or conditions. For example, they may have one or more of the following:

- **A Learning Disability:** A school-aged child may struggle with reading, spelling, writing, and math.

Prescribed Stimulant Use For ADHD Continues To Rise Steadily

The prescribed use of stimulant medications to treat attention deficit hyperactivity disorder (ADHD) rose slowly but steadily from 1996–2008, according to a study conducted by the National Institutes of Health (NIH) and the Agency for Healthcare Research and Quality (AHRQ). During the 1990s, stimulant prescription use increased significantly, going from a prevalence rate among youth of 0.6 percent in 1987 to 2.7 percent in 1997, with the rate stabilizing around 2.9 percent in 2002.

Recent reports suggest that the prescribed use of these medications and the diagnosis of ADHD have continued to rise. Based on the Health Resources and Services Administration's National Survey of Children's Health, the percentage of children age 4–17 years diagnosed with ADHD increased from 7.8 percent in 2003 to 9.5 percent in 2007.

"Stimulant medications work well to control ADHD symptoms, but they are only one method of treatment for the condition. Experts estimate that about 60 percent of children with ADHD are treated with medication," said co-author Benedetto Vitiello, MD, of NIH's National Institute of Mental Health (NIMH).

Overall, prescription use among 6- to 12-year-olds was highest (5.1 percent in 2008), but the fastest growth of prescribed use occurred among 13- to 18-year-olds (4.9 percent in 2008). "This continuous increase among teens likely reflects a recent realization that ADHD often persists as children age. They do not always grow out of their symptoms," said Dr. Vitiello.

Boys continued to be three times more likely to be prescribed a stimulant than girls, and use among white children continued to be higher than among black or Hispanic children. However, prescribed stimulant use is increasing among racial and ethnic minorities, likely suggesting more recognition of ADHD and acceptance of psychopharmacological treatment among these groups. In addition, rates were substantially lower in Western states compared to other regions of the nation, with no increase in recent years.

"These persistent differences in prescribed stimulant use related to age, racial and ethnic background, and geographical location indicate substantial variability in how families and doctors approach ADHD treatment throughout the United States," said AHRQ's Dr. Samuel Zuvekas.

The researchers concluded that, when comparing the rates of prescribed use with the estimated prevalence of ADHD diagnosis, it appears that many children with ADHD are not treated with stimulants. "The children with the most severe symptoms are more likely to be taking stimulants. Those with milder symptoms are more likely being treated with psychosocial treatments or other non-stimulant medications," they said.

Source: Excerpted from "Prescribed Stimulant Use for ADHD Continues to Rise Steadily," National Institute of Mental Health (www.nimh.nih.gov), August 2012.

- **Oppositional Defiant Disorder:** Kids with this condition, in which a child is overly stubborn or rebellious, often argue with adults and refuse to obey rules.

- **Conduct Disorder:** This condition includes behaviors in which the child may lie, steal, fight, or bully others. He or she may destroy property, break into homes, or carry or use weapons. These children or teens are also at a higher risk of using illegal substances. Kids with conduct disorder are at risk of getting into trouble at school or with the police.

- **Anxiety And Depression:** Treating ADHD may help to decrease anxiety or some forms of depression.

- **Bipolar Disorder:** Some children with ADHD may also have this condition in which extreme mood swings go from mania (an extremely high elevated mood) to depression in short periods of time.

- **Tourette Syndrome:** Very few children have this brain disorder, but, among those who do, many also have ADHD. People with Tourette syndrome have nervous tics, which can be evident as repetitive, involuntary movements, such as eye blinks, facial twitches, or grimacing, and/or as vocalizations, such as throat-clearing, snorting, sniffing, or barking out words inappropriately. These behaviors can be controlled with medication, behavioral interventions, or both.

ADHD also may coexist with a sleep disorder, bed-wetting, substance abuse, or other disorders or illnesses. Recognizing ADHD symptoms and seeking help early will lead to better outcomes for both affected children and their families.

Do teens with ADHD have special needs?

Most children with ADHD continue to have symptoms as they enter adolescence. Some children are not diagnosed with ADHD until they reach adolescence. This is more common among children with predominantly inattentive symptoms because they are not necessarily disruptive at home or in school. In these children, the disorder becomes more apparent as academic demands increase and responsibilities mount. For all teens, these years are challenging. But for teens with ADHD, these years may be especially difficult.

Although hyperactivity tends to decrease as a child ages, teens who continue to be hyperactive may feel restless and try to do too many things at once. They may choose tasks or activities that have a quick payoff, rather than those that take more effort, but provide bigger, delayed rewards. Teens with primarily attention deficits struggle with school and other activities in which they are expected to be more self-reliant.

Teens also become more responsible for their own health decisions. When a child with ADHD is young, parents are more likely to be responsible for ensuring that their child maintains treatment. But when the child reaches adolescence, parents have less control, and those with ADHD may have difficulty sticking with treatment.

What efforts are under way to improve treatment?

This is an exciting time in ADHD research. The expansion of knowledge in genetics, brain imaging, and behavioral research is leading to a better understanding of the causes of the disorder, how to prevent it, and how to develop more effective treatments for all age groups. Scientists continue to look for the biological basis of ADHD, and how differences in genes and brain structure and function may combine with life experiences to produce the disorder.

Chapter 42

Tourette Syndrome And Tics

What is Tourette syndrome?

Tourette syndrome (TS) is a neurological disorder characterized by repetitive, stereotyped, involuntary movements and vocalizations called tics. The disorder is named for Dr. Georges Gilles de la Tourette, the pioneering French neurologist who in 1885 first described the condition in an 86-year-old French noblewoman.

The early symptoms of TS are typically noticed first in childhood, with the average onset between the ages of three and nine years. TS occurs in people from all ethnic groups; males are affected about three to four times more often than females. It is estimated that 200,000 Americans have the most severe form of TS, and as many as one in 100 exhibit milder and less complex symptoms such as chronic motor or vocal tics. Although TS can be a chronic condition with symptoms lasting a lifetime, most people with the condition experience their worst tic symptoms in their early teens, with improvement occurring in the late teens and continuing into adulthood.

What are the symptoms?

Tics are classified as either simple or complex. Simple motor tics are sudden, brief, repetitive movements that involve a limited number of muscle groups. Some of the more common simple tics include eye blinking and other eye movements, facial grimacing, shoulder shrugging, and head or shoulder jerking. Simple vocalizations might include repetitive throat-clearing, sniffing, or grunting sounds. Complex tics are distinct, coordinated patterns of movements involving

About This Chapter: Excerpted from "Tourette Syndrome Fact Sheet," National Institute of Neurological Disorders and Stroke (www.ninds.nih.gov), October 2012.

several muscle groups. Complex motor tics might include facial grimacing combined with a head twist and a shoulder shrug. Other complex motor tics may actually appear purposeful, including sniffing or touching objects, hopping, jumping, bending, or twisting. Simple vocal tics may include throat-clearing, sniffing/snorting, grunting, or barking. More complex vocal tics include words or phrases. Perhaps the most dramatic and disabling tics include motor movements that result in self-harm such as punching oneself in the face or vocal tics including coprolalia (uttering socially inappropriate words such as swearing) or echolalia (repeating the words or phrases of others). However, coprolalia is only present in a small number (10–15 percent) of individuals with TS. Some tics are preceded by an urge or sensation in the affected muscle group, commonly called a premonitory urge. Some with TS will describe a need to complete a tic in a certain way or a certain number of times in order to relieve the urge or decrease the sensation.

Tics are often worse with excitement or anxiety and better during calm, focused activities. Certain physical experiences can trigger or worsen tics, for example tight collars may trigger neck tics, or hearing another person sniff or throat-clear may trigger similar sounds. Tics do not go away during sleep but are often significantly diminished.

What is the course of TS?

Tics come and go over time, varying in type, frequency, location, and severity. The first symptoms usually occur in the head and neck area and may progress to include muscles of the trunk and extremities. Motor tics generally precede the development of vocal tics and simple tics often precede complex tics. Most patients experience peak tic severity before the mid-teen years with improvement for the majority of patients in the late teen years and early adulthood. Approximately 10–15 percent of those affected have a progressive or disabling course that lasts into adulthood.

Can people with TS control their tics?

Although the symptoms of TS are involuntary, some people can sometimes suppress, camouflage, or otherwise manage their tics in an effort to minimize their impact on functioning. However, people with TS often report a substantial buildup in tension when suppressing their tics to the point where they feel that the tic must be expressed (against their will). Tics in response to an environmental trigger can appear to be voluntary or purposeful but are not.

What causes TS?

Although the cause of TS is unknown, current research points to abnormalities in certain brain regions (including the basal ganglia, frontal lobes, and cortex), the circuits that interconnect these regions, and the neurotransmitters (dopamine, serotonin, and norepinephrine) responsible for communication among nerve cells. Given the often complex presentation of TS, the cause of the disorder is likely to be equally complex.

What disorders are associated with TS?

Many individuals with TS experience additional neurobehavioral problems that often cause more impairment than the tics themselves. These include inattention, hyperactivity and impulsivity (attention deficit hyperactivity disorder—ADHD); problems with reading, writing, and arithmetic; and obsessive-compulsive symptoms such as intrusive thoughts/worries and repetitive behaviors. For example, worries about dirt and germs may be associated with repetitive hand washing, and concerns about bad things happening may be associated with ritualistic behaviors such as counting, repeating, or ordering and arranging. People with TS have also reported problems with depression or anxiety disorders, as well as other difficulties with living, that may or may not be directly related to TS. In addition, although most individuals with TS experience a significant decline in motor and vocal tics in late adolescence and early adulthood, the associated neurobehavioral conditions may persist. Given the range of potential complications, people with TS are best served by receiving medical care that provides a comprehensive treatment plan.

How is TS diagnosed?

TS is a diagnosis that doctors make after verifying that the patient has had both motor and vocal tics for at least one year. The existence of other neurological or psychiatric conditions can also help doctors arrive at a diagnosis. Common tics are not often misdiagnosed by knowledgeable clinicians. However, atypical symptoms or atypical presentations (for example, onset of symptoms in adulthood) may require specific specialty expertise for diagnosis. There are no blood, laboratory, or imaging tests needed for diagnosis. In rare cases, neuroimaging studies, such as magnetic resonance imaging (MRI) or computerized tomography (CT), electroencephalogram (EEG) studies, or certain blood tests may be used to rule out other conditions that might be confused with TS when the history or clinical examination is atypical.

It is not uncommon for patients to obtain a formal diagnosis of TS only after symptoms have been present for some time. The reasons for this are many. For families and physicians unfamiliar with TS, mild and even moderate tic symptoms may be considered inconsequential, part of a developmental phase, or the result of another condition. For example, parents may think that eye blinking is related to vision problems or that sniffing is related to seasonal allergies. Many patients are self-diagnosed after they, their parents, other relatives, or friends read or hear about TS from others.

How is TS treated?

Because tic symptoms often do not cause impairment, the majority of people with TS require no medication for tic suppression. However, effective medications are available for

---

Attention Woes In Kids With Tourette Syndrome Likely Caused By Co-Occurring Attention Deficit Hyperactivity Disorder (ADHD)

Co-occurring attention deficit hyperactivity disorder (ADHD) may be at the root of attention problems in children with Tourette syndrome (TS), according to National Institute of Mental Health (NIMH)-funded researchers. Their findings also support the theory that children with TS develop different patterns of brain activity in order to function at the same level as children without TS.

Background

Tourette syndrome is a chronic neurological disorder associated with repetitive, involuntary movements and vocalizations called tics. Many with TS also experience neurobehavioral problems such as inattention, hyperactivity, and impulsivity—symptoms that overlap with ADHD. In fact, researchers estimate that between 50–90 percent of youth with TS also have ADHD.

To explore the role of co-occurring ADHD in TS, Denis Sukhodolsky, PhD, of the Yale Child Study Center, and colleagues studied 236 children, of which:

- 56 had TS only
- 64 had ADHD only
- 45 had TS+ADHD
- 71 had neither and served as a comparison group

The researchers used well-known, standardized measures to evaluate the children's performance on tasks requiring:

- **Sustained Attention And Inhibitory Control:** Participants were shown various letters on a computer screen and told to press a button when they saw certain letters but not press the button when they saw a non-target letter.
- **Cognitive Inhibition:** Participants were shown an array of dots on sheets of paper and asked to name their color (red, green, and blue) as quickly as possible. In related tasks, participants were shown pages with similarly arrayed words ("red," "green," "blue") printed in black ink or a mismatched color of ink (such as "red" printed in green ink) and asked to read the words as quickly as possible.
- **Fine Motor Control:** Participants placed small pegs in a specially designed pegboard in 30-second trials using only their dominant hand, only their non-dominant hand, and both hands at the same time.

those whose symptoms interfere with functioning. Neuroleptics (drugs that may be used to treat psychotic and non-psychotic disorders) are the most consistently useful medications for tic suppression; a number are available but some are more effective than others (for example, haloperidol and pimozide).

- **Visual-Motor Integration:** Participants copied 24 geometric designs, presented in order of increasing difficulty.

Results Of The Study

Children with TS+ADHD showed similar problems with sustained attention as children with ADHD only. However, unlike those with ADHD only, children with TS+ADHD performed at the same level as the comparison group on all other tasks.

Children with TS only performed at the same level as the comparison group in tasks involving response inhibition and visual-motor integration. They performed at a slightly lower level than comparison children on the fine motor control task. Girls with TS only scored higher than boys with TS only on fine motor control tasks using their dominant hands.

Significance

The study helps to identify brain functions specific to particular disorders and the mechanisms underlying these functions. Similarities in performance between children with TS+ADHD and those with ADHD only suggest that co-occurring ADHD may underlie attention problems in children who have TS, according to the researchers.

The researchers also noted that the children with TS only didn't show impairment in response inhibition, lending support to a theory that such children develop compensatory brain mechanisms in an effort to control involuntary tics. Past imaging studies have shown that, during tasks involving response inhibition, children with TS have greater than normal activity in brain areas associated with cognitive control.

Differences in fine motor skills between girls and boys with TS may indicate differing developmental pathways and patterns of brain growth between the sexes. Because problems with fine motor control in childhood are associated with more severe tics in adulthood, the researchers highlighted this finding as an area for further study.

What's Next

Future studies may help advance the understanding of how TS arises and changes in brain growth and functioning that are associated with the disorder.

Source: Excerpted from "Attention Woes in Kids With Tourette Syndrome Likely Caused by Co-Occurring ADHD," National Institute of Mental Health (www.nimh.nih.gov), February 2013.

Unfortunately, there is no one medication that is helpful to all people with TS, nor does any medication completely eliminate symptoms. In addition, all medications have side effects. Many neuroleptic side effects can be managed by initiating treatment slowly and reducing the dose when side effects occur. The most common side effects of neuroleptics include sedation, weight gain, and cognitive dulling. Neurological side effects such as tremor, dystonic reactions (twisting movements or postures), parkinsonian-like symptoms, and other dyskinetic (involuntary) movements are less common and are readily managed with dose reduction.

Discontinuing neuroleptics after long-term use must be done slowly to avoid rebound increases in tics and withdrawal dyskinesias. One form of dyskinesia called tardive dyskinesia is a movement disorder distinct from TS that may result from the chronic use of neuroleptics. The risk of this side effect can be reduced by using lower doses of neuroleptics for shorter periods of time.

Other medications may also be useful for reducing tic severity, but most have not been as extensively studied or shown to be as consistently useful as neuroleptics. Additional medications with demonstrated efficacy include alpha-adrenergic agonists such as clonidine and guanfacine. These medications are used primarily for hypertension but are also used in the treatment of tics. The most common side effect from these medications that precludes their use is sedation. However, given the lower side effect risk associated with these medications, they are often used as first-line agents before proceeding to treatment with neuroleptics.

Effective medications are also available to treat some of the associated neurobehavioral disorders that can occur in patients with TS. Recent research shows that stimulant medications such as methylphenidate and dextroamphetamine can lessen ADHD symptoms in people with TS without causing tics to become more severe. However, the product labeling for stimulants currently contraindicates the use of these drugs in children with tics/TS and those with a family history of tics. Scientists hope that future studies will include a thorough discussion of the risks and benefits of stimulants in those with TS or a family history of TS and will clarify this issue. For obsessive-compulsive symptoms that significantly disrupt daily functioning, the serotonin reuptake inhibitors (clomipramine, fluoxetine, fluvoxamine, paroxetine, and sertraline) have been proven effective in some patients.

Behavioral treatments such as awareness training and competing response training can also be used to reduce tics. A recent National Institutes of Health (NIH)-funded, multi-center randomized control trial called Cognitive Behavioral Intervention for Tics, or CBIT, showed that training to voluntarily move in response to a premonitory urge can reduce tic symptoms. Other behavioral therapies, such as biofeedback or supportive therapy, have not been shown to reduce tic symptoms. However, supportive therapy can help a person with TS better cope with the disorder and deal with the secondary social and emotional problems that sometimes occur.

Is TS inherited?

Evidence from twin and family studies suggests that TS is an inherited disorder. Although early family studies suggested an autosomal dominant mode of inheritance (an autosomal dominant disorder is one in which only one copy of the defective gene, inherited from one parent, is necessary to produce the disorder), more recent studies suggest that the pattern of inheritance is much more complex. Although there may be a few genes with substantial effects, it is also possible that many genes with smaller effects and environmental factors may play a role in the development of TS.

Genetic studies also suggest that some forms of ADHD and OCD are genetically related to TS, but there is less evidence for a genetic relationship between TS and other neurobehavioral problems that commonly co-occur with TS. It is important for families to understand that genetic predisposition may not necessarily result in full-blown TS; instead, it may express itself as a milder tic disorder or as obsessive-compulsive behaviors. It is also possible that the gene-carrying offspring will not develop any TS symptoms.

The gender of the person also plays an important role in TS gene expression. At-risk males are more likely to have tics and at-risk females are more likely to have obsessive-compulsive symptoms.

Genetic counseling of individuals with TS should include a full review of all potentially hereditary conditions in the family.

What is the prognosis?

Although there is no cure for TS, the condition in many individuals improves in the late teens and early 20s. As a result, some may actually become symptom-free or no longer need medication for tic suppression. Although the disorder is generally lifelong and chronic, it is not a degenerative condition. Individuals with TS have a normal life expectancy. TS does not impair intelligence. Although tic symptoms tend to decrease with age, it is possible that neurobehavioral disorders such as ADHD, OCD, depression, generalized anxiety, panic attacks, and mood swings can persist and cause impairment in adult life.

What is the best educational setting for children with TS?

Although students with TS often function well in the regular classroom, ADHD, learning disabilities, obsessive-compulsive symptoms, and frequent tics can greatly interfere with academic performance or social adjustment. After a comprehensive assessment, students should be placed in an educational setting that meets their individual needs. Students may require tutoring, smaller or special classes, and in some cases special schools.

All students with TS need a tolerant and compassionate setting that both encourages them to work to their full potential and is flexible enough to accommodate their special needs. This setting may include a private study area, exams outside the regular classroom, or even oral exams when the child's symptoms interfere with his or her ability to write. Untimed testing reduces stress for students with TS.

What research is being done?

Within the Federal government, the National Institute of Neurological Disorders and Stroke (NINDS), a part of the National Institutes of Health (NIH), is responsible for supporting and conducting research on the brain and nervous system. The NINDS and other NIH components, such as the National Institute of Mental Health, the Eunice Kennedy Shriver National Institute of Child Health and Human Development, the National Institute on Drug Abuse, and the National Institute on Deafness and Other Communication Disorders, support research of relevance to TS, either at NIH laboratories or through grants to major research institutions across the country. Another component of the Department of Health and Human Services, the Centers for Disease Control and Prevention (CDC), funds professional education programs as well as TS research.

Knowledge about TS comes from studies across a number of medical and scientific disciplines, including genetics, neuroimaging, neuropathology, clinical trials (medication and non-medication), epidemiology, neurophysiology, neuroimmunology, and descriptive/diagnostic clinical science.

Part Six
Mental Health Treatments

Chapter 43

Diagnosing Mental Illness

Research shows that half of all lifetime cases of mental illness begin by age 14. Scientists are discovering that changes in the body leading to mental illness may start much earlier, before any symptoms appear.

Through greater understanding of when and how fast specific areas of children's brains develop, we are learning more about the early stages of a wide range of mental illnesses that appear later in life. Helping young children and their parents manage difficulties early in life may prevent the development of disorders. Once mental illness develops, it becomes a regular part of your child's behavior and more difficult to treat. Even though we know how to treat (though not yet cure) many disorders, many children with mental illnesses are not getting treatment.

This chapter addresses common questions about diagnosis options for children with mental illnesses. Disorders affecting children may include anxiety disorders, attention deficit hyperactivity disorder (ADHD), autism spectrum disorders, bipolar disorder, depression, eating disorders, and schizophrenia.

What should I do if I am concerned about mental, behavioral, or emotional symptoms?

Talk to your doctor or health care provider. Ask questions and learn everything you can about the behavior or symptoms that worry you. If you are in school, ask the teacher if you have been showing worrisome changes in behavior. Share this with your doctor or health care provider. Keep in mind that every child is different. Even normal development, such as when

About This Chapter: Excerpted from "Treatment of Children with Mental Illness," National Institute of Mental Health (www.nimh.nih.gov), 2009.

children develop language, motor, and social skills, varies from child to child. Ask if you need further evaluation by a specialist with experience in adolescent behavioral problems. Specialists may include psychiatrists, psychologists, social workers, psychiatric nurses, and behavioral therapists. Educators may also help evaluate your symptoms.

How do I know if my problems are serious?

Not every problem is serious. In fact, many everyday stresses can cause changes in your behavior. It is important to be able to tell the difference between typical behavior changes and those associated with more serious problems. Pay special attention to behaviors that include:

- Problems across a variety of settings, such as at school, at home, or with peers

- Changes in appetite or sleep

- Social withdrawal, or fearful behavior toward things you are not afraid of

- Returning to behaviors more common in younger children, such as bed-wetting, for a long time

- Signs of being upset, such as sadness or tearfulness

- Signs of self-destructive behavior, such as head-banging, or a tendency to get hurt often

- Repeated thoughts of death

Can symptoms be caused by a death in the family, illness in a parent, family financial problems, divorce, or other events?

Yes. Every member of a family is affected by tragedy or extreme stress, even the youngest child. If it takes more than one month for you to get used to a situation, or if you have severe reactions, talk to your doctor.

Check your response to stress. Take note if you get better with time or if professional care is needed. Stressful events are challenging, but they give you a chance learn important ways to cope.

How are mental illnesses diagnosed?

Before diagnosing a mental illness, the doctor or specialist tries to rule out other possible causes for your behavior. The doctor will:

- Take a history of any important medical problems

Survey Finds More Evidence That Mental Disorders Often Begin In Youth

A September 2010 study using data from the National Institute of Mental Health (NIMH)-funded National Comorbidity Survey-Adolescent Supplement (NCS-A) found that about 20 percent of youth are affected by a mental disorder sometime in their lifetime. The NCS-A is a nationally representative, face-to-face survey of more than 10,000 teens ages 13 to 18. Parents or caregivers were also asked to complete a corroborating questionnaire after teens were interviewed. The NCS-A used criteria established by the American Psychiatric Association's *Diagnostic and Statistical Manual* (*DSM-IV*) to assess for a wide range of mental disorders including mood and anxiety disorders, behavior disorders like attention deficit hyperactivity disorder (ADHD), eating disorders, and substance use disorders.

In this most recent analysis, Kathleen Merikangas, PhD, of NIMH, Ron Kessler, PhD, of Harvard University, and colleagues examined the prevalence of mental disorders, as well as the severity of the disorders, within a 12-month period to estimate the rate of serious emotional disturbances (SED) in youth. SED was defined by the Substance Abuse and Mental Health Administration (SAMHSA) as a "mental, behavioral, or emotional disorder … that resulted in functional impairment which substantially interferes with or limits the child's role or functioning in family, school, or community activities."

Results Of The Study

The researchers found that about eight percent of all respondents had SED. Those with behavior disorders were most likely to be considered to have a severe disorder. Those with three or more coexisting disorders were also more likely to be severely affected. Similar to adults, anxiety disorders were the most common conditions in adolescents. Echoing many other studies, girls were more likely to have a mood or anxiety disorder or eating disorder, while boys were more likely to have a behavior disorder like ADHD or substance use disorder. Contrary to regional studies, this report showed a lower rate of depression among Hispanics compared to whites.

Significance

The findings in this study reflect the widely held belief that most psychiatric disorders first manifest in childhood or adolescence and tend to persist or recur throughout a person's life. The researchers conclude that the high prevalence rate of mental disorders in U.S. adolescents underscores the need for more research focused on changing the trajectory of mental disorders in youth.

What's Next

More research is needed to better understand the differences in prevalence rates among cultural and ethnic groups in different regions of the country.

Source: Excerpted from "Survey Finds More Evidence That Mental Disorders Often Begin in Youth," National Institute of Mental Health (nimh.nih.gov), August 2012.

- Take a history of the problem—how long you have seen the problem—as well as a history of your development

- Take a family history of mental disorders

- Ask if you have experienced physical or psychological traumas, such as a natural disaster, or situations that may cause stress, such as a death in the family

- Consider reports from parents and other caretakers or teachers

Will I get better with time?

Some adolescents get better with time. But other adolescents need ongoing professional help. Talk to your doctor or specialist about problems that are severe, continuous, and affect daily activities. Also, don't delay seeking help. Treatment may produce better results if started early.

What are my treatment options?

Once a diagnosis is made, your specialist will recommend a specific treatment. It is important to understand the various treatment choices, which often include psychotherapy or medication. Talk about the options with a health care professional who has experience treating the illness observed in you. Some treatment choices have been studied experimentally, and other treatments are a part of health care practice. In addition, not every community has every type of service or program.

Chapter 44

Consequences Of Not Receiving Treatment For Mental Illness

Most people don't think twice before going to a doctor if they have an illness such as bronchitis, asthma, diabetes, or heart disease. However, many people who have a mental illness don't get the treatment that would alleviate their suffering. Studies estimate that two-thirds of all young people with mental health problems are not receiving the help they need and that less than one-third of the children under age 18, who have a serious mental health problem, receive any mental health services. Mental illness in adults often goes untreated too. What are the consequences of letting mental illness go untreated?

In September 2000, the U.S. surgeon general held a conference on children's mental health. The former Surgeon General, Dr. David Satcher, emphasized the importance of mental health in children by stating, "Children and families are suffering because of missed opportunities for prevention and early identification, fragmented services, and low priorities for resources. Overriding all of this is the issue of stigma, which continues to surround mental illness."

The consequences of mental illness in children and adolescents can be substantial. Many mental health professionals speak of accrued deficits that occur when mental illness in children is not treated. To begin with, mental illness can impair a student's ability to learn. Adolescents whose mental illness is not treated rapidly and aggressively tend to fall further and further behind in school. They are more likely to drop out of school and are less likely to be fully functional members of society when they reach adulthood. We also now know that depressive disorders in young people confer a higher risk for illness and interpersonal and psychosocial difficulties that persist after the depressive episode is over. Furthermore, many adults who

About this chapter: Excerpted from "The Consequences of Not Treating Mental Illness," *The Science of Mental Illness*. Copyright © 2005 by BSCS. All rights reserved. Reprinted with permission. Information has been reviewed by David A. Cooke, MD, FACP, September 2013.

Many Children Are Not Receiving Needed Mental Health Services

Of nearly 7.4 million children in the United States diagnosed with emotional, behavioral, or developmental conditions, a disproportionate number do not get the mental health services they need because they are underinsured, according to a new report released by the Health Resources and Services Administration (HRSA). The study also finds that boys, adolescents, and children from low-income families are affected by conditions such as depression or attention deficit disorder at higher rates than other children, but that adequate health services for these children remain an unmet need.

The report, "The Mental and Emotional Well-Being of Children: A Portrait of States and the Nation 2007," identified seven emotional, behavioral, or developmental conditions: depression, anxiety, attention deficit disorder/attention deficit hyperactivity disorder, conduct disorders, autism spectrum disorders, developmental delay, and Tourette syndrome. Children with these conditions can benefit from a variety of therapies including counseling and medication.

"Accessing mental health services has always been a challenge," said HRSA Administrator Mary K. Wakefield PhD, RN. "HRSA is committed to ensuring that mental health is fully integrated into primary health care, and we're working diligently to address the challenge of meeting the mental health needs of America's children in vulnerable and underserved communities."

Additional findings include:

- Nearly 7.4 million of children in the United States are reported by their parents to have been diagnosed with emotional, behavioral, or developmental conditions.
    - Nearly two-thirds are boys
    - More than half are between the ages of 12 and 17 years
    - Nearly one-quarter have family incomes below the Federal poverty level
    - One-third of these children have also been diagnosed with a chronic physical condition
- Over 29 percent of diagnosed children with insurance were reported by their parents to have insurance that did not usually or always meet their needs.
- Over 40 percent of diagnosed children have more than one emotional, behavioral, or developmental condition.
- Almost 46 percent of children with one or more emotional, behavioral, or developmental conditions also had learning disabilities, compared to 2.7 percent of children without these conditions.

Source: Excerpted from "Many Children Not Receiving Needed Mental Health Services, Study Finds," Health Resources and Services Administration (www.hrsa.gov), October 2010.

suffer from mental disorders have problems that originated in childhood. Depression in youth may predict more severe illness in adult life. Attention deficit hyperactivity disorder (ADHD), once thought to affect children and adolescents only, may persist into adulthood and may be associated with social, legal, and occupational problems.

The high incidence of mental illness has a great impact on society. Depression alone causes employers to lose over $23 billion each year due to decreased productivity and absenteeism of employees. The Global Burden of Disease Study, conducted by the World Health Organization, assessed the burden of all diseases in units that measure lost years of healthy life due to premature death or disability (disability-adjusted life years, or DALYs). Over 15 percent of the total DALYs were due to mental illness. In 1996, the United States spent more than $69 billion for the direct treatment of mental illnesses. Indirect costs of mental illness due to lost productivity in the workplace, schools, or homes represented a $79 billion loss for the U.S. economy in 1990.

Treatment, including psychotherapy and medication management, is cost-effective for patients, their families, and society. The benefits include fewer visits to other doctors' offices, diagnostic laboratories, and hospitals for physical ailments that are based in psychological distress; reduced need for psychiatric hospitalization; fewer sick days and disability claims; and increased job stability. Conversely, the costs of not treating mental disorders can be seen in ruined relationships, job loss or poor job performance, personal anguish, substance abuse, unnecessary medical procedures, psychiatric hospitalization, and suicide.

Chapter 45

Treatment Of Children With Mental Illness

Research shows that half of all lifetime cases of mental illness begin by age 14. Scientists are discovering that changes in the body leading to mental illness may start much earlier, before any symptoms appear.

This chapter addresses common questions about treatment options for children with mental illnesses. Disorders affecting children may include anxiety disorders, attention deficit hyperactivity disorder (ADHD), autism spectrum disorders, bipolar disorder, depression, eating disorders, and schizophrenia.

Are there treatment options for children?

Yes. Once a diagnosis is made, your specialist will recommend a specific treatment. It is important to understand the various treatment choices, which often include psychotherapy or medication. Talk about the options with a health care professional who has experience treating the illness observed in you. Some treatment choices have been studied experimentally, and other treatments are a part of health care practice. In addition, not every community has every type of service or program.

What are psychotropic medications?

Psychotropic medications are substances that affect brain chemicals related to mood and behavior. In recent years, research has been conducted to understand the benefits and risks of using psychotropics in children. Still, more needs to be learned about the effects of

About This Chapter: Excerpted from "Treatment of Children with Mental Illness," National Institute of Mental Health (www.nimh.gov), February 2013.

psychotropics, especially in children under six years of age. While researchers are trying to clarify how early treatment affects a growing body, families and doctors should weigh the benefits and risks of medication. Each child has individual needs, and each child needs to be monitored closely while taking medications.

Are there treatments other than medications?

Yes. Psychosocial therapies can be very effective alone and in combination with medications. Psychosocial therapies are also called "talk therapies" or "behavioral therapy," and they help people with mental illness change behavior. Therapies that teach parents and children coping strategies can also be effective.

Cognitive behavioral therapy (CBT) is a type of psychotherapy that can be used with children. It has been widely studied and is an effective treatment for a number of conditions, such as depression, obsessive-compulsive disorder, and social anxiety. A person in CBT learns to change distorted thinking patterns and unhealthy behavior. Children can receive CBT with or without their parents, as well as in a group setting. CBT can be adapted to fit the needs of each child. It is especially useful when treating anxiety disorders.

Additionally, therapies for ADHD are numerous and include behavioral parent training and behavioral classroom management.

Some children benefit from a combination of different psychosocial approaches. An example is behavioral parent management training in combination with CBT for the child. In other cases, a combination of medication and psychosocial therapies may be most effective. Psychosocial therapies often take time, effort, and patience. However, sometimes children learn new skills that may have positive long-term benefits.

When is it a good idea to use psychotropic medications in children?

When the benefits of treatment outweigh the risks, psychotropic medications may be prescribed. Some children need medication to manage severe and difficult problems. Without treatment, these children would suffer serious or dangerous consequences. In addition, psychosocial treatments may not always be effective by themselves. In some instances, however, they can be quite effective when combined with medication.

Does medication affect young children differently than older children or adults?

Yes. Young children handle medications differently than older children and adults. The brains of young children change and develop rapidly. Studies have found that developing brains can be very sensitive to medications. There are also developmental differences in how children metabolize—how their bodies process—medications. Therefore, doctors should carefully consider the dosage or how much medication to give each child. Much more research is needed to determine the effects and benefits of medications in children of all ages. But keep in mind that serious untreated mental disorders themselves can harm brain development.

Also, it is important to avoid drug interactions. If you take medicine for asthma or cold symptoms, talk to your doctor or pharmacist. Drug interactions could cause medications to not work as intended or lead to serious side effects.

How should medication be included in an overall treatment plan?

Medication should be used with other treatments. It should not be the only treatment. Consider other services, such as family therapy, family support services, educational classes, and behavior management techniques. If your doctor prescribes medication, he or she should evaluate you regularly to make sure the medication is working. Children need treatment plans tailored to their individual problems and needs.

What medications are used for which kinds of childhood mental disorders?

Psychotropic medications include stimulants, antidepressants, anti-anxiety medications, antipsychotics, and mood stabilizers. Dosages approved by the U.S. Food and Drug Administration (FDA), for use in children, depend on body weight and age.

What does it mean if a medication is specifically approved for use in children?

When the FDA approves a medication, it means the drug manufacturer provided the agency with information showing the medication is safe and effective in a particular group of people. Based on this information, the drug's label lists proper dosage, potential side effects, and approved age. Medications approved for children follow these guidelines.

Many psychotropic medications have not been studied in children, which means they have not been approved by the FDA for use in children. But doctors may prescribe medications as they feel appropriate, even if those uses are not included on the label. This is called "off-label" use. Research shows that off-label use of some medications works well in some children. Other medications need more study in children. In particular, the use of most psychotropic medications has not been adequately studied in preschoolers.

More studies in children are needed before we can fully know the appropriate dosages, how a medication works in children, and what effects a medication might have on learning and development.

Why haven't many medications been tested in children?

In the past, medications were seldom studied in children because mental illness was not recognized in childhood. Also, there were ethical concerns about involving children in research. This led to a lack of knowledge about the best treatments for children. In clinical settings today, children with mental or behavioral disorders are being prescribed medications at increasingly early ages. The FDA has been urging that medications be appropriately studied in children, and Congress passed legislation in 1997 offering incentives to drug manufacturers to carry out such testing. These activities have helped increase research on the effects of medications in children.

Majority Of Youth With Mental Disorders May Not Be Receiving Sufficient Services

A substantial proportion of youth with severe mental disorders do not receive mental health care, according to data from an National Institute of Mental Health (NIMH)-funded survey.

Background

Kathleen Merikangas, PhD, of NIMH, and colleagues analyzed data from the National Comorbidity Study-Adolescent Supplement (NCS-A), a nationally representative, face-to-face survey of more than 10,000 teens ages 13 to 18. Previously published results found that about 20 percent of youth are affected by a severe mental disorder. For the most recent study, Merikangas and colleagues tracked the rate at which these youth reported having ever received services specifically to treat their disorder. They also were asked to specify what types of services they received and how often they received them.

Results

About 36 percent of youth with any lifetime mental disorder received services, and only half of these youth who were severely impaired by their mental disorder received professional mental health treatment. The majority (68 percent) of the children who did receive services had fewer than six visits with a provider over their lifetime.

Service use was highest among those with attention deficit hyperactivity disorder (ADHD)—60 percent—and behavior disorders like conduct disorder or oppositional defiant disorder (45 percent). Among those with mood disorders such as depression or bipolar disorder, 38 percent

---

There still are ethical concerns about testing medications in children. However, strict rules protect participants in research studies. Each study must go through many types of review before, and after it begins.

How do I work with my school?

If you are having problems in school, or if a teacher raises concerns, you can work with the school to find a solution. You may ask the school to conduct an evaluation to determine whether you qualify for special education services. However, not all children diagnosed with a mental illness qualify for these services.

Start by speaking with your teacher, school counselor, or the school nurse. These professionals can help you get an evaluation started. Also, each state has a Parent Training and Information Center and a Protection and Advocacy Agency that can help you and your parents

received services, and 18 percent of those with an anxiety disorder received services. In addition, 15 percent of those with a substance use disorder received services, and 13 percent of those with an eating disorder received services.

Girls were more likely to receive services for anxiety disorders, and boys were more likely to receive services for ADHD. Racial and ethnic minorities were less likely than non-Hispanic whites to receive treatment for any mood or anxiety disorder, and less likely to receive mental health treatment in general than their white counterparts.

Significance

The researchers conclude that despite recent programs designed to improve mental health services for youth, such as the State Children's Health Insurance Program and the federal Children's Mental Health Initiative, many children in need of mental health care still do not receive it. In addition, the relatively low number of treatment visits suggests that the few who are getting treatment may not have sufficient professional follow-up. Finally, ethnic disparities in mental health care, especially of mood and anxiety disorders, are still widespread.

What's Next

More efforts are needed to increase awareness of mood and anxiety disorders among ethnic minority communities, improve access to services, and improve the assessment skills of clinicians and pediatricians who are often the "front line" treatment providers of youth with mental disorders.

Source: Excerpted from "Majority of Youth with Mental Disorders May Not Be Receiving Sufficient Services," National Institute of Mental Health (www.nimh.gov), August 2012.

request the evaluation. The evaluation must be conducted by a team of professionals who assess all areas related to the suspected disability using a variety of tools and measures.

What resources are available from the school?

Once you have been evaluated, there are several options you, depending on the specific needs. If special education services are needed, and if you are eligible under the Individuals with Disabilities Education Act (IDEA), the school district must develop an "individualized education program" specifically for you within 30 days.

If you are not eligible for special education services, you are still entitled to "free appropriate public education," available to all public school children with disabilities under Section 504 of the *Rehabilitation Act of 1973*. You are entitled to this regardless of the nature or severity your disability.

The U.S. Department of Education's Office for Civil Rights enforces Section 504 in programs and activities that receive Federal education funds.

What other resources are available?

Children with mental illness need guidance and understanding from their parents and teachers. This support can help you achieve your full potential and succeed in school. Before you were diagnosed, frustration, blame, and anger may have built up within a family. Parents and children may need special help to undo these unhealthy interaction patterns. Mental health professionals can counsel you and your family to help everyone develop new skills, attitudes, and ways of relating to each other.

Parents can also help by taking part in parenting skills training. This helps parents learn how to handle difficult situations and behaviors. Training encourages parents to share a pleasant or relaxing activity with their child, to notice and point out what their child does well, and to praise their child's strengths and abilities. Parents may also learn to arrange family situations in more positive ways. Also, parents may benefit from learning stress-management techniques to help them deal with frustration and respond calmly to their child's behavior.

Sometimes, the whole family may need counseling. Therapists can help family members find better ways to handle disruptive behaviors and encourage behavior changes. Finally, support groups help parents and families connect with others who have similar problems and concerns. Groups often meet regularly to share frustrations and successes, to exchange information about recommended specialists and strategies, and to talk with experts.

How can families of children with mental illness get support?

Like other serious illnesses, taking care of a child with mental illness is hard on the parents, family, and other caregivers. Caregivers often must tend to the medical needs of their loved ones, and also deal with how it affects their own health. The stress that caregivers are under may lead to missed work or lost free time. It can strain relationships with people who may not understand the situation and lead to physical and mental exhaustion.

Stress from caregiving can make it hard to cope with your loved one's symptoms. One study shows that if a caregiver is under enormous stress, his or her loved one has more difficulty sticking to the treatment plan. It is important to look after your own physical and mental health. You may also find it helpful to join a local support group.

Where can I go for help?

If you are unsure where to go for help, ask your family doctor. Others who can help are:

- Mental health specialists, such as psychiatrists, psychologists, social workers, or mental health counselors

- Health maintenance organizations

- Community mental health centers

- Hospital psychiatry departments and outpatient clinics

- Mental health programs at universities or medical schools

- State hospital outpatient clinics

- Family services, social agencies, or clergy

- Peer support groups

- Private clinics and facilities

- Employee assistance programs

- Local medical and/or psychiatric societies

You can also check the phone book under "mental health," "health," "social services," "hotlines," or "physicians" for phone numbers and addresses. An emergency room doctor can also provide temporary help and can tell you where and how to get further help.

Chapter 46

Finding A Therapist Who Can Help You Heal

Therapy can be an effective treatment for mental and emotional problems. But in order to reap its benefits, it's important to choose the right therapist—someone you trust who makes you feel cared for and has the experience to help you make changes for the better in your life. A good therapist helps you to become stronger and more self-aware. But your therapist cannot do the work for you. In order to make the most of your sessions, you must be an active participant.

How Therapy And Counseling Can Help

Talking about your thoughts and feelings with a supportive person makes you feel better. It can be very healing, in and of itself, to voice your worries or talk about something that's weighing on your mind. And it feels good to be listened to—to know that someone else cares about you and wants to help.

It can be very helpful to talk about your problems to close friends and family members. But sometimes, we need help that the people around us aren't able to provide. When you need extra support, an outside perspective, or some expert guidance, talking to a therapist or counselor can help. While the support of friends and family is important, therapy is different. Therapists are professionally-trained listeners who can help you get to the root of your problems, overcome emotional challenges, and make positive changes in your life.

About This Chapter: "Finding a Therapist Who Can Help You Heal," by Melinda Smith, MA, and Jeanne Segal, PhD, updated August 2013. © 2013 Helpguide.org. All rights reserved. Reprinted with permission. Helpguide provides a detailed list of references and resources for this article, with links to related Helpguide topics and information from other websites. For a complete list of these resources, go to http://www.helpguide.org/mental/psychotherapy_therapist_counseling.htm.

You don't have to be diagnosed with a mental health problem to benefit from therapy. Many people in therapy seek help for everyday concerns: relationship problems, job stress, or self-doubt, for example. Others turn to therapy during difficult times, such as a divorce.

Why Therapy And Not Medication?

The thought of being able to solve your problems with taking a pill each day can sound appealing. If only it was that easy! Mental and emotional problems have multiple causes, and medication is not a one-stop cure.

Medication may help ease certain symptoms, but it comes with side effects. Furthermore, it cannot solve the "big picture" problems. Medication won't fix your relationships, help you figure out what to do with your life, or give you insight into why you continue to do things you know are bad for you.

Therapy can be time consuming and challenging, as uncomfortable emotions and thoughts often arise as part of the treatment process. However, therapy provides long-lasting benefits that go beyond symptom relief. Therapy gives you the tools for transforming your life—for relating better to others, building the life you want for yourself, and coping with whatever curveballs come your way.

Myths About Therapy

- **I don't need a therapist. I'm smart enough to solve my own problems.** We all have our blind spots. Intelligence has nothing to do with it. A good therapist doesn't tell you what to do or how to live your life. He or she will give you an experienced, outside perspective and help you gain insight into yourself so you can make better choices.

- **Therapy is for crazy people.** Therapy is for people who have enough self-awareness to realize they need a helping hand, and want to learn tools and techniques to become more self-confident and emotionally balanced.

- **All therapists want to talk about is my parents.** While exploring family relationships can sometimes clarify thoughts and behaviors later in life, that is not the sole focus of therapy. The primary focus is what you need to change unhealthy patterns and symptoms in your life. Therapy is not about blaming your parents or dwelling on the past.

- **Therapy is self-indulgent. It's for whiners and complainers.** Therapy is hard work. Complaining won't get you very far. Improvement in therapy comes from taking a hard look at yourself and your life, and taking responsibility for your own actions. Your therapist will help you, but ultimately you're the one who must do the work.

Finding The Right Therapist For You

Finding the right therapist will probably take some time and work, but it's worth the effort. The connection you have with your therapist is essential. You need someone who you can trust—someone you feel comfortable talking to about difficult subjects and intimate secrets, someone who will be a partner in your recovery.

Therapy won't be effective unless you have this bond, so take some time at the beginning to find the right person. It's okay to shop around and to ask questions when interviewing potential therapists.

- **Experience matters.** One of the main reasons for seeing a therapist, rather than simply talking to a friend, is experience. Look for a therapist who is experienced in treating the problems that you have. Often, therapists have special areas of focus, such as depression or eating disorders. Experienced therapists have seen the problems you're facing again and again, which broadens their view and gives them more insight. And for some problems, such as trauma or post-traumatic stress disorder (PTSD), seeing a specialist is absolutely essential.

- **Learn about different treatment orientations.** Many therapists do a blend of orientations. However, it's a good idea to learn about the different treatment types, because that can affect your therapist's way of relating and suggested length of treatment.

- **Check licensing.** Credentials aren't everything, but if you're paying for a licensed professional, make sure the therapist holds a current license and is in good standing with the state regulatory board. Regulatory boards vary by state and by profession. Also check for complaints against the therapist.

- **Trust your gut.** Even if your therapist looks great on paper, if the connection doesn't feel right—if you don't trust the person or feel like they truly care—go with another choice. A good therapist will respect this choice and should never pressure you or make you feel guilty.

Questions To Ask Yourself When Choosing A Therapist

What's most important in a therapist or counselor is a sense of connection, safety, and support. Ask yourself the following questions:

- Does it seem like the therapist truly cares about you and your problems?
- Do you feel as if the therapist understands you?
- Does the therapist accept you for who you are?

- Would you feel comfortable revealing personal information to this individual?

- Do you feel as if you can be honest and open with this therapist? That you don't have to hide or pretend you're someone that you're not?

- Is the therapist a good listener? Does he or she listen without interrupting, criticizing, or judging? Pick up on your feelings and what you're really saying? Make you feel heard?

Types Of Therapy And Therapists

There are so many types of therapies and therapists; it might feel a little overwhelming to get started. Just remember that no one type of therapy is best, any more than any style of car is best. It all depends on your individual preferences and needs.

It is true that certain techniques are more useful than others in dealing with specific types of problems (phobias, for example). But in general, research about the "best" type of therapy always reaches the same conclusion: The philosophy behind the therapy is much less important than the relationship between you and your therapist.

If you feel comfortable and trusting in that relationship, the model of therapy, like your car, is just the vehicle that will help you move ahead to lead a more fulfilling life, regardless of the circumstances that brought you to therapy.

Common Types Of Therapy

Most therapists don't limit themselves to one specific type of therapy, instead blending different types in order to best fit the situation at hand. This can offer many powerful tools for the therapist to use. However, therapists often have a general orientation that guides them.

Individual Therapy: Individual therapy explores negative thoughts and feelings, as well as the harmful or self-destructive behaviors that might accompany them. Individual therapy may delve into the underlying causes of current problems (such as unhealthy relationship patterns or a traumatic experience from your past), but the primary focus is on making positive changes in the here and now.

Family Therapy: Family therapy involves treating more than one member of the family at the same time to help the family resolve conflicts and improve interaction. It is often based on the premise that families are a system. If one role in the family changes all are affected and need to change their behaviors as well.

Group Therapy: Group therapy is facilitated by a professional therapist, and involves a group of peers working on the same problem, such as anxiety, depression, or substance abuse, for example. Group therapy can be a valuable place to practice social dynamics in a safe environment and get inspiration and ideas from peers who are struggling with the same issues.

Couples Therapy (Marriage Counseling): Couples therapy involves the two people in a committed relationship. People go to couples therapy to learn how to work through their differences, communicate better, and problem-solve challenges in the relationship.

Types Of Therapists And Counselors

The following types of mental health professionals have advanced training in therapy and are certified by their respective boards. Many professional organizations provide online searches for qualified professionals. You may also want to double check with your state regulatory board to make sure the therapist's license is up to date and there are no ethical violations listed.

However, keep in mind that lay counselors—members of the clergy, life coaches, etc.—may be able to provide you with a supportive, listening ear. It's not always the credentials that determine the quality of the therapy.

Common Types Of Mental Health Professionals

- **Psychologist:** Psychologists have a doctoral degree in psychology (PhD or PsyD) and are licensed in clinical psychology.

- **Social Worker:** Licensed Clinical Social Workers (LCSWs) have a Master's degree in social work (MSW) along with additional clinical training.

- **Marriage And Family Therapist:** Marriage and Family Therapists (MFTs) have a Master's degree and clinical experience in marriage and family therapy.

- **Psychiatrists:** A psychiatrist is a physician (MD or DO) who specializes in mental health. Because they are medical doctors, psychiatrists can prescribe medication.

What To Expect In Therapy Or Counseling

Every therapist is different, but there are usually some similarities to how therapy is structured. Normally, sessions will last about an hour, and often be about once a week, although for more intensive therapy they maybe more often. Therapy is normally conducted in the therapist's office, but therapists also work in hospitals and nursing homes, and in some cases will do home visits.

Expect a good fit between you and your therapist. Don't settle for bad fit. You may need to see one or more therapists until you experience feeling understood and accepted.

- **Therapy is a partnership.** Both you and your therapist contribute to the healing process. You're not expected to do the work of recovery all by yourself, but your therapist can't do it for you either. Therapy should feel like a collaboration.

- **Therapy will not always feel pleasant.** Painful memories, frustrations or feelings might surface. This is a normal part of therapy and your therapist will guide you through this process. Be sure to communicate with your therapist about how you are feeling.

- **Therapy should be a safe place.** While there will be times when you'll feel challenged or when you're facing unpleasant feelings, you should always feel safe. If you're starting to feel overwhelmed or you're dreading your therapy sessions, talk to your therapist.

Your First Therapy Sessions

The first session or two of therapy is a time for mutual connection, a time for the therapist to learn about you and your issues. The therapist may ask for a mental and physical health history.

It's also a good idea to talk to the therapist about what you hope to achieve in therapy. Together, you can set goals and benchmarks that you can use to measure your progress along the way.

This is also an important time for you to be evaluating your connection with your therapist. Do you feel like your therapist cares about your situation, and is invested in your recovery? Do you feel comfortable asking questions and sharing sensitive information? Remember, your feelings as well as your thoughts are important, so if you are feeling uncomfortable, don't hesitate to consider another therapist.

How Long Does Therapy Last?

Everyone's treatment is different. How long therapy lasts depends on many factors. You may have complicated issues, or a relatively straightforward problem that you want to address. Some therapy treatment types are short term, while others may be longer. Practically, you might also be limited by your insurance coverage.

However, discussing the length of therapy is important to bring up with your therapist at the beginning. This will give you an idea of starting goals to work towards and what you want to accomplish. Don't be afraid to revisit this issue at any time as therapy progresses, as goals often are modified or changed during treatment.

Making The Most Of Therapy And Counseling

To make the most of therapy, you need to put what you're learning in your sessions into practice in your real life. Fifty minutes in therapy each week isn't going to fix you; it's how you use what you've learned with the rest of your time. Here are some tips for getting the most out of your therapy:

- **Make healthy lifestyle changes.** There are many things you can do in your daily life to support your mood and improve your emotional health. Reach out to others for support. Get plenty of exercise and sleep. Eat well. Make time for relaxation and play. The list goes on…

- **Don't expect the therapist to tell you what to do.** You and your therapists are partners in your recovery. Your therapist can help guide you and make suggestions for treatment, but only you can make the changes you need to move forward.

- **Make a commitment to your treatment.** Don't skip sessions unless you absolutely have to. If your therapist gives you homework in between sessions, be sure to do it. If you find yourself skipping sessions or are reluctant to go, ask yourself why. Are you avoiding painful discussion? Did last session touch a nerve? Talk about your reluctance with your therapist.

- **Share what you are feeling.** You will get the most out of therapy if you are open and honest with your therapist about your feelings. If you feel embarrassed or ashamed, or something is too painful to talk about, don't be afraid to tell your therapist. Slowly, you can work together to get at the issues.

Is Therapy Working?

You should be able to tell within a session or two whether you and your therapist are a good fit. But sometimes, you may like your therapist but feel like you aren't making progress. It's important to evaluate your progress to make sure you're getting what you need from therapy.

A word of caution: There is no smooth, fast road to recovery. It's a process that's full of twists, turns, and the occasional backtrack. Sometimes, what originally seemed like a straightforward problem turns into a more complicated issue. Be patient and don't get discouraged over temporary setbacks. It's not easy to break old, entrenched patterns.

Remember that growth is difficult, and you won't be a new person overnight. But you should notice positive changes in your life. Your overall mood might be improving, for example. You may feel more connected to family and friends. Or a crisis that might have overwhelmed you in the past doesn't throw you as much this time.

Tips For Evaluating Your Progress In Therapy

Is your life changing for the better? Look at different parts of your life: work, home, your social life.

- Are you meeting the goals you and your therapist have set?

- Is therapy challenging you? Is it stretching you beyond your comfort zone?

- Do you feel like you're starting to understand yourself better?

- Do you feel more confident and empowered?

- Are your relationships improving?

Your therapist should work with you, reevaluating your goals and progress as necessary. However, remember that therapy isn't a competition. You are not a failure if you don't meet your goals in the number of sessions you originally planned. Focus instead on overall progress and what you've learned along the way.

When To Stop Therapy Or Counseling

When to stop therapy depends on you and your individual situation. Ideally, you will stop therapy when you and your therapist have decided that you have met your goals. However, you may feel at some point that you have got what you need out of therapy, even if your therapist feels differently.

Leaving therapy can be difficult. Remember that the therapeutic relationship is a strong bond, and ending this relationship is a loss—even if treatment has been successful. Talk about this with your therapist. These feelings are normal. It's not uncommon for people to go back briefly to a therapist from time to time as needs arise.

As Long As You Continue To Progress In Therapy, It's An Option

Some people continue to go to therapy on an ongoing basis. That's okay, especially if you don't have other people to turn to for support in your life. Ideally, your therapist will be able to help you develop outside sources of support, but that's not always possible. If therapy meets an important need in your life and the expense is not an issue, continuing indefinitely is a legitimate choice.

Signs That You May Need To Change Therapists

- You don't feel comfortable talking about something.

- Your therapist is dismissive of your problems or concerns.

- Your therapist seems to have a personal agenda.

- Your therapist does more talking than listening.

- Your therapist tells you what to do and how to live your life.

Paying For Therapy And Counseling

In the U.S., for example, many insurance companies provide limited coverage for psychotherapy—often as few as 6–12 sessions. Read through your plan carefully to see what benefits you have. Some types of mental health professionals might not be covered. You may need a referral through your primary care physician.

Also keep in mind that some therapists do not accept insurance, only payment directly from the patient. Sometimes these therapists will accept sliding scale payments, where you pay what you can afford for each session. Don't be afraid to ask what arrangements can be made if you feel the therapist could be a good fit for you.

In other countries, insurance and eligibility requirements vary.

Affordable Therapy And Counseling Options

Take a look around your community for service agencies or organizations that may offer psychotherapy at discounted rates. Senior centers, family service agencies, and mental health clinics are good places to start. Many offer affordable options, including sliding payment scales.

Agencies that involve interns in training also can be an option for quality therapy. An intern may be a good choice for you if the intern is enthusiastic, empathetic, and has quality supervisory training. However, an intern's time at the agency is limited, so when the training is finished, you either need to stop the therapy or find another therapist.

Another possible way to obtain affordable therapy is to try bartering with a therapist or mental health clinic. A few clinics and health centers across the U.S. already encourage bartering services, swapping health care for carpentry, plumbing, or hairdressing services, for example. If you have a useful skill or are willing to volunteer your time, it may be worth trying to strike a deal.

Chapter 47

Going To A Therapist: What To Expect

Eric went to therapy a couple of years ago when his parents were getting divorced. Although he no longer goes, he feels the two months he spent in therapy helped him get through the tough times as his parents worked out their differences.

Melody began seeing her therapist a year ago when she was being bullied at school. She still goes every two weeks because she feels therapy is really helping to build her self-esteem.

Britt just joined a therapy group for eating disorders led by her school's psychologist, and her friend Dana said she'd go with her.

When our parents were in school, very few kids went to therapy. Now it's much more common and also more accepted. Lots of teens wonder if therapy could help them.

What is therapy?

Therapy isn't just for mental health. You've probably heard people discussing other types of medical therapy, such as physical therapy or chemotherapy. But the word "therapy" is most often used to mean psychotherapy (sometimes called "talk therapy")—in other words, psychological help to deal with stress or problems.

Psychotherapy is a process that's a lot like learning. Through therapy, people learn about themselves. They discover ways to overcome difficulties, develop inner strengths or skills, or make changes in themselves or their situations. Often, it feels good just to have a person to vent to, and other times it's useful to learn different techniques to help deal with stress.

About This Chapter: "Going To A Therapist," September 2010, reprinted with permission from www.kidshealth .org. This information was provided by KidsHealth®, one of the largest resources online for medically reviewed health information written for parents, kids, and teens. For more articles like this, visit www.KidsHealth.org, or www.TeensHealth.org. Copyright © 1995–2013 The Nemours Foundation. All rights reserved.

Some Reasons Teens Go To Therapists

When teens are going through a rough time, such as family troubles or problems in school, they might feel more supported if they talk to a therapist. They may be feeling sad, angry, or overwhelmed by what's been happening—and need help sorting out their feelings, finding solutions to their problems, or just feeling better. That's when therapy can help.

Just a few examples of situations in which therapy can help are when someone:

- Feels sad, depressed, worried, shy, or just stressed out
- Is dieting or overeating for too long or it becomes a problem (eating disorders)
- Cuts, burns, or self-injures
- Is dealing with an attention problem, such as attention deficit hyperactivity disorder (ADHD) or a learning problem
- Is coping with a chronic illness (such as diabetes or asthma) or a new diagnosis of a serious problem such as HIV, cancer, or a sexually transmitted disease (STD)
- Is dealing with family changes such as separation and divorce, or family problems such as alcoholism or addiction
- Is trying to cope with a traumatic event, death of a loved one, or worry over world events
- Has a habit he or she would like to get rid of, such as nail biting, hair pulling, smoking, or spending too much money, or getting hooked on medications, drugs, or pills
- Wants to sort out problems like managing anger or coping with peer pressure
- Wants to build self-confidence or figure out ways to make more friends

In short, therapy offers people support when they are going through difficult times.

Deciding to seek help for something you're going through can be really hard. It may be your idea to go to therapy or it might not. Sometimes parents or teachers bring up the idea first because they notice that someone they care about is dealing with a difficult situation, is losing weight, or seems unusually sad, worried, angry, or upset. Some people in this situation might welcome the idea or even feel relieved. Others might feel criticized or embarrassed and unsure if they'll benefit from talking to someone.

Sometimes people are told by teachers, parents, or the courts that they have to go see a therapist because they have been behaving in ways that are unacceptable, illegal, self-destructive, or dangerous. When therapy is someone else's idea, a person may at first feel like resisting the whole idea. But learning a bit more about what therapy involves and what to expect can help make it seem OK.

A psychotherapist (therapist, for short) is a person who has been professionally trained to help people deal with stress or other problems. Psychiatrists, psychologists, social workers, counselors, and school psychologists are the titles of some of the licensed professionals who work as therapists. The letters following a therapist's name (for example, MD, PhD, PsyD, EdD, MA, LCSW, LPC) refer to the particular education and degree that therapist has received.

Some therapists specialize in working with a certain age group or on a particular type of problem. Other therapists treat a mix of ages and issues. Some work in hospitals, clinics, or counseling centers. Others work in schools or in psychotherapy offices, often called a "private practice" or "group practice."

What do therapists do?

Most types of therapy include talking and listening, building trust, and receiving support and guidance. Sometimes therapists may recommend books for people to read or work through. They may also suggest keeping a journal. Some people prefer to express themselves using art or drawing. Others feel more comfortable just talking.

When a person talks to a therapist about which situations might be difficult for them or what stresses them out, this helps the therapist assess what is going on. The therapist and client then usually work together to set therapy goals and figure out what will help the person feel better or get back on track.

It might take a few meetings with a therapist before people really feel like they can share personal stuff. It's natural to feel that way. Trust is an essential ingredient in therapy—after all, therapy involves being open and honest about sensitive topics like feelings, ideas, relationships, problems, disappointments, and hopes. A therapist understands that people sometimes take a while to feel comfortable sharing personal information.

Most of the time, a person meets with a therapist one on one, which is known as individual therapy. Sometimes, though, a therapist might work with a family (called family therapy) or a group of people who all are dealing with similar issues (called group therapy or a support group). Family therapy gives family members a chance to talk together with a therapist about problems that involve them all. Group therapy and support groups help people give and receive support and learn from each other and their therapist by discussing the issues they have in common.

What happens during therapy?

If you see a therapist, he or she will talk with you about your feelings, thoughts, relationships, and important values. At the beginning, therapy sessions are focused on discussing what you'd like to work on and setting goals. Some of the goals people in therapy may set include things like:

- Improving self-esteem and gaining confidence

- Figuring out how to make more friends

- Feeling less depressed or less anxious

- Improving grades at school

- Learning to manage anger and frustration

- Making healthier choices (for example, about relationships or eating) and ending self-defeating behaviors

During the first visit, your therapist will probably ask you to talk a bit about yourself. Depending on your age, the therapist will also likely meet with a parent or caregiver and ask you to review information regarding confidentiality.

The first meeting can last longer than the usual "therapy hour" and is often called an "intake interview." This helps the therapist understand you better, and gives you a chance to see if you feel comfortable with the therapist. The therapist will probably ask about problems, concerns, and symptoms that you may be having, or the problems that parents or teachers are concerned about.

After one or two sessions, the therapist may talk to you about his or her understanding of what is going on with you, how therapy could help, and what the process will involve. Together, you and your therapist will decide on the goals for therapy and how frequently to meet. This may be once a week, every other week, or once a month.

With a better understanding of your situation, the therapist might teach you new skills or help you to think about a situation in a new way. For example, therapists can help people develop better relationship skills or coping skills, including ways to build confidence, express feelings, or manage anger.

Sticking to the schedule you agree on with your therapist and going to your appointments will ensure you have enough time with your therapist to work out your concerns. If your therapist suggests a schedule that you don't think you'll be able to keep, be up front about it so you can work out an alternative.

How private is it?

Therapists respect the privacy of their clients and they keep things they're told confidential. A therapist won't tell anyone else—including parents—about what a person discusses in his or her sessions unless that person gives permission. The only exception is if therapists believe their clients may harm themselves or others.

If the issue of privacy and confidentiality worries you, be sure to ask your therapist about it during your first meeting. It's important to feel comfortable with your therapist so you can talk openly about your situation.

Does it mean I'm crazy?

No. In fact, many people in your class have probably seen a therapist at some point—just like students often see tutors or coaches for extra help with schoolwork or sports. Getting help in dealing with emotions and stressful situations is as important to your overall health as getting help with a medical problem like asthma or diabetes.

There's nothing wrong with getting help with problems that are hard to solve alone. In fact, it's just the opposite. It takes a lot of courage and maturity to look for solutions to problems instead of ignoring or hiding them and allowing them to become worse. If you think that therapy could help you with a problem, ask an adult you trust—like a parent, school counselor, or doctor—to help you find a therapist.

A few adults still resist the idea of therapy because they don't fully understand it or have outdated ideas about it. A couple of generations ago, people didn't know as much about the mind or the mind-body connection as they do today, and people were left to struggle with their problems on their own. It used to be that therapy was only available to those with the most serious mental health problems, but that's no longer the case.

Therapy is helpful to people of all ages and with problems that range from mild to much more serious. Some people still hold onto old beliefs about therapy, such as thinking that teens "will grow out of" their problems. If the adults in your family don't seem open to talking about therapy, mention your concerns to a school counselor, coach, or doctor.

You don't have to hide the fact that you're going to a therapist, but you also don't have to tell anyone if you'd prefer not to. Some people find that talking to a few close friends about their therapy helps them to work out their problems and feel like they're not alone. Other people choose not to tell anyone, especially if they feel that others won't understand. Either way, it's a personal decision.

What can a person get out of therapy?

What someone gets out of therapy depends on why that person is there. For example, some people go to therapy to solve a specific problem, others want to begin making better choices, and others want to start to heal from a loss or a difficult life situation.

Therapy can help people feel better, be stronger, and make good choices as well as discover more about themselves. Those who work with therapists might learn about motivations that lead them to behave in certain ways or about inner strengths they have. Maybe you'll learn new coping skills, develop more patience, or learn to like yourself better. Maybe you'll find new ways to handle problems that come up or new ways to handle yourself in tough situations.

People who work with therapists often find that they learn a lot about themselves and that therapy can help them grow and mature. Lots of people discover that the tools they learn in therapy when they're young make them feel stronger and better able to deal with whatever life throws at them even as adults. If you are curious about the therapy process, talk to a counselor or therapist to see if you could benefit.

Chapter 48

Counseling And Therapy: Methods Of Treatment

Psychotherapy Is Talk Therapy

Psychotherapy, or "talk therapy," is a way to treat people with a mental disorder by helping them understand their illness. It teaches people strategies and gives them tools to deal with stress and unhealthy thoughts and behaviors. Psychotherapy helps patients manage their symptoms better and function at their best in everyday life.

Sometimes psychotherapy alone may be the best treatment for a person, depending on the illness and its severity. Other times, psychotherapy is combined with medications. Therapists work with an individual or families to devise an appropriate treatment plan.

Different Types Of Psychotherapy

Many kinds of psychotherapy exist. There is no "one-size-fits-all" approach. In addition, some therapies have been scientifically tested more than others. Some people may have a treatment plan that includes only one type of psychotherapy. Others receive treatment that includes elements of several different types. The kind of psychotherapy a person receives depends on his or her needs.

This chapter explains several of the most commonly used psychotherapies. However, it does not cover every detail about psychotherapy. Patients should talk to their doctor or a psychotherapist about planning treatment that meets their needs.

About This Chapter: Excerpted from "Psychotherapies," National Institute of Mental Health (www.nimh.nih.gov), 2008. Information has been reviewed by David A. Cooke, MD, FACP, September 2013.

Cognitive Behavioral Therapy

Cognitive behavioral therapy (CBT) is a blend of two therapies: cognitive therapy (CT) and behavioral therapy. CT was developed by psychotherapist Aaron Beck, MD, in the 1960s. CT focuses on a person's thoughts and beliefs, and how they influence a person's mood and actions, and aims to change a person's thinking to be more adaptive and healthy. Behavioral therapy focuses on a person's actions and aims to change unhealthy behavior patterns.

CBT helps a person focus on his or her current problems and how to solve them. Both patient and therapist need to be actively involved in this process. The therapist helps the patient learn how to identify distorted or unhelpful thinking patterns, recognize and change inaccurate beliefs, relate to others in more positive ways, and change behaviors accordingly.

CBT can be applied and adapted to treat many specific mental disorders.

CBT For Depression

Many studies have shown that CBT is a particularly effective treatment for depression, especially minor or moderate depression. Some people with depression may be successfully treated with CBT only. Others may need both CBT and medication. CBT helps people with depression restructure negative thought patterns. Doing so helps people interpret their environment and interactions with others in a positive and realistic way. It may also help a person recognize things that may be contributing to the depression and help him or her change behaviors that may be making the depression worse.

CBT For Anxiety Disorders

CBT for anxiety disorders aims to help a person develop a more adaptive response to a fear. A CBT therapist may use "exposure" therapy to treat certain anxiety disorders, such as a specific phobia, post-traumatic stress disorder, or obsessive compulsive disorder. Exposure therapy has been found to be effective in treating anxiety-related disorders; it works by helping a person confront a specific fear or memory while in a safe and supportive environment. The main goals of exposure therapy are to help the patient learn that anxiety can lessen over time and give him or her tools to cope with fear or traumatic memories.

A recent study sponsored by the Centers for Disease Control and Prevention concluded that CBT is effective in treating trauma-related disorders in children and teens.

CBT For Bipolar Disorder

People with bipolar disorder usually need to take medication, such as a mood stabilizer. But CBT is often used as an added treatment. The medication can help stabilize a person's mood so that he or she is receptive to psychotherapy and can get the most out of it. CBT can help a person cope with bipolar symptoms and learn to recognize when a mood shift is about to occur. CBT also helps a person with bipolar disorder stick with a treatment plan to reduce the chances of relapse (e.g., when symptoms return).

CBT For Eating Disorders

Eating disorders can be very difficult to treat. However, some small studies have found that CBT can help reduce the risk of relapse in adults with anorexia who have restored their weight. CBT may also reduce some symptoms of bulimia, and it may also help some people reduce binge-eating behavior.

CBT For Schizophrenia

Treating schizophrenia with CBT is challenging. The disorder usually requires medication first. But research has shown that CBT, as an add-on to medication, can help a patient cope with schizophrenia. CBT helps patients learn more adaptive and realistic interpretations of events. Patients are also taught various coping techniques for dealing with "voices" or other hallucinations. They learn how to identify what triggers episodes of the illness, which can prevent or reduce the chances of relapse.

CBT for schizophrenia also stresses skill-oriented therapies. Patients learn skills to cope with life's challenges. The therapist teaches social, daily functioning, and problem-solving skills. This can help patients with schizophrenia minimize the types of stress that can lead to outbursts and hospitalizations.

Dialectical Behavior Therapy

Dialectical behavior therapy (DBT), a form of CBT, was developed by Marsha Linehan, PhD. At first, it was developed to treat people with suicidal thoughts and actions. It is now also used to treat people with borderline personality disorder (BPD). BPD is an illness in which suicidal thinking and actions are more common.

The term "dialectical" refers to a philosophic exercise in which two opposing views are discussed until a logical blending or balance of the two extremes—the middle way—is found. In keeping with that philosophy, the therapist assures the patient that the patient's behavior and feelings are valid and understandable. At the same time, the therapist coaches the patient to understand that it is his or her personal responsibility to change unhealthy or disruptive behavior.

DBT emphasizes the value of a strong and equal relationship between patient and therapist. The therapist consistently reminds the patient when his or her behavior is unhealthy or disruptive—when boundaries are overstepped—and then teaches the skills needed to better deal with future similar situations. DBT involves both individual and group therapy. Individual sessions are used to teach new skills, while group sessions provide the opportunity to practice these skills.

Research suggests that DBT is an effective treatment for people with BPD. A recent National Institute of Mental Health (NIMH) funded study found that DBT reduced suicide attempts by half compared to other types of treatment for patients with BPD.

Interpersonal Therapy

Interpersonal therapy (IPT) is most often used on a one-on-one basis to treat depression or dysthymia (a more persistent but less severe form of depression). The current manual-based form of IPT used today was developed in the 1980s by Gerald Klerman, MD, and Myrna Weissman, MD.

IPT is based on the idea that improving communication patterns and the ways people relate to others will effectively treat depression. IPT helps identify how a person interacts with other people. When a behavior is causing problems, IPT guides the person to change the behavior. IPT explores major issues that may add to a person's depression, such as grief, or times of upheaval or transition. Sometimes IPT is used along with antidepressant medications.

IPT varies depending on the needs of the patient and the relationship between the therapist and patient. Basically, a therapist using IPT helps the patient identify troubling emotions and their triggers. The therapist helps the patient learn to express appropriate emotions in a healthy way. The patient may also examine relationships in his or her past that may have been affected by distorted mood and behavior. Doing so can help the patient learn to be more objective about current relationships.

Studies vary as to the effectiveness of IPT. It may depend on the patient, the disorder, the severity of the disorder, and other variables. In general, however, IPT is found to be effective in treating depression.

A variation of IPT called interpersonal and social rhythm therapy (IPSRT) was developed to treat bipolar disorder. IPSRT combines the basic principles of IPT with behavioral psychoeducation designed to help patients adopt regular daily routines and sleep/wake cycles, stick with medication treatment, and improve relationships. Research has found that when IPSRT is combined with medication, it is an effective treatment for bipolar disorder. IPSRT is as effective as other types of psychotherapy combined with medication in helping to prevent a relapse of bipolar symptoms.

Family-Focused Therapy

Family-focused therapy (FFT) was developed by David Miklowitz, PhD, and Michael Goldstein, PhD, for treating bipolar disorder. It was designed with the assumption that a patient's relationship with his or her family is vital to the success of managing the illness. FFT includes family members in therapy sessions to improve family relationships, which may support better treatment results.

Therapists trained in FFT work to identify difficulties and conflicts among family members that may be worsening the patient's illness. Therapy is meant to help members find more effective ways to resolve those difficulties. The therapist educates family members about their loved one's disorder, its symptoms and course, and how to help their relative manage it more effectively. When families learn about the disorder, they may be able to spot early signs of a relapse and create an action plan that involves all family members. During therapy, the therapist will help family members recognize when they express unhelpful criticism or hostility toward their relative with bipolar disorder. The therapist will teach family members how to communicate negative emotions in a better way. Several studies have found FFT to be effective in helping a patient become stabilized and preventing relapses.

FFT also focuses on the stress family members feel when they care for a relative with bipolar disorder. The therapy aims to prevent family members from "burning out" or disengaging from the effort. The therapist helps the family accept how bipolar disorder can limit their relative. At the same time, the therapist holds the patient responsible for his or her own well-being and actions to a level that is appropriate for the person's age.

Generally, the family and patient attend sessions together. The needs of each patient and family are different, and those needs determine the exact course of treatment. However, the main components of a structured FFT usually include: Family education on bipolar disorder; building communication skills to better deal with stress; and solving problems together as a family.

It is important to acknowledge and address the needs of family members. Research has shown that primary caregivers of people with bipolar disorder are at increased risk for illness themselves. For example, a 2007 study based on results from the NIMH-funded Systematic Treatment Enhancement Program for Bipolar Disorder (STEP-BD) trial found that primary caregivers of participants were at high risk for developing sleep problems and chronic conditions, such as high blood pressure. However, the caregivers were less likely to see a doctor for their own health issues. In addition, a 2005 study found that 33 percent of caregivers of bipolar patients had clinically significant levels of depression.

Psychotherapies For Children And Adolescents

Psychotherapies can be adapted to the needs of children and adolescents, depending on the mental disorder. For example, the NIMH-funded Treatment of Adolescents with Depression Study (TADS) found that CBT, when combined with antidepressant medication, was the most effective treatment over the short term for teens with major depression. CBT by itself was also an effective treatment, especially over the long term. Studies have found that individual and group-based CBT are effective treatments for child and adolescent anxiety disorders. Other studies have found that IPT is an effective treatment for child and adolescent depression.

Psychosocial treatments that involve a child's parents and family also have been shown to be effective, especially for disruptive disorders such as conduct disorder or oppositional defiant disorder. Some effective treatments are designed to reduce the child's problem behaviors and im-prove parent-child interactions. Focusing on behavioral parent management training, parents are taught the skills they need to encourage and reward positive behaviors in their children. Similar training helps parents manage their child's attention deficit/hyperactivity disorder (ADHD). This approach, which has been shown to be effective, can be combined with approaches directed at children to help them learn problem-solving, anger management and social interaction skills.

Family-based therapy may also be used to treat adolescents with eating disorders. One type is called the Maudsley approach, named after the Maudsley Hospital in London, where the approach was developed. This type of outpatient family therapy is used to treat anorexia nervosa in adolescents. It considers the active participation of parents to be essential in the recovery of their teen. The Maudsley approach proceeds through three phases:

- **Weight Restoration:** Parents become fully responsible for ensuring that their teen eats. A therapist helps parents better understand their teen's disease. Parents learn how to avoid criticizing their teen, but they also learn to make sure that their teen eats.

- **Returning Control Over Eating To The Teen:** Once the teen accepts the control par-ents have over his or her eating habits, parents may begin giving up that control. Parents are encouraged to help their teen take more control over eating again.

- **Establishing Healthy Adolescent Identity:** When the teen has reached and main-tained a healthy weight, the therapist helps him or her begin developing a healthy sense of identity and autonomy.

Several studies have found the Maudsley approach to be successful in treating teens with anorexia. Currently a large-scale, NIMH-funded study on the approach is under way.

Other Types Of Therapies

In addition to the therapies listed, many more approaches exist. Some types have been scientifically tested more than others. Also, some of these therapies are constantly evolving. They are often combined with more established psychotherapies. A few examples of other therapies are described here:

- **Psychodynamic Therapy:** Historically, psychodynamic therapy was tied to the principles of psychoanalytic theory, which asserts that a person's behavior is affected by his or her unconscious mind and past experiences. Now therapists who use psychodynamic therapy rarely include psychoanalytic methods. Rather, psychodynamic therapy helps people gain greater self-awareness and understanding about their own actions. It helps patients identify and explore how their nonconscious emotions and motivations can influence their behavior. Sometimes ideas from psychodynamic therapy are interwoven with other types of therapy, like CBT or IPT, to treat various types of mental disorders. Research on psychodynamic therapy is mixed. However, a review of 23 clinical trials involving psychodynamic therapy found it to be as effective as other established psychotherapies.

- **Light Therapy:** Light therapy is used to treat seasonal affective disorder (SAD), a form of depression that usually occurs during the autumn and winter months, when the amount of natural sunlight decreases. Scientists think SAD occurs in some people when their bodies' daily rhythms are upset by short days and long nights. Research has found that the hormone melatonin is affected by this seasonal change. Melatonin normally works to regulate the body's rhythms and responses to light and dark. During light therapy, a person sits in front of a "light box" for periods of time, usually in the morning. The box emits a full spectrum light, and sitting in front of it appears to help reset the body's daily rhythms. Also, some research indicates that a low dose of melatonin, taken at specific times of the day, can also help treat SAD.

Other types of therapies sometimes used in conjunction with the more established therapies include:

- **Expressive Or Creative Arts Therapy:** Expressive or creative arts therapy is based on the idea that people can help heal themselves through art, music, dance, writing, or other expressive acts. One study has found that expressive writing can reduce depression symptoms among women who were victims of domestic violence. It also helps college students at risk for depression.

- **Animal-Assisted Therapy:** Working with animals, such as horses, dogs, or cats, may help some people cope with trauma, develop empathy, and encourage better communication. Companion animals are sometimes introduced in hospitals, psychiatric wards, nursing homes, and other places where they may bring comfort and have a mild therapeutic effect. Animal-assisted therapy has also been used as an added therapy for children with mental disorders. Research on the approach is limited, but a recent study found it to be moderately effective in easing behavioral problems and promoting emotional well-being.

- **Play Therapy:** This therapy is used with children. It involves the use of toys and games to help a child identify and talk about his or her feelings, as well as establish communication with a therapist. A therapist can sometimes better understand a child's problems by watching how he or she plays. Research in play therapy is minimal.

Research Is Underway

Researchers are continually studying ways to better treat mental disorders with psychotherapy, and many NIMH-funded studies are underway.

Finding A Psychotherapist

Your family doctor can help you find a psychotherapist.

Chapter 49

Common Mental Health Medications

Medications are used to treat the symptoms of mental disorders such as schizophrenia, depression, bipolar disorder (sometimes called manic-depressive illness), anxiety disorders, and attention deficit-hyperactivity disorder (ADHD). Sometimes medications are used with other treatments such as psychotherapy. This chapter describes the types of medications used to treat mental disorders and the possible side effects of medications.

This chapter does not provide information about diagnosing mental disorders. Choosing the right medication, medication dose, and treatment plan should be based on a person's individual needs and medical situation, and under a doctor's care.

Information about medications is frequently updated, so check with the U.S. Food and Drug Administration (FDA) for the latest information on warnings, patient medication guides, or newly approved medications. Throughout this chapter you will see two names for medications—the generic name and in parenthesis, the trade name. An example is: fluoxetine (Prozac).

Understanding Psychiatric Medications

Psychiatric medications treat mental disorders. Sometimes called psychotropic or psycho-therapeutic medications, they have changed the lives of people with mental disorders for the better. Many people with mental disorders live fulfilling lives with the help of these medications. Without them, people with mental disorders might suffer serious and disabling symptoms.

Medications treat the symptoms of mental disorders. They cannot cure the disorder, but they make people feel better so they can function.

About This Chapter: Excerpted from "Mental Health Medications," National Institute of Mental Health (www .nimh.nih.gov), February 2012.

Medications work differently for different people. Some people get great results from medications and only need them for a short time. For example, a person with depression may feel much better after taking a medication for a few months, and may never need it again. People with disorders like schizophrenia or bipolar disorder, or people who have long-term or severe depression or anxiety may need to take medication for a much longer time.

Some people get side effects from medications and other people don't. Doses can be small or large, depending on the medication and the person. Factors that can affect how medications work in people include:

- Type of mental disorder, such as depression, anxiety, bipolar disorder, and schizophrenia
- Age, sex, and body size
- Physical illnesses
- Habits like smoking and drinking
- Liver and kidney function
- Genetics
- Other medications and herbal/vitamin supplements
- Diet
- Whether medications are taken as prescribed

Medications To Treat Schizophrenia

Antipsychotic medications are used to treat schizophrenia and schizophrenia-related disorders. Some of these medications have been available since the mid-1950s. They are also called conventional "typical" antipsychotics. Some of the more commonly used medications include chlorpromazine (Thorazine), haloperidol (Haldol), perphenazine, and fluphenazine.

In the 1990s, new antipsychotic medications were developed. These new medications are called second generation, or "atypical" antipsychotics.

One of these medications was clozapine (Clozaril). It is a very effective medication that treats psychotic symptoms, hallucinations, and breaks with reality, such as when a person believes he or she is the president. But clozapine can sometimes cause a serious problem called agranulocytosis, which is a loss of the white blood cells that help a person fight infection. Therefore, people who take clozapine must get their white blood cell counts checked every week or two.

Other atypical antipsychotics were developed. All of them are effective. Agranulocytosis is less likely to occur with these medications than with clozapine, but it has been reported. These include:

- Risperidone (Risperdal)
- Quetiapine (Seroquel)
- Aripiprazole (Abilify)
- Olanzapine (Zyprexa)
- Ziprasidone (Geodon)
- Paliperidone (Invega)

Side Effects

Some people have side effects when they start taking these medications. Most side effects go away after a few days and often can be managed successfully. People who are taking antipsychotics should not drive until they adjust to their new medication. Side effects of many antipsychotics include:

- Drowsiness
- Blurred vision
- Sensitivity to the sun
- Menstrual problems for women
- Dizziness when changing positions
- Rapid heartbeat
- Skin rashes

Atypical antipsychotic medications can cause major weight gain and changes in a person's metabolism. This may increase a person's risk of getting diabetes and high cholesterol. A person's weight, glucose levels, and lipid levels should be monitored regularly by a doctor while taking an atypical antipsychotic medication.

Typical antipsychotic medications can cause side effects related to physical movement, such as:

- Rigidity
- Tremors
- Persistent muscle spasms
- Restlessness

Long-term use of typical antipsychotic medications may lead to a condition called tardive dyskinesia (TD). TD causes muscle movements a person can't control. The movements commonly happen around the mouth. TD can range from mild to severe, and in some people the problem cannot be cured. Sometimes people with TD recover partially or fully after they stop taking the medication.

Response

Antipsychotics are usually pills that people swallow, or liquid they can drink. Some antipsychotics are shots that are given once or twice a month.

Symptoms of schizophrenia, such as feeling agitated and having hallucinations, usually go away within days. Symptoms like delusions usually go away within a few weeks. After about six weeks, many people will see a lot of improvement.

People respond in different ways to antipsychotic medications, and no one can tell beforehand how a person will respond. Sometimes a person needs to try several medications before finding the right one. Doctors and patients can work together to find the best medication or medication combination, and dose.

Some people may have a relapse—their symptoms come back or get worse. Usually, relapses happen when people stop taking their medication, or when they only take it sometimes. Some people stop taking the medication because they feel better or they may feel they don't need it anymore. But no one should stop taking an antipsychotic medication without talking to his or her doctor. When a doctor says it is okay to stop taking a medication, it should be gradually tapered off, never stopped suddenly.

Interactions

Antipsychotics can produce unpleasant or dangerous side effects when taken with certain medications. For this reason, all doctors treating a patient need to be aware of all the medications that person is taking. Doctors need to know about prescription and over-the-counter medicine, vitamins, minerals, and herbal supplements. People also need to discuss any alcohol or other drug use with their doctor.

Medications To Treat Depression

Depression is commonly treated with antidepressant medications. Antidepressants work to balance some of the natural chemicals in our brains. These chemicals are called neurotransmitters, and they affect our mood and emotional responses. Antidepressants work on neurotransmitters such as serotonin, norepinephrine, and dopamine.

The most popular types of antidepressants are called selective serotonin reuptake inhibitors (SSRIs). These include:

- Fluoxetine (Prozac)
- Citalopram (Celexa)
- Sertraline (Zoloft)
- Paroxetine (Paxil)
- Escitalopram (Lexapro)

Other types of antidepressants are serotonin and norepinephrine reuptake inhibitors (SNRIs). SNRIs are similar to SSRIs and include venlafaxine (Effexor) and duloxetine (Cymbalta). Another antidepressant that is commonly used is bupropion (Wellbutrin). Bupropion, which works on the neurotransmitter dopamine, is unique in that it does not fit into any specific drug type.

Side Effects

Antidepressants may cause mild side effects that usually do not last long. Any unusual reactions or side effects should be reported to a doctor immediately.

The most common side effects associated with SSRIs and SNRIs include headache, which usually goes away within a few days; nausea (feeling sick to your stomach), which usually goes away within a few days; sleeplessness or drowsiness, which may happen during the first few weeks but then goes away (sometimes the medication dose needs to be reduced or the time of day it is taken needs to be adjusted to help lessen these side effects.); agitation (feeling jittery); and sexual problems, which can affect both men and women.

Response

People taking antidepressants need to follow their doctors' directions. The medication should be taken in the right dose for the right amount of time. It can take three or four weeks until the medicine takes effect. Some people take the medications for a short time, and some people take them for much longer periods. People with long-term or severe depression may need to take medication for a long time.

Once a person is taking antidepressants, it is important not to stop taking them without the help of a doctor. Sometimes people taking antidepressants feel better and stop taking the medication too soon, and the depression may return. When it is time to stop the medication, the doctor will help the person slowly and safely decrease the dose. It's important to give the body time to adjust to the change. People don't get addicted, or "hooked," on the medications, but stopping them abruptly can cause withdrawal symptoms.

FDA Warning On Antidepressants

Antidepressants are safe and popular, but some studies have suggested that they may have unintentional effects, especially in young people. In 2005, the U.S. Food and Drug Administration (FDA) decided to adopt a "black box" warning label—the most serious type of warning—on all antidepressant medications. The warning says there is an increased risk of suicidal thinking or attempts in children and adolescents taking antidepressants. In 2007, the FDA proposed that makers of all antidepressant medications extend the warning to include young adults up through age 24.

The warning also says that patients of all ages taking antidepressants should be watched closely, especially during the first few weeks of treatment. Possible side effects to look for are depression that gets worse, suicidal thinking or behavior, or any unusual changes in behavior such as trouble sleeping, agitation, or withdrawal from normal social situations. Families and caregivers should report any changes to the doctor. To find the latest information visit the FDA website (www.fda.gov).

Medications To Treat Bipolar Disorder

Bipolar disorder, also called manic-depressive illness, is commonly treated with mood stabilizers. Sometimes, antipsychotics and antidepressants are used along with a mood stabilizer.

Mood Stabilizers

People with bipolar disorder usually try mood stabilizers first. In general, people continue treatment with mood stabilizers for years. Lithium is a very effective mood stabilizer. It was the first mood stabilizer approved by the FDA in the 1970s for treating both manic and depressive episodes.

Anticonvulsant medications also are used as mood stabilizers. They were originally developed to treat seizures, but they were found to help control moods as well. One anticonvulsant commonly used as a mood stabilizer is valproic acid, also called divalproex sodium (Depakote). For some people, it may work better than lithium. Other anticonvulsants used as mood stabilizers are carbamazepine (Tegretol), lamotrigine (Lamictal), and oxcarbazepine (Trileptal).

Atypical Antipsychotics

Atypical antipsychotic medications are sometimes used to treat symptoms of bipolar disorder. Often, antipsychotics are used along with other medications.

Antipsychotics used to treat people with bipolar disorder include:

- Olanzapine (Zyprexa), which helps people with severe or psychotic depression—often accompanied by a break with reality, hallucinations, or delusions

- Aripiprazole (Abilify)

- Risperidone (Risperdal)

- Ziprasidone (Geodon)

- Clozapine (Clozaril), which is often used for people who do not respond to lithium or anticonvulsants

Antidepressants

Antidepressants are sometimes used to treat symptoms of depression in bipolar disorder. Fluoxetine (Prozac), paroxetine (Paxil), or sertraline (Zoloft) are a few that are used. However, people with bipolar disorder should not take an antidepressant on its own. Doing so can cause the person to rapidly switch from depression to mania, which can be dangerous. To prevent this problem, doctors give patients a mood stabilizer or an antipsychotic along with an anti-depressant.

Side Effects

Treatments for bipolar disorder have improved over the last 10 years. But everyone responds differently to medications. If you have any side effects, tell your doctor right away. He or she may change the dose or prescribe a different medication.

Different medications for treating bipolar disorder may cause different side effects. Some medications used for treating bipolar disorder have been linked to unique and serious symptoms.

Lithium can cause several side effects, and some of them may become serious. If a person with bipolar disorder is being treated with lithium, he or she should visit the doctor regularly to check the levels of lithium in the blood, and make sure the kidneys and the thyroid are working normally.

Valproic acid may cause damage to the liver or pancreas, so people taking it should see their doctors regularly. Also, valproic acid may increase testosterone (a male hormone) levels in teenage girls and lead to a condition called polycystic ovarian syndrome (PCOS). PCOS is a disease that can affect fertility and make the menstrual cycle become irregular, but symptoms tend to go away after valproic acid is stopped. It also may cause birth defects in women who are pregnant.

Lamotrigine can cause a rare but serious skin rash that needs to be treated in a hospital. In some cases, this rash can cause permanent disability or be life-threatening.

In addition, valproic acid, lamotrigine, carbamazepine, oxcarbazepine and other anticonvulsant medications have an FDA warning. The warning states that their use may increase the risk of suicidal thoughts and behaviors. People taking anticonvulsant medications for bipolar or other illnesses should be closely monitored for new or worsening symptoms of depression, suicidal thoughts or behavior, or any unusual changes in mood or behavior. People taking these medications should not make any changes without talking to their health care professional.

Response

There is no cure for bipolar disorder, but treatment works for many people. Treatment works best when it is continuous, rather than on and off. However, mood changes can happen even when there are no breaks in treatment. Patients should be open with their doctors about treatment. Talking about how treatment is working can help it be more effective.

It may be helpful for people or their family members to keep a daily chart of mood symptoms, treatments, sleep patterns, and life events. This chart can help patients and doctors track the illness. Doctors can use the chart to treat the illness most effectively.

Because medications for bipolar disorder can have serious side effects, it is important for anyone taking them to see the doctor regularly to check for possibly dangerous changes in the body.

Medications To Treat Anxiety Disorders

Antidepressants, anti-anxiety medications, and beta-blockers are the most common medications used for anxiety disorders. Anxiety disorders include obsessive compulsive disorder (OCD), post-traumatic stress disorder (PTSD), generalized anxiety disorder (GAD), panic disorder, and social phobia.

Antidepressants

Antidepressants were developed to treat depression, but they also help people with anxiety disorders. SSRIs such as fluoxetine (Prozac), sertraline (Zoloft), escitalopram (Lexapro), paroxetine (Paxil), and citalopram (Celexa) are commonly prescribed for panic disorder, OCD, PTSD, and social phobia. The SNRI venlafaxine (Effexor) is commonly used to treat GAD.

Are herbal medicines used to treat depression?

The herbal medicine St. John's wort has been used for centuries in many folk and herbal remedies. Today in Europe, it is used widely to treat mild-to-moderate depression. In the United States, it is one of the top-selling botanical products.

The National Institutes of Health (NIH) conducted a clinical trial to determine the effectiveness of treating adults who have major depression with St. Johns wort. The study included 340 people diagnosed with major depression. One-third of the people took the herbal medicine, one-third took an SSRI, and one-third took a placebo, or "sugar pill." The people did not know what they were taking. The study found that St. John's wort was no more effective than the placebo in treating major depression. A study currently in progress is looking at the effectiveness of St. John's wort for treating mild or minor depression.

Other research has shown that St. John's wort can dangerously interact with other medications, including those used to control human immunodeficiency virus (HIV). On February 10, 2000, the FDA issued a Public Health Advisory letter stating that the herb appears to interfere with certain medications used to treat heart disease, depression, seizures, certain cancers, and organ transplant rejection. Also, St. Johns wort may interfere with oral contraceptives.

Because St. John's wort may not mix well with other medications, people should always talk with their doctors before taking it or any herbal supplement.

Source: Excerpted from "Mental Health Medications," National Institute of Mental Health (www.nimh.nih.gov), February 2012.

The antidepressant bupropion (Wellbutrin) is also sometimes used. When treating anxiety disorders, antidepressants generally are started at low doses and increased over time.

Benzodiazepines (Anti-Anxiety Medications)

The anti-anxiety medications called benzodiazepines can start working more quickly than antidepressants. The ones used to treat anxiety disorders include:

- Clonazepam (Klonopin), which is used for social phobia and GAD
- Lorazepam (Ativan), which is used for panic disorder
- Alprazolam (Xanax), which is used for panic disorder and GAD

Beta-Blockers

Beta-blockers control some of the physical symptoms of anxiety, such as trembling and sweating. Propranolol (Inderal) is a beta-blocker usually used to treat heart conditions and high blood pressure. The medicine also helps people who have physical problems related to anxiety. For example, when a person with social phobia must face a stressful situation, such as giving a speech, or attending an important meeting, a doctor may prescribe a beta-blocker. Taking the medicine for a short period of time can help the person keep physical symptoms under control.

Side Effects

The most common side effects for benzodiazepines are drowsiness and dizziness. Other possible side effects include upset stomach, blurred vision, headache, confusion, grogginess, and nightmares.

Common side effects from beta-blockers include fatigue, cold hands, dizziness, and weakness. In addition, beta-blockers generally are not recommended for people with asthma or diabetes because they may worsen symptoms.

Response

People can build a tolerance to benzodiazepines if they are taken over a long period of time and may need higher and higher doses to get the same effect. Some people may become dependent on them. To avoid these problems, doctors usually prescribe the medication for short periods, a practice that is especially helpful for people who have substance abuse problems or who become dependent on medication easily. If people suddenly stop taking benzodiazepines, they may get withdrawal symptoms, or their anxiety may return. Therefore, they should be tapered off slowly.

Medications To Treat ADHD

Attention deficit hyperactivity disorder (ADHD) occurs in both children and adults. ADHD is commonly treated with stimulants, such as:

- Methylphenidate (Ritalin, Metadate, Concerta, Daytrana)

- Amphetamine (Adderall)

- Dextroamphetamine (Dexedrine, Dextrostat)

In 2002, the FDA approved the nonstimulant medication atomoxetine (Strattera) for use as a treatment for ADHD. In February 2007, the FDA approved the use of the stimulant lisdexamfetamine dimesylate (Vyvanse) for the treatment of ADHD in children ages 6–12 years.

Side Effects

Most side effects are minor and disappear when dosage levels are lowered. The most common side effects include decreased appetite, sleep problems, stomachaches, and headaches.

A few children develop sudden, repetitive movements or sounds called tics. These tics may or may not be noticeable. Changing the medication dosage may make tics go away. Some children also may appear to have a personality change, such as appearing "flat" or without emotion.

FDA Warning On Possible Rare Side Effects

In 2007, the FDA required that all makers of ADHD medications develop Patient Medication Guides. The guides must alert patients to possible heart and psychiatric problems related to ADHD medicine

Forms Of ADHD Medications

Stimulant medications can be short-acting or long-acting, and can be taken in different forms such as a pill, patch, or powder. Long-acting, sustained and extended release forms allow children to take the medication just once a day before school.

Safety of ADHD medications

Stimulant medications are safe when given under a doctor's supervision. Some children taking them may feel slightly different or "funny."

Some parents worry that stimulant medications may lead to drug abuse or dependence, but there is little evidence of this. Research shows that teens with ADHD who took stimulant medications were less likely to abuse drugs than those who did not take stimulant medications.

Adding Psychotherapy To Medication Treatment Improves Outcomes In Pediatric OCD

Research shows that youth with obsessive compulsive disorder (OCD), who are already taking antidepressant medication, may benefit by adding a type of psychotherapy called cognitive behavior therapy (CBT). Among 124 children ages 7–17, researchers compared three treatment options:

- Medication management only (MM), prescribed and managed by a physician (an antidepressant known as a selective serotonin reuptake inhibitor, or SSRI)

- MM plus Instructional CBT (MM+I-CBT), a shorter, less intensive version of CBT administered by the prescribing physician

- MM plus CBT (MM+CBT) provided by a trained CBT therapist, including a type of therapy called exposure plus response prevention (ERP), in which children are exposed to feared situations and taught how to respond to the resulting anxiety without engaging in compulsions

After 12 weeks of treatment, nearly 69 percent of those receiving MM+CBT had responded to treatment, compared to 34 percent receiving MM+I-CBT and 30 percent receiving MM. Those receiving MM+CBT showed more improvement in all respects, compared to those receiving MM and MM+I-CBT.

The findings are consistent with other studies demonstrating that ERP is an effective treatment strategy for OCD, both alone and in combination with SSRIs. The researchers conclude that the full version of CBT with ERP should be widely disseminated as opposed to a brief version that may not be effective.

The researchers were unsure why there was so little difference in treatment response between the MM group and the MM+I-CBT group. They reasoned that the I-CBT was generally ineffective because it was brief and less intensive than the CBT. It also did not include key treatment components that are central to the full CBT protocol, such as exposure practices during the treatment sessions themselves. Future efforts should focus on making the full CBT with ERP more widely available in community settings, they concluded.

Source: Excerpted from "Adding Psychotherapy To Medication Treatment Improves Outcomes In Pediatric OCD," National Institute of Mental Health (www.nimh.nih.gov), August 2012.

Special Needs Of Adolescents Taking Psychiatric Medications

Most medications used to treat young people with mental illness are safe and effective. However, many medications have not been studied or approved for use with children. Researchers are not sure how these medications affect a child's growing body. Still, a doctor can give a young person an FDA-approved medication on an "off-label" basis. This means that the doctor prescribes the medication to help the patient even though the medicine is not approved for the specific mental disorder or age. For these reasons, it is important to watch young people who take these medications. Young people may have different reactions and side effects than adults.

Questions To Ask Your Doctor

You and your family can help your doctor find the right medications for you. The doctor needs to know your medical history; family history; information about allergies; other medications, supplements or herbal remedies you take; and other details about your overall health. You or a family member should ask the following questions when a medication is prescribed:

- What is the name of the medication?
- What is the medication supposed to do?
- How and when should I take it?
- How much should I take?
- What should I do if I miss a dose?
- When and how should I stop taking it?
- Will it interact with other medications I take?
- Do I need to avoid any types of food or drink while taking the medication? What should I avoid?
- Should it be taken with or without food?
- Is it safe to drink alcohol while taking this medication?
- What are the side effects? What should I do if I experience them?
- Is the Patient Package Insert for the medication available?

After taking the medication for a short time, tell your doctor how you feel, if you are having side effects, and any concerns you have about the medicine.

Chapter 50

Antidepressants: What You Need To Know About Depression Medication

Depression is a serious disorder that can cause significant problems in mood, thinking, and behavior at home, in school, and with peers. It is estimated that major depressive disorder (MDD) affects about five percent of adolescents.

Research has shown that, as in adults, depression in children and adolescents is treatable. Certain antidepressant medications, called selective serotonin reuptake inhibitors (SSRIs), can be beneficial to children and adolescents with MDD. Certain types of psychological therapies also have been shown to be effective. However, our knowledge of antidepressant treatments in youth, though growing substantially, is limited compared to what we know about treating depression in adults.

Recently, there has been some concern that the use of antidepressant medications themselves may induce suicidal behavior in youths. Following a thorough and comprehensive review of all the available published and unpublished controlled clinical trials of antidepressants in children and adolescents, the U.S. Food and Drug Administration (FDA) issued a public warning in October 2004 about an increased risk of suicidal thoughts or behavior (suicidality) in children and adolescents treated with SSRI antidepressant medications. In 2006, an advisory committee to the FDA recommended that the agency extend the warning to include young adults up to age 25.

More recently, results of a comprehensive review of pediatric trials conducted between 1988 and 2006 suggested that the benefits of antidepressant medications likely outweigh their risks to children and adolescents with major depression and anxiety disorders. The study, partially funded by National Institute of Mental Health (NIMH), was published in the April 18, 2007, issue of the *Journal of the American Medical Association*.

About This Chapter: Excerpted from "Antidepressant Medications for Children and Adolescents: Information for Parents and Caregivers," National Institute of Mental Health (www.nimh.nih.gov), February 2013.

What did the FDA review find?

In the FDA review, no completed suicides occurred among nearly 2,200 children treated with SSRI medications. However, about four percent of those taking SSRI medications experienced suicidal thinking or behavior, including actual suicide attempts—twice the rate of those taking placebo, or sugar pills.

In response, the FDA adopted a "black box" label warning indicating that antidepressants may increase the risk of suicidal thinking and behavior in some children and adolescents with MDD. A black-box warning is the most serious type of warning in prescription drug labeling.

The warning also notes that children and adolescents taking SSRI medications should be closely monitored for any worsening in depression, emergence of suicidal thinking or behavior, or unusual changes in behavior, such as sleeplessness, agitation, or withdrawal from normal social situations. Close monitoring is especially important during the first four weeks of treatment. SSRI medications usually have few side effects in children and adolescents, but for unknown reasons, they may trigger agitation and abnormal behavior in certain individuals.

What do we know about antidepressant medications?

The SSRIs include:

- Fluoxetine (Prozac)

- Sertraline (Zoloft)

- Paroxetine (Paxil)

- Citalopram (Celexa)

- Escitalopram (Lexapro)

- Fluvoxamine (Luvox)

Another antidepressant medication, venlafaxine (Effexor), is not an SSRI but is closely related.

SSRI medications are considered an improvement over older antidepressant medications because they have fewer side effects and are less likely to be harmful if taken in an overdose, which is an issue for patients with depression already at risk for suicide. They have been shown to be safe and effective for adults.

However, use of SSRI medications among children and adolescents ages 10–19 has risen dramatically in the past several years. Fluoxetine (Prozac) is the only medication approved by the FDA for use in treating depression in children ages eight and older. The other SSRI medications and the SSRI-related antidepressant venlafaxine have not been approved for treatment of depression in children or adolescents, but doctors still sometimes prescribe them to children on an "off-label" basis. In June 2003, however, the FDA recommended that paroxetine not be used in children and adolescents for treating MDD.

Fluoxetine can be helpful in treating childhood depression, and can lead to significant improvement of depression overall. However, it may increase the risk for suicidal behaviors in a small subset of adolescents. As with all medical decisions, doctors and families should weigh the risks and benefits of treatment for each individual patient.

What should be done for a child with depression?

A child or adolescent with MDD should be carefully and thoroughly evaluated by a doctor to determine if medication is appropriate. Psychotherapy often is tried as an initial treatment for mild depression. Psychotherapy may help to determine the severity and persistence of the depression and whether antidepressant medications may be warranted. Types of psychotherapies include "cognitive behavioral therapy," which helps people learn new ways of thinking and behaving, and "interpersonal therapy," which helps people understand and work through troubled personal relationships.

Those who are prescribed an SSRI medication should receive ongoing medical monitoring. Children already taking an SSRI medication should remain on the medication if it has been helpful, but should be carefully monitored by a doctor for side effects. Parents should promptly seek medical advice and evaluation if a child or adolescent experiences suicidal thinking or behavior, nervousness, agitation, irritability, mood instability, or sleeplessness that either emerges or worsens during treatment with SSRI medications.

Once started, treatment with these medications should not be abruptly stopped. Although they are not habit-forming or addictive, abruptly ending an antidepressant can cause withdrawal symptoms or lead to a relapse. Families should not discontinue treatment without consulting their doctor.

All treatments can be associated with side effects. Families and doctors should carefully weigh the risks and benefits, and maintain appropriate follow-up and monitoring to help control for the risks.

What does research tell us?

An individual's response to a medication cannot be predicted with certainty. It is extremely difficult to determine whether SSRI medications increase the risk for completed suicide, especially because depression itself increases the risk for suicide and because completed suicides, especially among children and adolescents, are rare. Most controlled trials are too small to detect for rare events such as suicide (thousands of participants are needed). In addition, controlled trials typically exclude patients considered at high risk for suicide.

One major clinical trial, the NIMH-funded Treatment for Adolescents with Depression Study (TADS), has indicated that a combination of medication and psychotherapy is the most effective treatment for adolescents with depression. The clinical trial of 439 adolescents

Teens With Treatment-Resistant Depression More Likely To Get Better With Switch To Combination Therapy

Teens with difficult-to-treat depression who do not respond to a first antidepressant medication are more likely to get well if they switch to another antidepressant medication and add psychotherapy rather than just switching to another antidepressant, according to a large, multi-site trial funded by the National Institute of Mental Health (NIMH).

"The findings should be encouraging for families with a teen who has been struggling with depression for some time," said lead researcher David Brent, MD, of the University of Pittsburgh. "Even if a first attempt at treatment is unsuccessful, persistence will pay off. Being open to trying new evidence-based medications or treatment combinations is likely to result in improvement."

Adolescents with treatment-resistant depression have unique needs, for which standard treatments do not always work.

"About 40 percent of adolescents with depression do not adequately respond to a first treatment course with an antidepressant medication, and clinicians have no solid guidelines on how to choose subsequent treatments for these patients," said NIMH Director Thomas R. Insel, MD.

Brent and colleagues conducted testing at six regionally dispersed clinics with 334 adolescents ages 12–18. The teens in the study all had major depression and had not responded to a previous two-month course of a selective serotonin reuptake inhibitor (SSRI), a type of antidepressant. The teens were randomly assigned to one of four interventions for 12 weeks:

- Switch to another SSRI—paroxetine (Paxil), citalopram (Celexa) or fluoxetine (Prozac)
- Switch to a different SSRI plus cognitive behavioral therapy (CBT), a type of psychotherapy that emphasizes problem-solving and behavior change
- Switch to venlafaxine (Effexor)—another type of antidepressant called a serotonin and norepinephrine reuptake inhibitor (SNRI)
- Switch to venlafaxine plus CBT

The researchers chose to compare SSRIs with an SNRI because some studies on adults have found

ages 12–17 with MDD compared four treatment groups—one that received a combination of fluoxetine and CBT, one that received fluoxetine only, one that received CBT only, and one that received a placebo only. After the first 12 weeks, 71 percent responded to the combination treatment of fluoxetine and CBT, 61 percent responded to the fluoxetine only treatment, 43 percent responded to the CBT only treatment, and 35 percent responded to the placebo treatment.

At the beginning of the study, 29 percent of the TADS participants were having clinically significant suicidal thoughts. Although the rate of suicidal thinking decreased among all

---

that venlafaxine is more effective than an SSRI in managing treatment-resistant depression.

About 55 percent of those who switched to either type of medication and added CBT responded, while 41 percent of those who switched to another medication alone responded. There were no differences in response between those who switched to an SSRI and those who switched to an SNRI, nor were there differences in response among the three SSRIs tested.

Unlike similar studies on adolescent depression, the test called TORDIA (for Treatment of SSRI-Resistant Depression in Adolescents) did not exclude teens who were thinking about suicide or had attempted suicide. They were included, so that TORDIA would mirror real-world treatment situations—and its findings would be readily applicable to community settings.

More than half of the participants expressed suicidal thinking and behavior (suicidality) before treatment began, and all teens were monitored weekly for side effects related to suicidality and predictive symptoms like hostility and irritability.

None of the TORDIA treatment groups, however, showed any measurable effects on suicidality, a finding consistent with other studies that have discovered suicidality does not necessarily subside when the depression does. The researchers reiterated the need for new treatments that specifically prevent or alleviate suicidality.

Although none of the medications seemed to be superior over the others, venlafaxine was associated with more adverse effects, such as skin infections and cardiovascular side effects. The researchers concluded that because venlafaxine had a greater potential for side effects, switching to another SSRI should be considered first.

The findings echo those of the NIMH-funded Treatment for Adolescents with Depression Study (TADS), which concluded that depressed teens benefited most from a combination of medication and psychotherapy over both the short and long terms. They are also consistent with results from the NIMH-funded Systematic Treatment Alternatives to Relieve Depression (STAR*D) study, which showed that adults with persistent depression can get well after trying several treatment strategies.

Source: Excerpted from "Teens With Treatment-Resistant Depression More Likely To Get Better With Switch To Combination Therapy," National Institute of Mental Health (www.nimh.nih.gov), 2013.

the treatment groups, those in the fluoxetine/CBT combination treatment group showed the greatest reduction in suicidal thinking.

Researchers are working to better understand the relationship between antidepressant medications and suicide. So far, results are mixed. One study, using national Medicaid files, found that among adults, the use of antidepressants does not seem to be related to suicide attempts or deaths. However, the analysis found that the use of antidepressant medications may be related to suicide attempts and deaths among children and adolescents.

Another study analyzed health plan records for 65,103 patients treated for depression. It found no significant increase among adults and young people in the risk for suicide after starting treatment with newer antidepressant medications.

A third study analyzed suicide data from the National Vital Statistics and commercial prescription data. It found that among children ages 5–14, suicide rates from 1996 to 1998 were actually lower in areas of the country with higher rates of SSRI antidepressant prescriptions. The relationship between the suicide rates and the SSRI use rates, however, is unclear.

New NIMH-funded research will help clarify the complex interplay between suicide and antidepressant medications. In addition, the NIMH-funded Treatment of Resistant Depression in Adolescents (TORDIA) study, will investigate how best to treat adolescents whose depression is resistant to the first SSRI medication they have tried. Finally, NIMH also is supporting the Treatment of Adolescent Suicide Attempters (TASA) study, which is investigating the treatment of adolescents who have attempted suicide. Treatments include antidepressant medications, CBT or both.

Chapter 51

Electroconvulsive Therapy (ECT)

What is electroconvulsive therapy (ECT)?

Electroconvulsive therapy (ECT) is one of the most studied and most effective treatments for selected severe mental illness such as major depression with psychotic feature. ECT has received much attention in the mainstream media: both negative and positive. While ECT carries long history of negative connotations, it can be a life-saving procedure for many people and is a relatively safe procedure that is only performed under the supervision of trained healthcare professionals. In some illnesses, ECT can be up to 90 percent effective in reducing the severity of symptoms. ECT has important risks to weigh as well, including the medical risks of the procedure itself (typically small) and problems with memory that may continue after the treatments end (sometimes related to the number of treatments).

ECT is a treatment of choice for over tens of thousands of Americans each year. Since it was first performed, ECT has become safer and more successful in helping people who require immediate treatment, people who cannot be treated with psychiatric medications, and people who have not responded to other psychiatric treatments. While it carries significant risks, many potential consequences of ECT can be prevented by a thorough consultation with a non-psychiatric medical doctor prior to beginning treatment. The cognitive and memory side-effects of ECT are usually not permanent, but it is advised that any person considering treatment with ECT discuss this and other issues with their psychiatrist.

ECT is regularly performed in hospitals by a medical team that consists of psychiatrists, anesthesiologists, nurses, and other healthcare professionals. ECT begins when an anesthesiologist

About This Chapter: This chapter is reprinted from "Electroconvulsive Therapy (ECT) Fact Sheet," July 2012, © NAMI, the National Alliance on Mental Illness, www.nami.org.

administers medications to cause the patient to lose consciousness. This ensures that the patient will not experience any physical pain associated with their treatment. The psychiatrist will then use a machine that delivers an electrical shock to the patient's brain. This causes the patient to experience a controlled seizure that lasts in most situations for less than one to two minutes.

The seizure causes activation of neurons throughout the brain and changes in many of the chemicals in a person's brain. It is thought that these actions then result in a decrease in the symptoms of mental illness. Usually ECT is "unilateral" in that a seizure is started only on one side of the brain. Sometimes when people are not responding to this treatment alone, ECT is done "bilaterally" and seizures are started on both sides of the brain. This can be more effective but also carries a greater risk of side-effects, especially memory and cognitive-related side effects.

Depending on their illness, most people will have between four and six treatments before their symptoms show significant improvement. Most patients will continue to have regular treatments until their symptoms are significantly decreased. Some patients will then continue to have "maintenance ECT" on a less frequent schedule (for example, once per week, once every other week, or once per month).

Who will benefit from treatment with ECT?

Treatment with ECT is highly effective and works rapidly when compared with other psychiatric treatments for the right conditions. While some antidepressants may take between two to three months to have a complete effect, some people who are treated with ECT may begin to feel better within one week of beginning their treatment.

ECT is specifically valuable in the treatment of severe depression and depression with psychosis. In some patients who do not improve with multiple medication treatments, ECT may be the only treatment that effectively controls their symptoms. ECT is often used in patients with severe suicidal thoughts or behaviors as it works significantly faster than other treatments to decrease these distressing symptoms. It can also work to reverse complex symptoms of mania that may have been treatment resistant. ECT can be employed for a presentation known at catatonia. It is not indicated [suggested] for anxiety disorders, substance abuse disorders, and personality disorders.

What are the risks of ECT?

As it is now practiced, ECT is a much safer procedure than it was in earlier decades. In fact, while ECT may be associated with significant side-effects, the most common side-effects of ECT are headaches and muscle pain that normally go away shortly after each treatment.

Cognitive and memory side-effects may require regular assessment by a clinician. As with any other medical or surgical procedure requiring anesthesia, there are risks associated with receiving the sedating medications involved in anesthesia. Therefore, ECT may not be recommended in people with other severe medical illnesses including heart, lung, and neurological diseases.

Many patients undergoing ECT will notice that they have some trouble with their thinking around the time that they are receiving treatment with ECT. The most common symptom is being confused following the procedure. In most people, this lasts for less than a few hours and is the result of having had a seizure and having received anesthesia.

Somewhere between one-quarter to two-thirds of people receiving ECT will have memory problems as a result of ECT. Some people will experience trouble forming new memories and remembering things that happen after they start receiving ECT but usually disappears within a few days to weeks of stopping treatment. Some people will experience trouble remembering things that happened to them before they started ECT and this often lasts longer. The risks of ECT are substantial but so is its power to reverse life threatening symptoms for selected severe mental illnesses.

Chapter 52

Transcranial Magnetic Stimulation

Transcranial magnetic stimulation (TMS) is a relatively new treatment for major depression that is being investigated by a number of scientists across the world. At the current time, the Food and Drug Administration (FDA) has only officially cleared TMS for a single indication: treatment-resistant depression. TMS, as a generic procedure, has not been approved by the FDA. Rather, a specific device that performs TMS, the NeuroStar, was cleared by the FDA in October 2008 for clinical use in treatment-resistant depression.

TMS is an outpatient intervention which could be an option for individuals diagnosed with major depression who have not responded to trials of antidepressant medications at an adequate dose and duration. In clinical trials, individuals had been treated with an average of five medication treatment attempts, one of which was at an adequate dose and duration. TMS has not been thoroughly studied for people who have failed two or more adequate trials of antidepressants or for people who have not been on antidepressants. TMS is not indicated for individuals who have bipolar disorder, depression with psychosis, or individuals with a high risk of suicide.

Each session of TMS consists of a session lasting approximately 40 minutes conducted in an outpatient office using a specific technology. The procedure, given daily, occurs over a four- to six-week period. The TMS device sends magnetic pulses to the frontal left side of the brain which generates weak electrical currents. These magnetic pulses are similar to what one would experience in getting a magnetic resonance image (MRI) of their brain.

About This Chapter: Information in this chapter is reprinted from "Transcranial Magnetic Stimulation (TMS) Fact Sheet," August 2012, © NAMI, the National Alliance on Mental Illness, www.nami.org.

The theory of the treatment is that the resulting electrical currents activate neurotransmitters implicated in the symptoms of depression—serotonin, norepinephrine, and dopamine. Studies have shown that the frontal left side of the brain is an area that can be underactive in individuals with major depression, hence the rationale for the site of the stimulation.

In a randomized, controlled clinical trial with individuals who had not adequately benefited from prior antidepressant medication, patients treated with TMS experienced a significantly greater improvement in symptoms than patients treated with placebo. In an open-label trial, which is most like real-world clinical practice, 54 percent of individuals treated with TMS experienced a significant improvement in symptoms. While these studies suggest that TMS may be quite beneficial, other studies have suggested otherwise—that TMS may not have a substantial benefit as opposed to placebo treatment.

TMS requires no anesthesia or sedation, has a low rate (about five percent) of discontinuation due to adverse effects (most commonly headache) and has no systemic side effects—as opposed to oral antidepressant therapy which can be associated with sexual side effects, weight gain, nausea, constipation, or dry mouth. Medical devices such as pacemakers or metal objects in one's head prevent the use of TMS. Seizure risk can be raised by TMS, yet TMS has not been frequently shown to cause seizures in individuals without an underlying seizure disorder. As this is a newer treatment, there are no long-term studies of the effects of TMS. Another important consideration is that TMS may not be covered by medical insurance in some cases and can be expensive if coverage is not part of the health plan.

Like all new treatments, doctors are still sorting out best uses for TMS as well as its potential downsides. At this time, there is no evidence to support the use of "maintenance treatment" with TMS once the initial episode of treatment is over. Researchers and doctors are also trying to better assess when and if TMS can be an alternative to electroconvulsive therapy (ECT), which has more treatment intensity and side effects. It is safe to say we have more to learn about this intervention. Academic medical centers are most familiar with this intervention and may conduct research studies on TMS. Individuals interested in this—or any other new treatment—are encouraged to review any emerging information from research and clinical practice with their doctors.

Chapter 53

Complementary And Alternative Approaches To Mental Health Care

Natural And Herbal Supplements For Common Mental Disorders

Many medications for common mental disorders, although helpful, can cause unpleasant side effects that discourage patients from taking their prescribed dose. In recent years, there has been a great deal of interest in natural substances to treat the symptoms of depression, anxiety, and PMS—either to enhance the effects of prescription drugs or to use alone.

Studies show that a lack of certain nutrients may contribute to the development of mental disorders. Notably, essential vitamins, minerals, and omega-3 fatty acids are often deficient in the general population in America and other developed countries, and are exceptionally deficient in patients suffering from mental disorders.

Many experts believe that nutrition has the potential to affect the symptoms and severity of depression. Supplements including omega-3 fatty acids, vitamins C and E, and folate have been investigated.

Omega-3 fatty acids such as eicosapentaenoic acid (EPA) and docosahexaenoic acid (DHA) might have an impact on depression because these compounds are widespread in the brain. The evidence is not fully conclusive, but omega-3 supplements are an option. One to two grams of omega-3 fatty acids daily is the generally accepted dose for healthy individuals, but for patients with mental disorders, up to three grams has been shown to be safe and effective.

About This Chapter: Information in this chapter is reprinted from "Natural And Herbal Supplements For Common Mental Disorders," by Jane Collingwood, © 2013 Psych Central (www.psychcentral.com). All rights reserved. Reprinted with permission.

Supplements that contain amino acids have been found to reduce symptoms, possibly because they are converted to neurotransmitters in the brain that help alleviate depression. For example, serotonin is made using the amino acid tryptophan. Dietary supplements that contain tyrosine or phenylalanine, later converted into dopamine and norepinephrine, are also available.

Deficiencies of magnesium and the B vitamin folate have been linked to depression. Trials suggest that patients treated with 0.8mg of folic acid per day or 0.4mg of vitamin B12 per day will have reduced depression symptoms. Patients treated with 125 to 300mg of magnesium with each meal and at bedtime have shown rapid recovery from major depression.

Experts have looked at a range of herbal remedies and supplements for individuals with anxiety. The evidence supports the effectiveness of kava for mild to moderate anxiety disorders. Kava does, however, impact on other medicines metabolized by the liver.

St. John's wort, valerian, Sympathyl (a mixture of California poppy, hawthorn, and elemental magnesium), and passionflower have been investigated for anxiety but the studies have generally been small or inconsistent. Lower than average omega-3 levels have been reported in patients with anxiety, and supplementation with omega-3s appears to improve some symptoms. Zinc and chromium supplements may be helpful, as well as calcium and vitamin B6.

Trials of women with premenstrual syndrome (PMS) suggest that vitamin B6 "relieves overall premenstrual and depressive premenstrual symptoms." Dietary studies also indicate that calcium taken at 1,200 mg per day may be useful.

Four hundred IU per day of vitamin E has shown some effectiveness, and several other supplements are under investigation. These include magnesium, manganese and tryptophan.

Calcium supplementation is another promising option. Fluctuations in calcium levels may help explain some features of PMS. Tiredness, appetite changes, and depressive symptoms were significantly improved in one study of women receiving calcium, compared with placebo.

People with obsessive compulsive disorder (OCD) often benefit from selective serotonin reuptake inhibitors (SSRIs), so the nutrients that increase serotonin levels are likely to reduce symptoms. Again, the amino acid tryptophan is a precursor to serotonin, and tryptophan supplements can increase serotonin levels and treat OCD.

St. John's Wort has also been shown to benefit OCD symptoms. A dose of 900 mg per day of St. John's Wort has been found to improve OCD symptoms and is less likely to cause side effects, but it can interfere with some prescription medicines.

Dr. Shaheen E. Lakhan of the Global Neuroscience Initiative Foundation in Los Angeles says, "There is tremendous resistance from clinicians to using supplements as treatments, mostly due to their lack of knowledge on the subject. Others rather use prescription drugs that the drug companies and the FDA researches, monitors, and recalls if necessary.

Mindfulness Meditation Is Associated With Structural Changes In The Brain

According to a recent study, practicing mindfulness meditation appears to be associated with measurable changes in the brain regions involved in memory, learning, and emotion. Mindfulness meditation focuses attention on breathing to develop increased awareness of the present. Previous research has demonstrated that mindfulness mediation may reduce symptoms of anxiety, depression, and chronic pain, but little is known about its effects on the brain. The focus of the current study—published in the journal *Psychiatry Research: Neuroimaging*—was to identify brain regions that changed in participants enrolled in an eight-week mindfulness-based stress reduction program.

In this study, researchers from Massachusetts General Hospital, Bender Institute of Neuroimaging in Germany, and the University of Massachusetts Medical School, took magnetic resonance images of the brains of 16 participants, two weeks before and after they joined the meditation program. (Participants were physician- and self-referred individuals seeking stress reduction.) Researchers also took brain images of a control group of 17 non-meditators over a similar time period. Participants in the meditation group attended weekly sessions that included mindfulness training exercises and received audio recordings for guided meditation practice at home. They also kept track of how much time they practiced each day. Members of both groups completed a questionnaire, before and after joining the group, which measured five aspects of mindfulness: observing, describing, acting with awareness, non-judging of inner experience, and non-reactivity to inner experience.

Brain images in the meditation group revealed increases in gray matter concentration in the left hippocampus. The hippocampus is an area of the brain involved in learning, memory, and emotional control, and is suspected of playing a role in producing some of the positive effects of meditation. Gray matter also increased in four other brain regions (though not in the insula, a region that has shown changes in other meditation studies) in the meditation group. Responses to the questionnaire indicated improvements in three of the five aspects of mindfulness in the mediators, but not the control group.

The researchers concluded that these findings may represent an underlying brain mechanism associated with mindfulness-based improvements in mental health. Additional studies are needed to determine the associations between specific types of brain change and behavioral mechanisms thought to improve a variety of disorders.

Source: Excerpted from "Mindfulness Meditation Is Associated with Structural Changes in the Brain," National Center for Complementary and Alternative Medicine (nccam.nih.gov), January 2011.

"However, for some patients, prescription drugs do not have the efficacy of nutritional supplements, and they sometimes have far more dangerous side effects. So for clinicians to avoid these supplement therapies because of a lack of knowledge and unwillingness to use treatments not backed by drug companies and the FDA, they are compromising their patients' recovery."

Dr. Lakhan believes that psychiatrists should be aware of nutritional therapies, appropriate doses, and possible side effects in order to provide alternative and complementary treatments for their patients. "This may reduce the number of noncompliant patients suffering from mental disorders that choose not to take their prescribed medications," he adds.

Part Seven
Mental Wellness Topics For Teens

Chapter 54

Building Healthy Self-Esteem

Most people feel bad about themselves from time to time. Feelings of low self-esteem may be triggered by being treated poorly by someone else recently or in the past, or by a person's own judgments of him or herself. This is normal. However, low self-esteem is a constant companion for too many people—especially those who experience depression, anxiety, phobias, psychosis, delusional thinking, or who have an illness or a disability. If you are one of these people, you may go through life feeling bad about yourself needlessly. Low self-esteem keeps you from enjoying life, doing the things you want to do, and working toward personal goals.

You have a right to feel good about yourself. However, it can be very difficult to feel good about yourself when you are under the stress of having symptoms that are hard to manage, when you are dealing with a disability, when you are having a difficult time, or when others are treating you badly. At these times, it is easy to be drawn into a downward spiral of lower and lower self-esteem. For instance, you may begin feeling bad about yourself when someone insults you, you are under a lot of pressure at school, or you are having a difficult time getting along with someone in your family. Then you begin to give yourself negative self-talk, like "I'm no good." That may make you feel so bad about yourself that you do something to hurt yourself or someone else, such as getting drunk or yelling at your family and friends. By using the ideas and activities in this chapter, you can avoid doing things that make you feel even worse and do those things that will make you feel better about yourself.

This chapter will give you ideas on things you can do to feel better about yourself—to raise your self-esteem. The ideas have come from people like you—people who realize they have low self-esteem and are working to improve it.

About This Chapter: Excerpted from "Building Self-Esteem: A Self-Help Guide," Substance Abuse and Mental Health Services Administration (www.samhsa.gov), January 2002. Information has been reviewed by David A. Cooke, MD, FACP, September 2013.

As you begin to use the methods in this chapter (and other methods that you may think of to improve your self-esteem), you may notice that you have some feelings of resistance to positive feelings about yourself. This is normal. Don't let these feelings stop you from feeling good about yourself. They will diminish as you feel better and better about yourself. To help relieve these feelings, let your friends know what you are going through. Have a good cry, if you can. Do things to relax, such as meditating or taking a nice warm bath.

As you read this chapter and review the exercises, keep the following statement in mind: "I am a very special, unique, and valuable person. I deserve to feel good about myself."

Self-Esteem, Depression, And Other Illnesses

Before you begin to consider strategies and activities to help raise your self-esteem, it is important to remember that low self-esteem may be due to depression. Low self-esteem is a symptom of depression. To make things even more complicated, the depression may be a symptom of some other illness.

Have you felt sad consistently for several weeks but don't know why you are feeling so sad—such as, nothing terribly bad has happened, or maybe something bad has happened, but you haven't been able to get rid of the feelings of sadness? Is this accompanied by other changes, like wanting to eat all the time (or having no appetite), wanting to sleep all the time, or waking up very early and not being able to get back to sleep?

If you answered yes to either question, there are two things you need to do:

- See your doctor for a physical examination to determine the cause of your depression and to discuss treatment choices.

- Do some things that will help you to feel better right away like eating well; getting plenty of exercise and outdoor light; spending time with good friends; and doing fun things like going to a movie, painting a picture, playing a musical instrument, or reading a good book.

Things You Can Do Right Away—Every Day—To Raise Your Self-Esteem

Pay Attention To Your Own Needs And Wants

Listen to what your body, your mind, and your heart are telling you. For instance, if your body is telling you that you have been sitting down too long, stand up and stretch. If your heart is longing to spend more time with a special friend, do it. If your mind is telling you to clean up your basement, listen to your favorite music, or stop thinking bad thoughts about yourself, take those thoughts seriously.

Take Very Good Care Of Yourself

As you were growing up, you may not have learned how to take good care of yourself. In fact, much of your attention may have been on taking care of others, on just getting by, or on "behaving well." Begin today to take good care of yourself. Treat yourself as a wonderful parent would treat a small child or as one very best friend might treat another. If you work at taking good care of yourself, you will find that you feel better about yourself. Here are some ways to take good care of you:

- **Eat healthy foods.** Avoid junk foods (foods containing a lot of sugar, salt, or fat). A healthy daily diet is usually:

  - Five or six servings of vegetables and fruit

  - Six servings of whole grain foods like bread, pasta, cereal, and rice

  - Two servings of protein foods like beef, chicken, fish, cheese, cottage cheese, or yogurt

- **Exercise.** Moving your body helps you to feel better and improves your self-esteem. Arrange a time every day or as often as possible when you can get some exercise, preferably outdoors. You can do many different things. Taking a walk is the most common. You could run, ride a bicycle, play a sport, climb up and down stairs several times, put on a tape, or play the radio and dance to the music—anything that feels good to you. If you have a health problem that may restrict your ability to exercise, check with your doctor before beginning or changing your exercise habits.

- **Keep yourself clean.** Do personal hygiene tasks that make you feel better about yourself–things like taking a regular shower or bath, washing and styling your hair, trimming your nails, brushing and flossing your teeth.

  - Have a physical examination every year to make sure you are in good health.

  - Plan fun activities for yourself. Learn new things every day.

- **Take time to do things you enjoy.** You may be so busy, or feel so badly about yourself, that you spend little or no time doing things you enjoy--things like playing a musical instrument, doing a craft project, flying a kite, or going fishing. Make a list of things you enjoy doing. Then do something from that list every day. Add to the list anything new that you discover you enjoy doing.

- **Stop procrastinating.** Get something done that you have been putting off. Clean out that drawer. Wash that window. Write that letter. Pay that bill.

- **Use your special talents and abilities.** For instance, if you are good with your hands, then make things for yourself, family, and friends. If you like animals, consider having a pet or at least playing with friends' pets.

- **Dress well.** Dress in clothes that make you feel good about yourself. If you have little money to spend on new clothes, check out thrift stores in your area.

- **Give yourself rewards.** You are a great person. Listen to a CD or tape.

- **Spend time with people.** Spend time with those who make you feel good about yourself—people who treat you well. Avoid people who treat you badly.

- **Make your living space a place that honors the person you are.** Whether you live in a single room, a small apartment, or a large home, make that space comfortable and attractive for you. If you share your living space with others, have some space that is just for you--a place where you can keep your things and know that they will not be disturbed and that you can decorate any way you choose.

- **Display items that you find attractive.** You can also display items that remind you of your achievements and of the special times and special people in your life. If cost is a factor, use your creativity to think of inexpensive or free ways that you can add to the comfort and enjoyment of your space.

- **Make your meals a special time.** Turn off the television, radio, and stereo. Set the table, even if you are eating alone. Light a candle or put some flowers or an attractive object in the center of the table. Arrange your food in an attractive way on your plate. If you eat with others, encourage discussion of pleasant topics. Avoid discussing difficult issues at meals.

- **Take advantage of opportunities to learn.** Learn something new or improve your skills. Take a class or go to a seminar. Many adult education programs are free or very inexpensive. For those that are more costly, ask about a possible scholarship or fee reduction.

- **Begin doing those things that make you feel better about yourself.** Go on a diet, begin an exercise program, or keep your living space clean.

- **Do something nice for another person.** Smile at someone who looks sad. Say a few kind words to the check-out cashier. Help your spouse with an unpleasant chore. Take a meal to a friend who is sick. Send a card to an acquaintance. Volunteer for a worthy organization.

- **Make it a point to treat yourself well every day.** Before you go to bed each night, write about how you treated yourself well during the day.

You may be doing some of these things now. There will be others you need to work on. You will find that you will continue to learn new and better ways to take care of yourself. As you incorporate these changes into your life, your self-esteem will continue to improve.

Changing Negative Thoughts About Yourself To Positive Ones

You may be giving yourself negative messages about yourself. Many people do. These are messages that you learned when you were young. You learned from many different sources including other children, your teachers, family members, caregivers, even from the media, and from prejudice and stigma in our society.

Once you have learned them, you may have repeated these negative messages over and over to yourself, especially when you were not feeling well or when you were having a hard time. You may have come to believe them. You may have even worsened the problem by making up some negative messages or thoughts of your own. These negative thoughts or messages make you feel bad about yourself and lower your self-esteem.

Some examples of common negative messages that people repeat over and over to themselves include: "I am a jerk," "I am a loser," "I never do anything right," "No one would ever like me," "I am a klutz." Most people believe these messages—no matter how untrue or unreal they are. They come up immediately in the right circumstance, for instance: If you get a wrong answer, you think, "I am so stupid." They may include words like *should, ought,* or *must.* The messages tend to imagine the worst in everything, especially you, and they are hard to turn off or unlearn.

You may think these thoughts or give yourself these negative messages so often that you are hardly aware of them. Pay attention to them. Carry a small pad with you as you go about your daily routine for several days, and jot down negative thoughts about yourself whenever you notice them. Some people say they notice more negative thinking when they are tired, sick, or dealing with a lot of stress. As you become aware of your negative thoughts, you may notice more and more of them.

It helps to take a closer look at your negative thought patterns to check out whether or not they are true. You may want a close friend or counselor to help you with this. When you are in a good mood and when you have a positive attitude about yourself, ask yourself the following questions about each negative thought you have noticed:

- Is this message really true?

- Would a person say this to another person? If not, why am I saying it to myself?

- What do I get out of thinking this thought? If it makes me feel badly about myself, why not stop thinking it?

You could also ask someone else—someone who likes you and who you trust—if you should believe this thought about yourself. Often, just looking at a thought or situation in a new light helps.

The next step in this process is to develop positive statements you can say to yourself to replace these negative thoughts whenever you notice yourself thinking them. You can't think two thoughts at the same time. When you are thinking a positive thought about yourself, you can't be thinking a negative one. In developing these thoughts, use positive words like happy, peaceful, loving, enthusiastic, and warm. Avoid using negative words such as worried, frightened, upset, tired, bored, not, never, and can't.

Don't make a statement like "I am not going to worry anymore." Instead say "I focus on the positive" or whatever feels right to you. Substitute "it would be nice if" for "should." Always use the present tense as if the condition already exists ("I am healthy, I am well, I am happy, I have a good job"). Use I, me, or your own name.

You can do this by folding a piece of paper in half the long way to make two columns. In one column write your negative thought and in the other column write a positive thought that contradicts the negative thought as shown in Table 54.1.

You can work on changing your negative thoughts to positive ones by:

- Replacing the negative thought with the positive one every time you realize you are thinking the negative thought

Table 54.1 Replacing Negative Thoughts With Positive Ones

Negative Thought	Positive Thought
I am not worth anything.	I am a valuable person.
I have never accomplished anything.	I have accomplished many things.
I always make mistakes.	I do many things well.
I am a jerk.	I am a great person.
I don't deserve a good life.	I deserve to be happy and healthy.
I am stupid.	I am smart.

- Repeating your positive thought over and over to yourself, out loud whenever you get a chance and even sharing them with another person, if possible

- Writing them over and over

- Making signs that say the positive thought, hanging them in places where you would see them often-like on your refrigerator door or on the mirror in your bathroom—and repeating the thought to yourself several times when you see it

It helps to reinforce the positive thought if you repeat it over and over to yourself when you are deeply relaxed, like when you are doing a deep-breathing or relaxation exercise, or when you are just falling asleep or waking up.

Changing the negative thoughts you have about yourself to positive ones takes time and persistence. If you use the following techniques consistently for four to six weeks, you will notice that you don't think these negative thoughts about yourself as much. If they recur at some other time, you can repeat these activities. Don't give up. You deserve to think good thoughts about yourself.

Activities That Will Help You Feel Good About Yourself

Any of the following activities will help you feel better about yourself and reinforce your self-esteem over the long term. Read through them. Do those that seem most comfortable to you. You may want to do some of the other activities at another time. You may find it helpful to repeat some of these activities again and again.

Make Affirming Lists

Making lists, rereading them often, and rewriting them from time to time will help you to feel better about yourself. If you have a journal, you can write your lists there. If you don't, any piece of paper will do. Make a list of:

- At least five of your strengths (for example, persistence, courage, friendliness, creativity)

- At least five things you admire about yourself (for example, your good relationship with your brother or your spirituality)

- The five greatest achievements in your life so far, like recovering from a serious illness, doing well in school, or learning to use a computer

- At least 20 accomplishments—simple or advanced

- Ten ways you can "treat" or reward yourself that don't include food and don't cost anything (such as walking in woods, window-shopping, watching children playing on a playground, gazing at a baby's face or at a beautiful flower, or chatting with a friend)

- Ten things you can do to make yourself laugh

- Ten things you could do to help someone else

- Ten things that you do that make you feel good about yourself

Reinforcing A Positive Self-Image

To do this exercise, you will need a piece of paper, a pencil or pen, and a timer or clock. Any kind of paper will do, but if you have paper and pen you really like, that will be even better.

Set a timer for 10 minutes or note the time on your watch or a clock. Write your name across the top of the paper. Then, write everything positive and good you can think of about yourself. Include special attributes, talents, and achievements. You can use single words or sentences, whichever you prefer. You can write the same things over and over, if you want to emphasize them. Don't worry about spelling or grammar. Your ideas don't have to be organized. Write down whatever comes to mind. You are the only one who will see this paper. Avoid making any negative statements or using any negative words—only positive ones. When the 10 minutes are up, read the paper over to yourself. You may feel sad when you read it over because it is a new, different, and positive way of thinking about yourself—a way that contradicts some of the negative thoughts you may have had about yourself. Those feelings will diminish as you reread this paper. Read the paper over again several times. Put it in a convenient place—your pocket, purse, wallet, or the table beside your bed. Read it over to yourself at least several times a day to keep reminding yourself of how great you are! Find a private space and read it aloud. If you can, read it to a good friend or family member who is supportive.

Developing Positive Affirmations

Affirmations are positive statements that you can make about yourself that make you feel better about yourself. They describe ways you would like to feel about yourself all the time. They may not, however, describe how you feel about yourself right now. The following examples of affirmations will help you in making your own list of affirmations:

- I feel good about myself.

- I take good care of myself. I eat right, get plenty of exercise, do things I enjoy, get good health care, and attend to my personal hygiene needs.

- I spend my time with people who are nice to me and make me feel good about myself.

- I am a good person.

- I deserve to be alive.

- Many people like me.

Make a list of your own affirmations. Keep this list in a handy place, like your pocket or purse. You may want to make copies of your list so you can have them in several different places of easy access. Read the affirmations over and over to yourself, reading aloud whenever you can. Share them with others when you feel like it. Write them down from time to time. As you do this, the affirmations tend to gradually become true for you.

You gradually come to feel better and better about yourself.

Your Personal "Celebratory Scrapbook" And Place To Honor Yourself

Develop a scrapbook that celebrates you and the wonderful person you are. Include pictures of yourself at different ages, writings you enjoy, mementos of things you have done and places you have been, cards you have received, etc. Or set up a place in your home that celebrates "you." It could be on a bureau, shelf, or table. Decorate the space with objects that remind you of the special person you are. If you don't have a private space that you can leave set up, put the objects in a special bag, box, or your purse and set them up in the space whenever you do this work. Take them out and look at them whenever you need to bolster your self-esteem.

Appreciation Exercise

At the top of a sheet of paper write "I like _____ (your name) because:" Have friends, acquaintances, family members, etc., write an appreciative statement about you on it. When you read it, don't deny it or argue with what has been written, just accept it! Read this paper over and over. Keep it in a place where you will see it often.

Self-Esteem Calendar

Get a calendar with large blank spaces for each day. Schedule into each day some small thing you would enjoy doing, such as "go into a flower shop and smell the flowers," "call my sister," "draw a sketch of my cat," "buy a new CD," "tell my mom I love her," "bake brownies," "wear my favorite scent," etc. Now make a commitment to check your "enjoy life" calendar every day and do whatever you have scheduled for yourself.

Mutual Complimenting Exercise

Get together for 10 minutes with a person you like and trust. Set a timer for five minutes or note the time on a watch or clock. One of you begins by complimenting the other person—saying everything positive about the other person—for the first five minutes. Then, the other person does the same thing to that person for the next five minutes. Notice how you feel about yourself before and after this exercise. Repeat it often.

Self-Esteem Resources

Go to your library. Look up books on self-esteem. Read one or several of them. Try some of the suggested activities.

This chapter is just the beginning of the journey. As you work on building your self-esteem, you will notice that you feel better more and more often, that you are enjoying your life more than you did before, and that you are doing more of the things you have always wanted to do.

Chapter 55

Improving Mental Health

Your mental health is very important. You will not have a healthy body if you don't also take care of your mind. People depend on you. It's important for you to take care of yourself so that you can do the important things in life—whether it's working, learning, taking care of your family, volunteering, enjoying the outdoors, or whatever is important to you.

Good mental health helps you enjoy life and cope with problems. It offers a feeling of well-being and inner strength. Just as you take care of your body by eating right and exercising, you can do things to protect your mental health. In fact, eating right and exercising can help maintain good mental health. You don't automatically have good mental health just because you don't have mental health illness. You have to work to keep your mind healthy.

Nutrition And Mental Health

The food you eat can have a direct effect on your energy level, physical health, and mood. A "healthy diet" is one that has enough of each essential nutrient, contains many foods from all of the basic food groups, provides the right amount of calories to maintain a healthy weight, and does not have too much fat, sugar, salt, or alcohol.

By choosing foods that can give you steady energy, you can help your body stay healthy. (Visit choosemyplate.gov to help find personalized eating plans and other interactive tools to help you make good food choices.) This may also help your mind feel good. The same diet doesn't work for every person. In order to find the best foods that are right for you, talk to your

About This Chapter: Excerpted from "Good Mental Health," Office on Women's Health (www.womenshealth .gov), U.S. Department of Health and Human Services, April 2013.

health care professional. Some vitamins and minerals may help with the symptoms of depression. Experts are looking into how a lack of some nutrients—including folate, vitamin B12, calcium, iron, selenium, zinc, and omega-3—may contribute to depression in new mothers. Ask your doctor or another health care professional for more information.

Exercise And Mental Health

Regular physical activity is important to the physical and mental health of almost everyone, including older adults. Being physically active can help you continue to do the things you enjoy and stay independent as you age. Regular physical activity over long periods of time can produce long-term health benefits. That's why health experts say that everyone should be active every day to maintain their health.

If you are diagnosed with depression or anxiety, your doctor may tell you to exercise in addition to taking any medications or receiving counseling. This is because exercise has been shown to help with the symptoms of depression and anxiety. Your body makes certain chemicals, called endorphins, before and after you work out. They relieve stress and improve your mood. Exercise can also slow or stop weight gain, which is a common side effect of some medications used to treat mental health disorders.

Sleep And Mental Health

Your mind and body will feel better if you sleep well. Your body needs time every day to rest and heal. If you often have trouble sleeping—either falling asleep, or waking during the night and being unable to get back to sleep—one or several of the following ideas might be helpful to you:

- Go to bed at the same time every night and get up at the same time every morning. Avoid "sleeping in" (sleeping much later than your usual time for getting up). It will make you feel worse.

- Establish a bedtime "ritual" by doing the same things every night for an hour or two before bedtime so your body knows when it is time to go to sleep.

- Avoid caffeine, nicotine, and alcohol.

- Eat on a regular schedule and avoid a heavy meal prior to going to bed. Don't skip any meals.

- Eat plenty of dairy foods and dark green leafy vegetables.

- Exercise daily, but avoid strenuous or invigorating activity before going to bed.

- Play soothing music on a tape or CD that shuts off automatically after you are in bed.

- Try a turkey sandwich and a glass of milk before bedtime to make you feel drowsy.

- Try having a small snack before you go to bed, something like a piece of fruit and a piece of cheese, so you don't wake up hungry in the middle of the night. Have a similar small snack if you awaken in the middle of the night.

- Take a warm bath or shower before going to bed.

- Place a drop of lavender oil on your pillow.

- Drink a cup of herbal chamomile tea before going to bed.

You need to see your doctor if:

- You often have difficulty sleeping and the solutions listed above are not working for you

- You awaken during the night gasping for breath

- Your breathing stops when you are sleeping

- You snore loudly

- You wake up feeling like you haven't been asleep

- You fall asleep often during the day

Stress And Mental Health

Stress can happen for many reasons. Stress can be brought about by a traumatic accident, death, or emergency situation. Stress can also be a side effect of a serious illness or disease.

There is also stress associated with daily life, the workplace, and family responsibilities. It's hard to stay calm and relaxed in our hectic lives. With all we have going on in our lives, it seems almost impossible to find ways to de-stress. But it's important to find those ways. Your health depends on it.

Common symptoms of stress include:

- Headache

- Sleep disorders

- Difficulty concentrating

- Short-temper

- Upset stomach

- Dissatisfaction (with school and/or job)

- Low morale

- Depression

- Anxiety

Remember to always make time for you. It's important to care for yourself. Think of this as an order from your doctor, so you don't feel guilty! No matter how busy you are, you can try to set aside at least 15 minutes each day in your schedule to do something for yourself, like taking a bubble bath, going for a walk, or calling a friend.

Chapter 56

Dealing With Depression: Self-Help And Coping Tips

Depression drains your energy, hope, and drive, making it difficult to do what you need to feel better. But while overcoming depression isn't quick or easy, it's far from impossible. You can't beat it through sheer willpower, but you do have some control—even if your depression is severe and stubbornly persistent. The key is to start small and build from there. Feeling better takes time, but you can get there if you make positive choices for yourself each day.

The Road To Depression Recovery

Recovering from depression requires action, but taking action when you're depressed is hard. In fact, just thinking about the things you should do to feel better, like going for a walk or spending time with friends, can be exhausting.

It's the Catch-22 of depression recovery: The things that help the most are the things that are the most difficult to do. There's a difference, however, between something that's difficult and something that's impossible.

Start Small And Stay Focused

The key to depression recovery is to start with a few small goals and slowly build from there. Draw upon whatever resources you have. You may not have much energy, but you probably have enough to take a short walk around the block or pick up the phone to call a loved one.

Take things one day at a time and reward yourself for each accomplishment. The steps may seem small, but they'll quickly add up. And for all the energy you put into your depression recovery, you'll get back much more in return.

Depression Self-Help Tip 1: Cultivate Supportive Relationships

Getting the support you need plays a big role in lifting the fog of depression and keeping it away. On your own, it can be difficult to maintain perspective and sustain the effort required to beat depression, but the very nature of depression makes it difficult to reach out for help. However, isolation and loneliness make depression even worse, so maintaining your close relationships and social activities are important.

The thought of reaching out to even close family members and friends can seem overwhelming. You may feel ashamed, too exhausted to talk, or guilty for neglecting the relationship. Remind yourself that this is the depression talking. Your loved ones care about you and want to help.

- **Turn to trusted friends and family members.** Share what you're going through with the people you love and trust. Ask for the help and support you need. You may have retreated from your most treasured relationships, but they can get you through this tough time.

- **Try to keep up with social activities even if you don't feel like it.** Often when you're depressed, it feels more comfortable to retreat into your shell, but being around other people will make you feel less depressed.

- **Join a support group for depression.** Being with others dealing with depression can go a long way in reducing your sense of isolation. You can also encourage each other, give and receive advice on how to cope, and share your experiences.

Depression Self-Help Tip 2: Challenge Negative Thinking

Depression puts a negative spin on everything, including the way you see yourself, the situations you encounter, and your expectations for the future.

But you can't break out of this pessimistic mind frame by "just thinking positive." Happy thoughts or wishful thinking won't cut it. Rather, the trick is to replace negative thoughts with more balanced thoughts. Ways to challenge negative thinking, [include]:

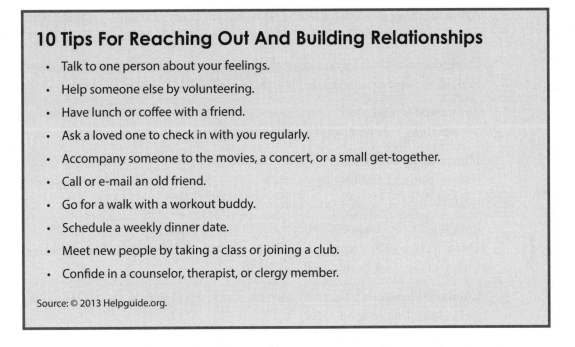

10 Tips For Reaching Out And Building Relationships

- Talk to one person about your feelings.
- Help someone else by volunteering.
- Have lunch or coffee with a friend.
- Ask a loved one to check in with you regularly.
- Accompany someone to the movies, a concert, or a small get-together.
- Call or e-mail an old friend.
- Go for a walk with a workout buddy.
- Schedule a weekly dinner date.
- Meet new people by taking a class or joining a club.
- Confide in a counselor, therapist, or clergy member.

Source: © 2013 Helpguide.org.

- **Think outside yourself.** Ask yourself if you'd say what you're thinking about yourself to someone else. If not, stop being so hard on yourself. Think about less harsh statements that offer more realistic descriptions.

- **Allow yourself to be less than perfect.** Many depressed people are perfectionists, holding themselves to impossibly high standards and then beating themselves up when they fail to meet them. Battle this source of self-imposed stress by challenging your negative ways of thinking

- **Socialize with positive people.** Notice how people who always look on the bright side deal with challenges, even minor ones, like not being able to find a parking space. Then consider how you would react in the same situation. Even if you have to pretend, try to adopt their optimism and persistence in the face of difficulty.

- **Keep a "negative thought log."** Whenever you experience a negative thought, jot down the thought and what triggered it in a notebook. Review your log when you're in a good mood. Consider if the negativity was truly warranted. Ask yourself if there's another way to view the situation. For example, let's say your boyfriend was short with you and you automatically assumed that the relationship was in trouble. It's possible, though, he's just having a bad day. Types of negative thinking that add to depression, [include]:

- **All-or-nothing thinking:** Looking at things in "black or white" categories, with no middle ground ("If I fall short of perfection, I'm a total failure.")

- **Overgeneralization:** Generalizing from a single negative experience, expecting it to hold true forever ("I can't do anything right.")

- **The mental filter:** Ignoring positive events and focusing on the negative; noticing the one thing that went wrong, rather than all the things that went right

- **Diminishing the positive:** Coming up with reasons why positive events don't count ("She said she had a good time on our date, but I think she was just being nice.")

- **Jumping to conclusions:** Making negative interpretations without actual evidence; [acting] like a mind reader ("He must think I'm pathetic.") or a fortune teller ("I'll be stuck in this dead end job forever.")

- **Emotional reasoning:** Believing that the way you feel reflects reality ("I feel like such a loser. I really am no good!")

- **"Shoulds" and "should nots":** Holding yourself to a strict list of what you should and shouldn't do, and beating yourself up if you don't live up to your rules

- **Labeling:** Labeling yourself based on mistakes and perceived shortcomings ("I'm a failure; an idiot; a loser.")

Depression Self-Help Tip 3: Take Care Of Yourself

In order to overcome depression, you have to take care of yourself. This includes following a healthy lifestyle, learning to manage stress, setting limits on what you're able to do, adopting healthy habits, and scheduling fun activities into your day.

- **Aim for eight hours of sleep.** Depression typically involves sleep problems. Whether you're sleeping too little or too much, your mood suffers. Get on a better sleep schedule by learning healthy sleep habits.

- **Expose yourself to a little sunlight every day.** Lack of sunlight can make depression worse. Make sure you're getting enough. Take a short walk outdoors, have your coffee outside, enjoy an al fresco meal, "people watch" on a park bench, or sit out in the garden. Aim for at least 15 minutes of sunlight a day to boost your mood. If you live somewhere with little winter sunshine, try using a light therapy box.

- **Keep stress in check.** Not only does stress prolong and worsen depression, but it can also trigger it. Figure out all the things in your life that stress you out. Examples include: work overload, unsupportive relationships, taking on too much, or health problems. Once you've identified your stressors, you can make a plan to avoid them or minimize their impact.

- **Practice relaxation techniques.** A daily relaxation practice can help relieve symptoms of depression, reduce stress, and boost feelings of joy and well-being. Try yoga, deep breathing, progressive muscle relaxation, or meditation.

- **Care for a pet.** While nothing can replace the human connection, pets can bring joy and companionship into your life and help you feel less isolated. Caring for a pet can also get you outside of yourself and give you a sense of being needed—both powerful antidotes to depression.

- **Do things you enjoy (or used to).** While you can't force yourself to have fun or experience pleasure, you can choose to do things that you used to enjoy. Pick up a former hobby or a sport you used to like. Express yourself creatively through music, art, or writing. Go out with friends. Take a day trip to a museum, the mountains, or the ballpark.

- **Push yourself to do things (even when you don't feel like it).** You might be surprised at how much better you feel once you're out in the world. Even if your depression doesn't lift immediately, you'll gradually feel more upbeat and energetic as you make time for fun activities.

Develop A Wellness Toolbox

Come up with a list of things that you can do for a quick mood boost. Include any strategies, activities, or skills that have helped in the past. The more "tools" for coping with depression, the better. Try and implement a few of these ideas each day, even if you're feeling good:

- Spend some time in nature.
- Read a good book.
- Take a long, hot bath.
- Play with a pet.
- Listen to music.

- List what you like about yourself.
- Watch a funny movie or TV show.
- Take care of a few small tasks.
- Write in your journal.
- Do something spontaneous.

Source: © 2013 Helpguide.org.

Depression Self-Help Tip 4: Get Regular Exercise

When you're depressed, exercising may be the last thing you feel like doing. But exercise is a powerful tool for dealing with depression. In fact, studies show that regular exercise can be as effective as antidepressant medication at increasing energy levels and decreasing feelings of fatigue.

Scientists haven't figured out exactly why exercise is such a potent antidepressant, but evidence suggests that physical activity triggers new cell growth in the brain, increases mood-enhancing neurotransmitters and endorphins, reduces stress, and relieves muscle tension—all things that can have a positive effect on depression.

To gain the most benefits, aim for 30 minutes of exercise per day. You can start small, though, as short 10-minute bursts of activity can have a positive effect on your mood. Here are a few easy ways to get moving:

- Take the stairs rather than the elevator.

- Park your car in the farthest spot in the lot.

- Take your dog for a walk.

- Pair up with an exercise partner.

- Walk while you're talking on the phone.

Exercise As An Antidepressant

The following exercise tips offer a powerful prescription for boosting mood:

- Exercise now…and again. A 10-minute walk can improve your mood for two hours. The key to sustaining mood benefits is to exercise regularly.

- Choose activities that are moderately intense. Aerobic exercise undoubtedly has mental health benefits, but you don't need to sweat strenuously to see results.

- Find exercises that are continuous and rhythmic (rather than intermittent). Walking, swimming, dancing, stationery biking, and yoga are good choices.

- Add a mind-body element. Activities such as yoga and tai chi rest your mind and increase your energy. You can also add a meditative element to walking or swimming by repeating a mantra (a word or phrase) as you move.

- Start slowly, and don't overdo it. More isn't better. Athletes who over train find their moods drop rather than lift.

Source: Adapted from Johns Hopkins Health Alerts, © 2013 Helpguide.org.

As a next step, try incorporating walks or some other enjoyable, easy form of exercise into your daily routine. The key is to pick an activity you enjoy, so you're more likely to keep up with it.

Depression Self-Help Tip 5: Eat A Healthy, Mood-Boosting Diet

Eat a healthy, mood-boosting diet. What you eat has a direct impact on the way you feel. Aim for a balanced diet of low-fat protein, complex carbohydrates, fruits and vegetables. Reduce your intake of foods that can adversely affect your brain and mood, such as caffeine, alcohol, trans fats, saturated fats, and foods with high levels of chemical preservatives or hormones (such as, certain meats).

- **Don't skip meals.** Going too long between meals can make you feel irritable and tired, so aim to eat something at least every three to four hours.

- **Minimize sugar and refined carbs.** You may crave sugary snacks, baked goods, or comfort foods such as pasta or French fries, but these "feel-good" foods quickly lead to a crash in mood and energy.

- **Focus on complex carbohydrates.** Foods such as baked potatoes, whole-wheat pasta, oatmeal, and whole grain breads can boost serotonin levels without a crash.

- **Boost your B vitamins.** Deficiencies in B vitamins such as folic acid and B-12 can trigger depression. To get more, take a B-complex vitamin supplement or eat more citrus fruit, leafy greens, beans, chicken, and eggs.

- **Try super-foods**. [Foods] rich in nutrients that can boost mood, such as bananas (magnesium to decrease anxiety, vitamin B6 to promote alertness, tryptophan to boost feel-good serotonin levels), brown rice (serotonin, thiamine to support sociability), and spinach (magnesium, folate to reduce agitation and improve sleep).

- **Consider taking a chromium supplement.** Some depression studies show that chromium picolinate reduces carbohydrate cravings, eases mood swings, and boosts energy. Supplementing with chromium picolinate is especially effective for people who tend to overeat and oversleep when depressed.

Omega-3 Fatty Acids Play An Essential Role In Stabilizing Mood

Foods rich in certain omega-3 fats called eicosapentaenoic acid (EPA) and docosahexaenoic acid (DHA) can give your mood a big boost. The best sources are fatty fish such as salmon, herring, mackerel, anchovies, sardines, and some cold-water fish oil supplements. Canned albacore tuna and lake trout can also be good sources, depending on how the fish were raised and processed. When cooking fish, grill or bake rather than fry.

You may hear a lot about getting your omega-3s from foods rich in alpha-linolenic acid (ALA) fatty acids, such as vegetable oils and nuts (especially walnuts), flax, soybeans, and tofu. Be aware that our bodies generally convert very little ALA into EPA and DHA, so you may not see as big of a benefit.

Some people avoid seafood because they worry about mercury or other possible toxins, but most experts agree that the benefits of eating one or two servings a week of cold-water fatty fish outweigh the risks.

Depression Self-Help Tip 6:
Know When To Get Additional Help

If you find your depression getting worse and worse, seek professional help. Needing additional help doesn't mean you're weak. Sometimes the negative thinking in depression can make you feel like you're a lost cause, but depression can be treated and you can feel better!

Don't forget about these self-help tips, though. Even if you're receiving professional help, these tips can be part of your treatment plan, speeding your recovery and preventing depression from returning.

Chapter 57

Coping With Stress

Everyone—adults, teens, and even children—experiences stress at times. Stress can be beneficial by helping people develop the skills they need to cope with and adapt to new and potentially threatening situations throughout life. However, the beneficial aspects of stress diminish when it is severe enough to overwhelm a person's ability to take care of themselves. Using healthy ways to cope and getting the right care and support can put problems in perspective and help stressful feelings and symptoms subside.

Stress is a condition that is often characterized by symptoms of physical or emotional tension. It is a reaction to a situation where a person feels threatened or anxious. Stress can be positive (for example, preparing for a wedding) or negative (for example, dealing with a natural disaster).

Sometimes, after experiencing a traumatic event that is especially frightening—including personal or environmental disasters, or being threatened with an assault—people have a strong and lingering stress reaction to the event. Strong emotions, jitters, sadness, or depression may all be part of this normal and temporary reaction to the stress of an overwhelming event.

Common reactions to a stressful event can include:

- Disbelief, shock, and numbness

- Feeling sad, frustrated, and helpless

- Fear and anxiety about the future

- Feeling guilty

About This Chapter: Excerpted from "Coping With Stress," Centers for Disease Control and Prevention (CDC; www.cdc.gov), April 2013, and "Feelin' Frazzled," BAM! Body and Mind, CDC, January 2013.

- Anger, tension, and irritability

- Difficulty concentrating and making decisions

- Crying

- Reduced interest in usual activities

- Wanting to be alone

- Loss of appetite

- Sleeping too much or too little

- Nightmares or bad memories

- Reoccurring thoughts of the event

- Headaches, back pains, and stomach problems

- Increased heart rate, difficulty breathing

- Smoking or use of alcohol or drugs

Healthy Ways To Cope With Stress

Feeling emotional and nervous or having trouble sleeping and eating can all be normal reactions to stress. Engaging in healthy activities and getting the right care and support can put problems in perspective and help stressful feelings subside in a few days or weeks. Some tips for beginning to feel better are:

- **Take care of yourself.** Eat healthy, well-balanced meals; exercise on a regular basis; get plenty of sleep; and give yourself a break if you feel stressed out.

- **Talk to others.** Share your problems and how you are feeling and coping with a parent, friend, counselor, doctor, or pastor.

- **Avoid drugs and alcohol.** Drugs and alcohol may seem to help with the stress. In the long run, they create additional problems and increase the stress you are already feeling.

- **Take a break.** If your stress is caused by a national or local event, take breaks from listening to the news stories, which can increase your stress.

- **Recognize when you need more help.** If problems continue or you are thinking about suicide, talk to a psychologist, social worker, or professional counselor.

Source: Excerpted from "Coping With Stress," CDC, April 2013.

Feeling Frazzled?

Finding yourself in a hectic situation, whether it's forgetting your homework or missing your ride home, can really stress you out. Are you looking for a safety net for those days that seem to get worse by the second? Could you really use some advice on how to de-stress both your body and your mind? Knowing how to deal can be half the battle! Check out the following tips to keep you cool, calm, and collected.

Put Your Body In Motion

Moving from the chair to the couch while watching TV is not being physically active! Physical activity is one of the most important ways to keep stress away by clearing your head and lifting your spirits. Physical activity also increases endorphin levels—the natural "feel-good" chemicals in the body which leave you with a naturally happy feeling. Whether you like full-fledged games of football, tennis, or roller hockey, or you prefer walks with family and friends, it's important to get up, get out, and get moving!

Fuel Up

Start your day off with a full tank—eating breakfast will give you the energy you need to tackle the day. Eating regular meals (this means no skipping dinner) and taking time to enjoy them (nope, eating in the car on the way to practice doesn't count) will make you feel better too.

Make sure to fuel up with fruits, vegetables, proteins (peanut butter, a chicken sandwich, or a tuna salad) and grains (wheat bread, pasta, or some crackers)—these will give you the power you need to make it through those hectic days.

Don't be fooled by the jolt of energy you get from sodas and sugary snacks—this only lasts a short time, and once it wears off, you may feel sluggish and more tired than usual. For that extra boost of energy to sail through history notes, math class, and after school activities, grab a banana, some string cheese, or a granola bar for some power-packed energy!

Laugh Out Loud (LOL!)

Some say that laughter is the best medicine—well, in many cases, it is! Did you know that it takes 15 facial muscles to laugh? Lots of laughing can make you feel good—and, that good feeling can stay with you even after the laughter stops. So, head off stress with regular doses of laughter by watching a funny movie or cartoons, reading a joke book (you may even learn some new jokes), or even make up your own riddles. Laughter can make you feel like a new person!

Everyone has those days when they do something really silly or stupid—instead of getting upset with yourself, laugh out loud! No one's perfect! Life should be about having fun. So, lighten up!

Have Fun With Friends

Being with people you like is always a good way to ditch your stress. Get a group together to go to the movies, shoot some hoops, or play a board game—or just hang out and talk. Friends can help you work through your problems and let you see the brighter side of things.

Spill To Someone You Trust

Instead of keeping your feelings bottled up inside, talk to someone you trust or respect about what's bothering you. It could be a friend, a parent, someone in your family, or a teacher. Talking out your problems and seeing them from a different view might help you figure out ways to deal with them. Just remember, you don't have to go it alone!

Tips For Coping With Stress

After a traumatic or violent event, it is normal to feel anxious about your safety and security. Even if you were not directly involved, you may worry about whether this type of event may someday affect you. How can you deal with these fears? Start by looking at the tips below for some ideas.

- **Talk to and stay connected to others.** This connection might be your parent, another relative, a friend, neighbor, teacher, coach, school nurse, counselor, family doctor, or member of your church or temple. Talking with someone can help you make sense out of your experience and figure out ways to feel better. If you are not sure where to turn, call your local crisis intervention center or a national hotline.

- **Get active.** Go for a walk, play sports, write a play or poem, play a musical instrument, or join an after-school program. Volunteer with a community group that promotes nonviolence or another school or community activity that you care about. Trying any of these can be a positive way to handle your feelings and to see that things are going to get better.

- **Take care of yourself.** As much as possible, try to get enough sleep, eat right, exercise, and keep a normal routine. It may be hard to do, but by keeping yourself healthy you will be better able to handle a tough time.

- **Take information breaks.** Pictures and stories about a disaster can increase worry and other stressful feelings. Taking breaks from the news, Internet, and conversations about the disaster can help calm you down.

Source: Excerpted from "Coping With Stress," CDC, April 2013.

Take Time To Chill

Pick a comfy spot to sit and read, daydream, or even take a snooze. Listen to your favorite music. Work on a relaxing project like putting together a puzzle or making jewelry.

Stress can sometimes make you feel like a tight rubber band—stretched to the limit! If this happens, take a few deep breaths to help yourself unwind. If you're in the middle of an impossible homework problem, take a break! Finding time to relax after (and sometimes during) a hectic day or week can make all the difference.

Catch Some Zzzzz...

Fatigue is a best friend to stress. When you don't get enough sleep, it's hard to deal—you may feel tired, cranky, or you may have trouble thinking clearly. When you're overtired, a problem may seem much bigger than it actually is. You may have a hard time doing a school assignment that usually seems easy, you don't do your best in sports or any physical activity, or you may have an argument with your friends over something really stupid.

Sleep is a big deal! Getting the right amount of sleep is especially important for kids your age. Because your body (and mind) is changing and developing, it requires more sleep to recharge for the next day. So don't resist, hit the hay!

Keep A Journal

If you're having one of those crazy days when nothing goes right, it's a good idea to write things down in a journal to get it off of your chest—like how you feel, what's going on in your life, and things you'd like to accomplish. You could even write down what you do when you're faced with a stressful situation, and then look back and think about how you handled it later. So, find a quiet spot, grab a notebook and pen, and start writing!

Get It Together

Too much to do but not enough time? Forgot your homework? Feeling overwhelmed or discombobulated? Being unprepared for school, practice, or other activities can make for a very stressful day! Getting everything done can be a challenge, but all you have to do is plan a little and get organized.

Lend A Hand

Get involved in an activity that helps others. It's almost impossible to feel stressed out when you're helping someone else. It's also a great way to find out about yourself and the special qualities you never knew you had! Signing up for a service project is a good idea, but helping others is as easy as saying hello, holding a door, or volunteering to keep a neighbor's pet. If you want to get involved in a more organized volunteer program, try working at a local recreation center, or helping with an after school program. The feeling you will get from helping others is greater than you can imagine!

Don't Sweat The Small Stuff

Try to pick a few really important things and let the rest slide—getting worked up over every little thing will only increase your stress. So, toughen up and don't let stressful situations get to you! Remember, you're not alone—everyone has stresses in their lives. It's up to you to choose how to deal with them.

Chapter 58

Coping With A Disaster Or Traumatic Event

If you've gone through a traumatic experience, you may be struggling with upsetting emotions, frightening memories, or a sense of constant danger. Or you may feel numb, disconnected, and unable to trust other people. When bad things happen, it can take a while to get over the pain and feel safe again. But with the right treatment, self-help strategies, and support, you can speed your recovery. Whether the traumatic event happened years ago or yesterday, you can heal and move on.

What Is Emotional And Psychological Trauma?

Emotional and psychological trauma is the result of extraordinarily stressful events that shatter your sense of security, making you feel helpless and vulnerable in a dangerous world.

Traumatic experiences often involve a threat to life or safety, but any situation that leaves you feeling overwhelmed and alone can be traumatic—even if it doesn't involve physical harm. It's not the objective facts that determine whether an event is traumatic, but your subjective emotional experience of the event. The more frightened and helpless you feel, the more likely you are to be traumatized.

Causes Of Emotional Or Psychological Trauma

An event will most likely lead to emotional or psychological trauma if:

About This Chapter: "Healing Emotional and Psychological Trauma: Symptoms, Treatment, and Recovery," by Lawrence Robinson, Melinda Smith, M.A., and Jeanne Segal, Ph.D., updated February 2013, © 2013 Helpguide.org. All rights reserved. Reprinted with permission. Helpguide provides a detailed list of references and resources for this article, with links to related Helpguide topics and information from other websites. For a complete list of these resources, go to http://www.helpguide.org/mental/emotional_psychological_trauma.htm.

- It happened unexpectedly.

- You were unprepared for it.

- You felt powerless to prevent it.

- It happened repeatedly.

- Someone was intentionally cruel.

- It happened in childhood.

Emotional and psychological trauma can be caused by single-blow, one-time events, such as a horrible accident, a natural disaster, or a violent attack. Trauma can also stem from ongoing, relentless stress, such as living in a crime-ridden neighborhood or struggling with cancer.

Risk Factors That Increase Your Vulnerability To Trauma

Not all potentially traumatic events lead to lasting emotional and psychological damage. Some people rebound quickly from even the most tragic and shocking experiences. Others are devastated by experiences that, on the surface, appear to be less upsetting.

A number of risk factors make people susceptible to emotional and psychological trauma. People are more likely to be traumatized by a stressful experience if they're already under a heavy stress load or have recently suffered a series of losses.

People are also more likely to be traumatized by a new situation if they've been traumatized before—especially if the earlier trauma occurred in childhood.

Childhood Trauma Increases The Risk Of Future Trauma

Experiencing trauma in childhood can have a severe and long-lasting effect. Children who have been traumatized see the world as a frightening and dangerous place. When childhood trauma is not resolved, this fundamental sense of fear and helplessness carries over into adulthood, setting the stage for further trauma.

Childhood trauma results from anything that disrupts a child's sense of safety and security, including:

- An unstable or unsafe environment

- Separation from a parent

- Serious illness

- Intrusive medical procedures

- Sexual, physical, or verbal abuse

- Domestic violence

- Neglect

- Bullying

Commonly Overlooked Causes Of Emotional And Psychological Trauma

- Falls or sports injuries
- Surgery (especially in the first three years of life)
- The sudden death of someone close
- A car accident
- The breakup of a significant relationship
- A humiliating or deeply disappointing experience
- The discovery of a life-threatening illness or disabling condition

Source: © 2013 Helpguide.org.

Symptoms Of Emotional And Psychological Trauma

Following a traumatic event, or repeated trauma, people react in different ways, experiencing a wide range of physical and emotional reactions. There is no "right" or "wrong" way to think, feel, or respond to trauma, so don't judge your own reactions or those of other people. Your responses are NORMAL reactions to ABNORMAL events.

Emotional and psychological symptoms of trauma [can include]:

- Shock, denial, or disbelief

- Anger, irritability, mood swings

- Guilt, shame, self-blame

- Feeling sad or hopeless

- Confusion, difficulty concentrating

- Anxiety and fear

- Withdrawing from others
- Feeling disconnected or numb

Physical symptoms of trauma [can include]:

- Insomnia or nightmares
- Being startled easily
- Racing heartbeat
- Aches and pains
- Fatigue
- Difficulty concentrating
- Edginess and agitation
- Muscle tension

These symptoms and feelings typically last from a few days to a few months, gradually fading as you process the trauma. But even when you're feeling better, you may be troubled from time to time by painful memories or emotions—especially in response to triggers such as an anniversary of the event or an image, sound, or situation that reminds you of the traumatic experience.

Grieving Is Normal Following Trauma

Whether or not a traumatic event involves death, survivors must cope with the loss, at least temporarily, of their sense of safety and security. The natural reaction to this loss is grief. Like people who have lost a loved one, trauma survivors go through a grieving process. This process, while inherently painful, is easier if you turn to others for support, take care of yourself, and talk about how you feel.

When To Seek Professional Help For Emotional Or Psychological Trauma

Recovering from a traumatic event takes time, and everyone heals at his or her own pace. But if months have passed and your symptoms aren't letting up, you may need professional help from a trauma expert. Seek help for emotional or psychological trauma if you're:

- Having trouble functioning at home, [school], or work

- Suffering from severe fear, anxiety, or depression

- Unable to form close, satisfying relationships

- Experiencing terrifying memories, nightmares, or flashbacks

- Avoiding more and more things that remind you of the trauma

- Emotionally numb and disconnected from others

- Using alcohol or drugs to feel better

Finding A Trauma Specialist

Working through trauma can be scary, painful, and potentially retraumatizing. Because of the risk of retraumatization, this healing work is best done with the help of an experienced trauma specialist.

Finding the right therapist may take some time. It's very important that the therapist you choose has experience treating trauma. But the quality of the relationship with your therapist is equally important. Choose a trauma specialist you feel comfortable with. Trust your instincts. If you don't feel safe, respected, or understood, find another therapist. There should be a sense of trust and warmth between you and your trauma therapist.

After meeting a potential trauma therapist, ask yourself these questions:

- Did you feel comfortable discussing your problems with the therapist?

- Did you feel like the therapist understood what you were talking about?

- Were your concerns taken seriously or were they minimized or dismissed?

- Were you treated with compassion and respect?

- Do you believe that you could grow to trust the therapist?

Treatment For Psychological And Emotional Trauma

In order to heal from psychological and emotional trauma, you must face and resolve the unbearable feelings and memories you've long avoided. Otherwise they will return again and again, unbidden and uncontrollable. Trauma treatment and healing involves:

- Processing trauma-related memories and feelings

- Discharging pent-up "fight-or-flight" energy

- Learning how to regulate strong emotions

- Building or rebuilding the ability to trust other people

Trauma Therapy Treatment Approaches

Trauma disrupts the body's natural equilibrium, freezing you in a state of hyperarousal and fear. In essence, your nervous system gets stuck in overdrive. Successful trauma treatment must address this imbalance and reestablish your physical sense of safety. The following therapies are commonly used in the treatment of emotional and psychological trauma:

Somatic Experiencing: Somatic experiencing takes advantage of the body's unique ability to heal itself. The focus of therapy is on bodily sensations, rather than thoughts and memories about the traumatic event. By concentrating on what's happening in your body, you gradually get in touch with trauma-related energy and tension. From there, your natural survival instincts take over, safely releasing this pent-up energy through shaking, crying, and other forms of physical release.

Eye Movement Desensitization And Reprocessing (EMDR): EMDR incorporates elements of cognitive-behavioral therapy with eye movements or other forms of rhythmic, left-right stimulation. These back-and-forth eye movements are thought to work by "unfreezing" traumatic memories, allowing you to resolve them.

Cognitive-Behavioral Therapy: Cognitive-behavioral therapy helps you process and evaluate your thoughts and feelings about a trauma. While cognitive-behavioral therapy doesn't treat the physiological effects of trauma, it can be helpful when used in addition to a body-based therapy such as somatic experiencing or EMDR.

Emotional And Psychological Trauma Recovery Tips

Recovering from emotional and psychological trauma takes time. Give yourself time to heal and to mourn the losses you've experienced. Don't try to force the healing process. Be patient with the pace of recovery. Finally, be prepared for difficult and volatile emotions. Allow yourself to feel whatever you're feeling without judgment or guilt.

Trauma Self-Help Strategy 1: Don't Isolate

Following a trauma, you may want to withdraw from others, but isolation makes things worse. Connecting to others will help you heal, so make an effort to maintain your relationships and avoid spending too much time alone.

- **Ask for support.** It's important to talk about your feelings and ask for the help you need. Turn to a trusted family member, friend, counselor, or clergyman.

- **Participate in social activities, even if you don't feel like it.** Do "normal" things with other people, things that have nothing to do with the traumatic experience. If you've retreated from relationships that were once important to you, make the effort to reconnect.

- **Join a support group for trauma survivors.** Being with others who are facing the same problems can help reduce your sense of isolation and hearing how others cope can help inspire you.

- **Volunteer.** As well as helping others, volunteering can be a great way to challenge the sense of helplessness that often accompanies trauma. Remind yourself of your strengths and reclaim your sense of power by comforting or helping others.

Trauma Self-Help Strategy 2: Stay Grounded

In order to stay grounded after a trauma, it helps to have a structured schedule to follow.

Stick to a daily routine, with regular times for waking, sleeping, eating, working, and exercise. Make sure to schedule time for relaxing and social activities, too.

Break large jobs into smaller, manageable tasks. Take pleasure from the accomplishment of achieving something, even it's a small thing.

Find activities that make you feel better and keep your mind occupied (reading, taking a class, cooking, playing with your kids or pets), so you're not dedicating all your energy and attention to focusing on the traumatic experience.

Staying Grounded: A Trauma Self-Help Exercise

If you are feeling disoriented, confused, or upset, you can do the following exercise:

- **Sit on a chair.** Feel your feet on the ground. Press on your thighs. Feel your behind on the seat and your back against the chair.
- **Look around you.** Pick six objects that have red or blue. This should allow you to feel in the present, more grounded, and in your body. Notice how your breath gets deeper and calmer.
- **Go outdoors.** You may want to go outdoors and find a peaceful place to sit on the grass. As you do, feel how your body can be held and supported by the ground.

Source: © 2013 Helpguide.org.

Allow yourself to feel what you feel when you feel it. Acknowledge your feelings about the trauma as they arise and accept them. Accepting your feelings is part of the grieving process and is necessary for healing.

Trauma Self-Help Strategy 3: Take Care Of Your Health

A healthy body increases your ability to cope with stress from a trauma.

- **Get plenty of sleep.** After a traumatic experience, worry or fear may disturb your sleep patterns. A lack of sleep can make your trauma symptoms worse and make it harder to maintain your emotional balance. Go to sleep and get up at the same time each day and aim for seven to nine hours of sleep each night.

- **Avoid alcohol and drugs.** Their use can worsen your trauma symptoms and exacerbate feelings of depression, anxiety, and isolation.

- **Exercise regularly.** Regular exercise boosts serotonin, endorphins, and other feel-good brain chemicals. It also boosts self-esteem and helps to improve sleep. For maximum results, aim for 30 to 60 minutes of activity on most days.

- **Eat a well-balanced diet.** Eating small, well-balanced meals throughout the day will help you keep your energy up and minimize mood swings. While you may be drawn to sugary foods for the quick boost they provide, complex carbohydrates are a better choice. Foods rich in certain omega-3 fats—such as salmon, walnuts, soybeans, and flaxseeds—can give your mood a boost.

- **Reduce stress.** Making time for rest and relaxation will help you bring your life back into balance. Try relaxation techniques such as meditation, yoga, or deep breathing exercises. Schedule time for activities that bring you joy—favorite hobbies or activities with friends, for example.

Helping Someone Deal With Emotional And Psychological Trauma

It can be difficult to know how to help a loved one who's suffered a traumatic or distressing experience, but your support can be a crucial factor in their recovery.

- **Be patient and understanding.** Healing from emotional or psychological trauma takes time. Be patient with the pace of recovery and remember that everyone's response to trauma is different. Don't judge your loved one's reaction against your own response or anyone else's.

- **Offer practical support.** [This will] help your loved one get back into a normal routine. That may mean help with collecting groceries or housework, for example, or simply being available to talk or listen.

- **Don't pressure your loved one into talking.** But, be available when they want to talk. Some trauma survivors find it difficult to talk about what happened. Don't force your loved one to open up but let them know you are there to listen whenever they feel ready.

- **Help your loved one to socialize and relax.** Encourage them to participate in physical exercise, seek out friends, and pursue hobbies and other activities that bring them pleasure. Take a fitness class together or set a regular lunch date with friends.

- **Don't take the trauma symptoms personally.** Your loved one may become angry, irritable, withdrawn, or emotionally distant. Remember that this is a result of the trauma and may not have anything to do with you or your relationship.

How Children React To Emotional And Psychological Trauma

Some common reactions to trauma and ways to help your child deal with them:

- **Regression:** Many children may try to return to an earlier stage when they felt safer and more cared for. Younger children may wet the bed or want a bottle; older children may fear being alone. It's important to be patient and comforting if [a] child responds this way.

- **Thinking The Event Is Their Fault:** Children younger than seven or eight tend to think that if something goes wrong, it must be their fault—no matter how irrational this may sound to an adult. Be sure [the] child understands that he [or she] did not cause the event.

- **Sleep Disorders:** Some children have difficulty falling to sleep; others wake frequently or have troubling dreams. If you can, give [the] child a stuffed animal, soft blanket, or flashlight to take to bed. Try spending extra time together in the evening, doing quiet activities or reading. Be patient. It may take a while before [the] child can sleep through the night again.

- **Feeling Helpless:** Being active in a campaign to prevent an event like this one from happening again, writing thank you letters to people who have helped, and caring for others can bring a sense of hope and control to everyone in the family.

Source: Sidran Institute, © 2013 Helpguide.org.

Helping A Child Recover From Trauma

It's important to communicate openly with children following trauma. Let them know that it's normal to feel scared or upset. [Children] may also look to you for cues on how they should respond to traumatic events, so let him or her see you dealing with symptoms of trauma in a positive way.

Chapter 59

Playing Helps Kids Learn And Grow

What would childhood be without time to play? Play, it turns out, is essential to growing up healthy. Research shows that active, creative play benefits just about every aspect of child development.

"Play is behavior that looks as if it has no purpose," says National Institutes of Health (NIH) psychologist Dr. Stephen Suomi. "It looks like fun, but it actually prepares for a complex social world." Evidence suggests that play can help boost brain function, increase fitness, improve coordination and teach cooperation.

Suomi notes that all mammals—from mice to humans—engage in some sort of play. His research focuses on rhesus monkeys. While he's cautious about drawing parallels between monkeys and people, his studies offer some general insights into the benefits of play.

Active, vigorous social play during development helps to sculpt the monkey brain. The brain grows larger. Connections between brain areas may strengthen. Play also helps monkey youngsters learn how to fit into their social group, which may range from 30–200 monkeys in three or four extended families.

Both monkeys and humans live in highly complex social structures, says Suomi. "Through play, rhesus monkeys learn to negotiate, to deal with strangers, to lose gracefully, to stop before things get out of hand, and to follow rules," he says. These lessons prepare monkey youngsters for life after they leave their mothers.

Play may have similar effects in the human brain. Play can help lay a foundation for learning the skills we need for social interactions. If human youngsters lack playtime, says Dr.

About This Chapter: Reprinted from "It's a Kid's Job: Playing Helps Kids Learn and Grow," *News in Health*, National Institutes of Health (www.nih.gov), June 2012.

Roberta Golinkoff, an infant language expert at the University of Delaware, "social skills will likely suffer. You will lack the ability to inhibit impulses, to switch tasks easily and to play on your own." Play helps young children master their emotions and make their own decisions. It also teaches flexibility, motivation, and confidence.

Kids don't need expensive toys to get a lot out of playtime. "Parents are children's most enriching plaything," says Golinkoff. Playing and talking to babies and children are vital for their language development. Golinkoff says that kids who talk with their parents tend to acquire a vocabulary that will later help them in school. "In those with parents who make a lot of demands, language is less well developed," she says. The key is not to take over the conversation, or you'll shut it down.

Unstructured, creative, physical play lets children burn calories and develops all kinds of strengths, such as learning how the world works. In free play, children choose the games, make the rules, learn to negotiate and release stress. Free play often involves fantasy. If children, say, want to learn about being a fireman, they can imagine and act out what a fireman does. And if something scary happens, free play can help defuse emotions by working them out.

"Sports are a kind of play, but it's not the kids calling the shots," says Golinkoff. It's important to engage in a variety of activities, including physical play, social play, and solitary play. "The key is that in free play, kids are making the decisions," says Golinkoff. You can't learn to make decisions if you're always told what to do.

Some experts fear that free play is becoming endangered. In the last two decades, children have lost an average of eight hours of free play per week. As media screens draw kids indoors, hours of sitting raise the risk for obesity and related diseases. When it comes to video games and other media, it is suggested by experts that parents should monitor content, especially violent content, and limit the amount of time children sit.

There's also been a national trend toward eliminating school recess. It's being pushed aside for academic study, including standardized test preparation. "Thousands of children have lost recess altogether," says child development expert Dr. Kathryn Hirsh-Pasek of Temple University. "Lack of recess has important consequences for young children who concentrate better when they come inside after a break from the schoolwork."

Many kids, especially those in low-income areas, lack access to safe places to play. This makes their school recess time even more precious. In response to these changes, some educators are now insisting that preschool and elementary school children have regular periods of active, free play with other children. The type of learning that happens during playtime is not always possible in the classroom. School recess is also important because of the growing number of obese children in the United States. Running around during recess can help kids stay at a healthy weight.

Play also may offer advantages within the classroom. In an NIH-funded study, Hirsh-Pasek, Golinkoff, and their colleagues found a link between preschoolers' math skills and their ability to copy models of two- and three-dimensional building block constructions. Play with building blocks—and block play alongside adults—can help build children's spatial skills so they can get an early start toward the later study of science, technology, engineering, or math.

"In a way, a child is becoming a young scientist, checking out how the world works," says Hirsh-Pasek. "We never outgrow our need to play." Older children, including teens, also need to play and daydream, which helps their problem-solving and creative imagination. Adults, too, need their breaks, physical activity and social interaction.

At the NIH Clinical Center in Bethesda, Maryland, "Recreation therapy services are seen as essential to the patients' recovery," says Donna Gregory, chief of recreational therapy. She and her team tailor activities for both children and adults. Games can get patients moving, even for just minutes at a time, which improves their functioning.

Medical play helps children cope with invasive procedures. A 2-year-old can be distracted with blowing bubbles; older kids can place their teddy bear in the magnetic resonance imaging (MRI) machine or give their doll a shot before they themselves get an injection. It gives kids a sense of control and supports their understanding in an age-appropriate, meaningful way.

Without play and recreation, people can become isolated and depressed. "There's therapeutic value in helping patients maintain what's important to them," says Gregory. "When you are physically and socially active, it gives life meaning."

Chapter 60

Dealing With Divorce

For many people, their parents' divorce marks a turning point in their lives, whether the divorce happened many years ago or is taking place right now.

About half the marriages in the United States today end in divorce, so plenty of kids and teens have to go through this. But when it happens to you, you can feel very alone and unsure of what it all means.

It may seem hard, but it is possible to cope with divorce—and have a good family life in spite of some changes divorce may bring.

Why Are My Parents Divorcing?

Parents divorce for many reasons. Usually divorce happens when couples feel they can no longer live together due to fighting and anger, or because the love they had when they married has changed. Divorce can also be because one parent falls in love with someone else, and sometimes it is due to a serious problem like drinking, abuse, or gambling. Sometimes nothing bad happens, but parents just decide to live apart.

Did you know it's really common for teens to think that their parents' divorce is somehow their fault? Just try to remember that parents' decisions to split up are to do with issues between them, and not because of something you might have done or not done.

Some kids feel guilty about what happened, or wish they had prevented arguments by cooperating more within the family, doing better with their behavior, or getting better grades.

About This Chapter: "Dealing With Divorce," August 2010, reprinted with permission from www.kidshealth .org. This information was provided by KidsHealth®, one of the largest resources online for medically reviewed health information written for parents, kids, and teens. For more articles like this, visit www.KidsHealth.org, or www.TeensHealth.org. Copyright © 1995–2013 The Nemours Foundation. All rights reserved.

But separation and divorce are a result of a couple's problems with each other, not with their kids. The decisions adults make about divorce are their own.

If your parents are divorcing, you may experience many feelings. Your emotions may change frequently, too. You may feel stressed out, angry, frustrated, or sad. You might feel protective of one parent or blame one for the situation. You may feel abandoned, afraid, worried, or guilty. You may also feel relieved, especially if there has been a lot of tension or fighting at home. These feelings are very typical and talking about them with a friend, family member, or trusted adult can really help.

How Will Divorce Change My Life?

Depending on what happens in your family, you might have to adjust to many changes. These could include things like moving, changing schools, spending time with both parents separately, and perhaps dealing with parents' unpleasant feelings about one another.

Your parents may go to court to determine custody arrangements. You could end up living with one parent most of the time and visiting the other, or your parents may split their time with you evenly. At the beginning, it means you might have to be flexible and might have more hassles to deal with for a while.

Some teens have to travel between parents, and that can create challenges both socially and practically. Over time you can figure out a new routine that works for all of you. Often, it takes a while for custody arrangements to be finalized. This can give people time to adapt to these big changes and let families figure out what works best.

Money matters may change for your parents, too. A parent who didn't work during the marriage may need to find a job to pay for rent or a mortgage. This might be something a parent is excited about, but he or she may also feel nervous or pressured about finances. There are also expenses associated with divorce, from lawyers' fees to the cost of moving to a new place to live.

Your family may not be able to afford all the things you were used to before the divorce. This is one of the difficult changes often associated with divorce. There can be good changes too—but how you cope with the stressful changes depends on your situation, your personality, and your support network.

What Parents And Teens Can Do To Make It Easier

Keep the peace. Dealing with divorce is easiest when parents get along. Teens find it especially hard when their parents fight and argue or act with bitterness toward each other. You can't do much to influence how your parents behave during a divorce, but you can ask them to do their best to call a truce to any bickering or unkind things they might be saying about each other.

No matter what problems a couple may face, as parents they need to handle visiting arrangements peacefully to minimize the stress their kids may feel. Letting your parents know that even though you know everyone is super-stressed, you don't want to get caught in the middle.

Be fair. Most teens say it's important that parents don't try to get them to "take sides." You need to feel free to hang out with and talk to each of your parents without the other parent acting jealous, hurt, or mad. It's unfair for anyone to feel that talking to one parent is being disloyal to the other or that the burden of one parent's happiness is on your shoulders.

When parents find it hard to let go of bitterness or anger, or if they are depressed about the changes brought on by divorce, they can find help from a counselor or therapist. This can help parents get past the pain divorce may have created, to find personal happiness, and to lift any burdens from their kids. Kids and teens can also benefit from seeing a family therapist or someone who specializes in helping them get through the stress of a family breakup. It might feel weird at first to talk to someone you don't know about personal feelings, but it can be really helpful to hear about how other teens in your situation have coped.

Keep in touch. Going back and forth between two homes can be tough, especially if parents live far apart. It can be a good idea to keep in touch with a parent you see less often because of distance. Even a quick email saying "I'm thinking of you" helps ease the feelings of missing each other. Making an effort to stay in touch when you're apart can keep both of you up to date on everyday activities and ideas.

Work it out. You may want both parents to come to special events, like games, meets, plays, or recitals. But sometimes a parent may find it awkward to attend if the other is present. It helps if parents can figure out a way to make this work, especially because you may need to feel the support and presence of both parents even more during divorce. You might be able to come up with an idea for a compromise or solution to this problem and suggest it to both parents.

Talk about the future. Many teens whose parents divorce worry that their own plans for the future could be affected. Some are concerned that the costs of divorce (like legal fees and expenses of two households) might mean there will be less money for college or other things.

Pick a good time to tell your parents about your concerns—when there's enough time to sit down with one or both parents to discuss how the divorce will affect you. Don't worry about putting added stress on your parents, just try to pick a good time to talk when everyone

369

is feeling calm. It's better to bring your concerns into the open than to keep them to yourself and let worries or resentment build. There are solutions for most problems and advisors and counselors who can help teens and their parents find those solutions.

Figure out your strengths. How do you deal with stress? Do you get angry and take it out on siblings, friends, or yourself? Or are you someone who is a more of a pleaser who puts others first? Do you tend to avoid conflict altogether and just hope that problems will magically disappear?

A life-changing event like a divorce can put people through some tough times, but it can also help them learn about their strengths, and put in place some new coping skills. For example, how can you cope if one parent bad-mouths another? Sometimes staying quiet until the anger has subsided and then discussing it calmly with your mom or dad can help. You may want to tell them you have a right to love both your parents, no matter what they are doing to each other.

If you need help figuring out your strengths or how to cope—like from a favorite aunt or from your school counselor—ask for it! And if you find it hard to confront your parents, try writing them a letter. Figure out what works for you.

Live your life. Sometimes during a divorce, parents may be so caught up in their own changes it can feel like your own life is on hold. In addition to staying focused on your own plans and dreams, make sure you participate in as many of your normal activities as possible. When things are changing at home, it can really help to keep some things, such as school activities and friends, the same.

If things get too hard at home, see if you can stay with a friend or relative until things calm down. Take care of yourself by eating right and getting regular exercise—two great stress busters! Figure out what's important to you—spending time with friends, working hard at school, writing or drawing, or being great at basketball. Finding your inner strength and focusing on your own goals can really help your stress levels.

Let others support you. Talk about your feelings and reactions to the divorce with someone you trust. If you're feeling down or upset, let your friends and family members support you. These feelings usually pass. If they don't, and if you're feeling depressed or stressed out, or if it's hard to concentrate on your normal activities, let a counselor or therapist help you. Your parents, school counselor, or a doctor or other health professional can help you find one.

Many communities and schools have support groups for kids and teens whose parents have divorced. It can really help to talk with other people your age who are going through similar experiences.

Bringing Out The Positive

There will be ups and downs in the process, but teens can cope successfully with their parents' divorce and the changes it brings. You might even discover some unexpected positives. Many teens find their parents are actually happier after the divorce or they may develop new and better ways of relating to both parents when they have separate time with each one.

Some teens learn compassion and caring skills when a younger brother or sister needs their support and care. Siblings who are closer in age may form tighter bonds, learning to count on each other more because they're facing the challenges of their parents' divorce together.

Coping well with divorce also can bring out strength and maturity. Some become more responsible, better problem solvers, better listeners, or better friends. Looking back on the experience, lots of people say that they learned coping skills they never knew they had and feel stronger and more resilient as a result of what they went through.

Many movies have been made about divorce and stepfamilies—some with happy endings, some not. That's how it is in real life too. But most teens who go through a divorce learn (sometimes to their surprise) that they can make it through this difficult situation successfully.

Giving it time, letting others support you along the way, and keeping an eye on the good things in your life can make all the difference.

Chapter 61

Dealing With Grief

What is grief?

Grief is the normal response of sorrow, emotion, and confusion that comes from losing someone or something important to you. It is a natural part of life. Grief is a typical reaction to death, divorce, job loss, a move away from family and friends, or loss of good health due to illness.

How does grief feel?

Just after a death or loss, you may feel empty and numb, as if you are in shock. You may notice physical changes such as trembling, nausea, trouble breathing, muscle weakness, dry mouth, or trouble sleeping and eating.

You may become angry—at a situation, a particular person, or just angry in general. Almost everyone in grief also experiences guilt. Guilt is often expressed as "I could have, I should have, and I wish I would have" statements.

People in grief may have strange dreams or nightmares, be absent-minded, withdraw socially, or lack the desire to return to work. While these feelings and behaviors are normal during grief, they will pass.

How long does grief last?

Grief lasts as long as it takes you to accept and learn to live with your loss. For some people, grief lasts a few months. For others, grieving may take years. The length of time spent grieving is different for each person. There are many reasons for the differences, including personality,

About This Chapter: Excerpted from "How to Deal With Grief," Substance Abuse and Mental Health Services Administration (www.samhsa.gov), January 2001. Information has been reviewed by David A. Cooke, MD, FACP, September 2013.

health, coping style, culture, family background, and life experiences. The time spent grieving also depends on your relationship with the person lost and how prepared you were for the loss.

How will I know when I'm done grieving?

Every person who experiences a death or other loss must complete a four-step grieving process:

1. Accept the loss.

2. Work through and feel the physical and emotional pain of grief.

3. Adjust to living in a world without the person or item lost.

4. Move on with life.

The grieving process is over only when a person completes the four steps.

What if these feelings won't go away?

If you recently experienced a death or other loss, feelings of grief are part of a normal reaction. But if these feelings persist with no lifting mood, ask for help.

How does grief differ from depression?

Depression is more than a feeling of grief after losing someone or something you love. Clinical depression is a whole body disorder. It can take over the way you think and feel. Symptoms of depression include:

- A sad, anxious, or "empty" mood that won't go away
- Loss of interest in what you used to enjoy
- Low energy, fatigue, feeling "slowed down"
- Changes in sleep patterns
- Loss of appetite, weight loss, or weight gain
- Trouble concentrating, remembering, or making decisions
- Feeling hopeless or gloomy
- Feeling guilty, worthless, or helpless
- Thoughts of death or suicide or a suicide attempt
- Recurring aches and pains that don't respond to treatment

Source: SAMHSA (www.samhsa.gov), January 2001.

Chapter 62

Getting Along With Family And Friends

Someone took your seat at lunch or pushed ahead of you in line. Your best friend wants you to let her cheat off your test paper. A guy in math class called you...something not so nice. Sometimes it seems like life is a sea of problems—and your ship is sinking. The information in this chapter can help you handle the things that make you crazy. (Well, not all of them. You'll still have homework.)

In every situation, everyone sees things differently and wants to do things their way. And it's normal for people to believe they are right, which leads to disagreements. Problems are never fun—but they can help you to have a good discussion and you can work things out. Clearing the air will help you learn more about your friends, your family, and even yourself. Solving problems in the right way also can help you get through them quickly and easily—and stop them from getting out of control (or even violent).

Some kids deal with problems or situations by avoiding them. They might always give in to other people, or just pretend the problems aren't there. Others confront problems head on and try to make other people see it their way or do what they want. The best way to work through problems is by understanding how the other person feels. What's your style? Are you totally cool or hot headed?

The good news is that your style isn't set in stone—you can exchange it for one that works better! The same thing doesn't work for every situation—so try something new if your old way isn't cutting it. Everyone — can learn how to deal better with situations, people, or things that make them mad. Realize that anger is a reaction and that your reaction to a situation determines

About This Chapter: Excerpted from "BAM! Guide To Getting Along," Centers for Disease Control and Prevention (www.cdc.gov), January 2013.

the outcome. In other words, you can choose how you respond to things that upset you. How you look at a situation can determine whether you become angry or not. By recognizing the chain of reactions that builds up to anger, you can break the cycle and keep your cool, even in the hottest situations.

If sparks do start to fly, you have the power to put out the fire. The next time you have an issue on your hands, don't explode or let someone walk all over you. If you feel like you're about to lose it, put it on simmer, and use these tips to cool down:

1. Take some deep breaths and concentrate on relaxing your body with each breath.

2. Count to 10 slowly.

3. Think before you react. (What are consequences of your actions?)

4. Keep your voice "low and slow."

5. Get away. Remove yourself from the situation—leave the room for a minute or take a short walk.

Iron Out Your Issues

No plan will magically solve every problem or situation, but here are some ideas that have worked like a charm for other people.

Take A Moment

Stepping back from the whole mess gives everyone a chance to cool down and think. When you're having a problem with someone, first take some time to understand your own thoughts and feelings. What's really the issue? For example, do you feel like you're not getting enough respect? What do you want? Why?

When Is A Conflict Not A Conflict At All?

When you stop it before it starts. Lots of times, problems start when someone doesn't understand where another person is coming from. (Remember the last time someone got mad at you for what seemed like no reason?) So, if you're confused about why someone is acting weird or mean, find out why. Talk, e-mail, instant message (IM),or send a text message. When they tell you, listen—really listen. And if someone tries to make you mad on purpose, just ignore them or ask them why. No one controls your feelings but you!

Source: "BAM! Guide To Getting Along," Centers for Disease Control and Prevention (www.cdc.gov), January 2013.

Next, find a time to work out the problem with the other person. Pick a quiet place where it's easy to talk. Make sure to give yourself enough time. (Out by the school buses 15 minutes before soccer practice probably isn't a good choice!)

Set The Tone

The "tone" is the mood of the talk. When you wake up in a bad mood, it can spoil the whole day, right? You want to make sure that your talk at least starts off with a good mood. Just saying "Let's work this out" can make a huge difference!

Agree On The Problem

Take turns telling your sides of the story. You can't solve a problem if you don't really understand everything that's going on.

- **When it's your turn:** See how calm you can be. Speak softly, slowly, and firmly. No threats (like "If you don't shut up, I'll..."), because they can raise the problem to a whole new level-a bad one. No need to get all excited or mad! Try giving your point of view this way: "I feel ____(angry, sad, or upset) when you____ (take my stuff without permission, call me a name, or leave me out) because___ (you should ask first, it hurts my feelings, or makes me feel lonely)." This really works to get people to listen, because they don't feel like you're judging them. Check out the difference. You could say "You're always late to pick me up!" or "I feel embarrassed when you pick me up late because all of my friends leave right on time and it seems like no one remembered me." You can also try just stating the facts. Instead of saying "You're a thief!" try "Maybe you picked up my shirt by mistake."

- **When it's the other person's turn:** Let them explain. Listen. Don't interrupt. Try to understand where they're coming from. Show that you hear them. When people aren't getting along, each person is part of the problem—but most of us tend to blame the other person. When you've done something wrong, be ready to say you're sorry.

The goal is to decide together what the real issues are. Do not pass "Go" until you do that. It's huge!

Think Of Solutions

Take turns coming up with ways to solve the problem. Get creative. Usually, there are lots possible solutions. Next, talk about the good and bad points of each one.

Make A Deal

Choose a solution that you both can agree on. Pick an idea that you both think will work. Get into the specifics—talk about exactly who will do what and when you'll do it. Everyone should give something.

Stick Like Glue

Keep your word and stick to what you agreed to. Give your compromise a chance. See if it sent your problem up in smoke or if the fires are still burning.

Know When To Get Help

Sometimes a problem gets really serious. If you aren't talking and you don't trust each other, you might need another person to step in. If it looks like the problem might turn into a fight, it's definitely time to get help. Someone like a teacher, parent, or religious advisor can help calm things down so you can safely talk out the problem with the other person.

Can't Solve It?

Sometimes that's okay. Just agree to disagree. You can still get along even if you don't see eye-to-eye on a certain thing.

More Than One Way

What could you do if the girl who sits next to you in science class keeps whispering to you? It's distracting and you both keep getting in trouble! If you talk to "chatty Cathy" after class, you might find out that she's whispering to you because she doesn't understand what's going on in class. Together, you might come up with these ideas that might solve the problem:

- She could try not to talk to you in class, and you could ignore her to make sure she doesn't!
- She could ask the teacher more questions in class instead of turning to you for help.
- She could whisper to somebody else when she's confused.
- You could help her with the assignments before or after class.
- Both of you could go to the teacher and explain the situation.

After you have some ideas, the next step is to decide which will work...and which won't.

Source: "BAM! Guide To Getting Along," Centers for Disease Control and Prevention (www.cdc.gov), January 2013.

Getting Along With Parents And Guardians

Kim has been fighting with her parents a lot lately. She thinks her parents' rules are unfair. They tell her she needs to listen and follow their rules.

Like Kim, your relationship with your parents or guardians may be confusing right now. As you get older, you can do more things on your own. You also have more freedom to spend time with other people—like friends or crushes. You may feel you are ready to choose where you go and what you do. But, you need to follow your parents' or guardians' rules. They make rules because they care about you and want you to be safe. Their rules may make you angry, though, and you may find that you're fighting with them more than you used to.

Each family is unique and special. No matter what type of family you have, sometimes there will be tough times as you grow up. Keep in mind, your parents or guardians make rules because they love you and want to keep you safe. It's important to listen to them and follow their rules.

Stepparents

Learning to get along with a stepparent is hard for some teens. A new stepparent can make you worry about how you fit into the family—and whether your parent loves you as much as they did before. There may be times when you feel sad and upset, even if you like your stepparent. A new stepparent can mean new rules in your house, and sometimes new siblings, too.

How To Deal With Fights With Your Parents And Guardians

- **Talk about the rules.** Talk about things ahead of time so that you will be able to tell what they will say yes or no to before you make plans. Ask your parents or guardians to tell you the reason for each rule. Ask if you can tell them how the rules make you feel. See if they will listen to your ideas about what the rules should be. They may be willing to use your ideas when making rules.

- **Try to stay calm.** Don't yell or stomp your feet when your parents or guardians say no. If you listen to what they say, you will show them that you are growing up.

- **Follow the rules.** If your parents or guardians tell you to be home at a certain time, be home at that time. If you are going to be late, call and tell them so they don't worry about you. If you follow the rules, they may let you come home later in the future.

- **Pick your battles.** Cleaning your room is no fun, but it's most likely not worth fighting about. Everyone has to do it!

- **Spend time with your family.** Some teens fight with their parents or guardians over how much time they spend with their friends. Talk it over and make some special family time. There are lots of things your family can do together—like going on a hike, a bike ride, or going to the beach.

Source: Excerpted from "Parents, Stepparents, Grandparents, and Guardians," September 2009, and "How To Deal With Fights With Your Parents/Guardians," June 2008, Office on Women's Health (www.girlshealth.gov).

Cool Rules

Ever notice how quickly people get angry? It seems like people can go from totally happy to totally ticked off in no time at all. In fact, the feeling of anger is actually a series of reactions that happen in just 1/30th of a second.

The amazing thing about anger is that it's not a basic emotion like, say, happiness. It is actually a secondary emotion and it is supposed to help keep you safe and protect you from danger—the old "fight or flight" thing! But if it gets out of hand (or if you try to ignore it), it can lead to some serious issues. Break the chain with this simple way to remember how to deal with anger:

- **Stop it at the first spark.** Lots of things can trigger anger, like losing a soccer game, having to deal with your bossy little sister, or your computer crashing when you're in the middle of instant messaging your pals or writing a school paper. The important thing is to figure out what is really making you angry. Is it the same thing every time or do different things bring you to the boiling point? If it is always the same situation, person, or thing, try to avoid it. And if you can't avoid them (because you know your little sister isn't going anywhere), think of different ways you can keep from getting angry. Instead of hurling the computer out the window, think about how you avoid it crashing to begin with, like not having your e-mail and a game going at the same time. If losing the soccer game has got your goat, use your anger as motivation to improve your skills.

- **What's it all mean?** Good job on figuring out how to spot the things you know make you angry. But, your little sister is still driving you nuts. Since she's staying put, you've got to figure out a way to handle your anger that won't make things worse. This brings us to the second link in the chain. To avoid it, all you need to do is try to look at things from her point of view—you're older and she wants to hang with you because she thinks you're cool. With that in mind, it's easier to keep your cool. Spend some time just with her so that she won't need to stalk you when all your friends are over. You might even find out that she's not half bad. By changing the way you deal with her and understanding her point of view, you can break the anger chain before you even notice you're mad!

- **You are still furious.** You've tried to change your reactions to the things that you know make you crazy, you're busy looking at everything from everyone else's point of view, but you can still feel your temperature is raising. Well, that's your body responding to your feelings. You get hot and your muscles might start to tighten and you start breathing harder. Don't let it get the best of you—there are things you can do to stay in control. Take some deep breaths, focus on relaxing your muscles, and slow down!

- **Now, you're talking to yourself.** The next link in the chain comes when you catch yourself thinking or saying something in reaction to what's happening to make you mad. We've all done it. We think things like "He's so stupid" or say to a friend "You're always so mean!" before we can stop ourselves. If you catch yourself doing this, take a minute to think. Try to remember that you are dealing with a person who may not know how you feel. Stay calm. Lashing back won't get you anywhere. So try to talk to your friend, let him know he hurt your feelings, and then try to move on.

- **Learn from the past.** History plays a part in how you deal with anger. The way you feel in a situation depends on your background. You may be used to people keeping their feelings in and not talking about them, or you may be used to people exploding and yelling when they are angry. Neither of these reactions is necessarily good. People who bottle up their feelings can end up exploding later, or become depressed. People who vent and yell just tend to keep the anger cycle in motion. The trick is to deal with your anger so that you can learn how to not get riled up in the first place. Try these suggestions to help you stay calm, cool, and collected:

  - Go for a walk.

  - Write down your feelings on a piece of paper, then tear it up and throw it away.

  - Face the mirror and practice talking to the person that you are mad at.

That's The Way The Story Ends...

Isn't it amazing how many things come in between the first spark and being really mad? The whole chain happens so fast because we train ourselves to react in a certain way without even knowing we're doing it. But if you learn to recognize the steps in between, you can break the chain before you lose your cool. No matter how hard you try, you won't be able to avoid getting angry in every situation. You just have to decide the best way to respond. Anger doesn't have to be negative—if you handle it the right way it can actually clue you in to dangerous situations and make you a stronger person. Remember these tips to help you keep your cool:

- Avoid letting your anger or other angry people control you.

- Never use your body or voice to hurt others.

- Get away from the situation so your feelings don't overwhelm you.

- Evaluate your choices. Think before you react.

- Remember, you are responsible for your own choices. No one can make you angry, you allow yourself to become angry. And you can choose not to get angry too.

Chapter 63

Running Away Doesn't Solve Problems

When you were little, did you ever run away? Maybe you packed up your backpack and made it down the driveway or around the corner to your friend's backyard. But after a little while, you forgot why you were running away and it was getting dark out, so you went home.

We hope that was the last time you thought about running away because there's a big difference between thinking about running away (or walking a few blocks down the street) and actually running away.

Running away is a serious problem. According to the National Runaway Switchboard, an organization that takes calls and helps kids who have run away or are thinking of running away, one in seven kids between the ages of 10 and 18 will run away at some point. And there are one million to three million runaway and homeless kids living on the streets in the United States.

Why Kids Run Away

Remember how you felt the last time you got in a big fight with your parents or one of your brothers or sisters? That kind of anger and hurt can be what pushes someone to run away from home.

In fact, most kids run away due to problems with their families. Some kids run away because of one terrible argument. Some even decide to leave without ever having a fight. They might have done something they're ashamed of, and they're afraid to tell their parents.

Other reasons kids run away include:

- Abuse (violence in the family)
- Parents separating or divorcing or the arrival of a new stepparent
- Death in the family
- Birth of a new baby in the family
- Family financial worries
- Kids or parents drinking alcohol or taking drugs
- Problems at school
- Peer pressure
- Failing or dropping out of school

These are problems faced by lots of kids and teens—and there are ways to deal with all of these problems besides running away. Kids who think about running away might not know how to solve tough problems or don't have adults to help them. Sometimes a really big problem can make it seem like running away is the only choice.

Unfortunately, the problems kids hope to escape by running away are replaced by other—sometimes even bigger—problems of life on the streets.

The Reality Of Running Away

When you think about running away, you probably imagine that there will be no more rules, no parent to tell you what to do, no more fights. Sounds great and exciting, right?

In reality, running away is anything but fun. Kids and teens who run away face new problems like not having any money, food to eat, a safe place to sleep, or anyone to look out for them.

People with no home and no money become desperate, doing anything just to meet their basic needs. Because of this, they often find themselves in risky situations that would be frightening, even for adults. Runaway kids get involved in dangerous crimes much more often than kids who live at home.

Kids who live on the streets often have to steal to meet basic needs. Many take drugs or alcohol to get through the day because they become so depressed and feel that no one cares about them. Some are forced to do things they wouldn't normally do to make money. The number of kids with human immunodeficiency virus (HIV) or acquired immunodeficiency syndrome (AIDS) and other diseases is higher on streets, too, because these kids might use intravenous (IV) drugs or have unprotected sex (often for money).

Runaway Prevention

Let's face it—stress is a part of life, even for kids—but being able to deal with problems with confidence, hope, and practical solutions makes kids less likely to run away.

To build your problem-solving skills, try to:

- **Know your emotions.** Try to understand what you are feeling inside and use words to describe it.

- **Express your emotions.** Don't be afraid to tell those close to you how you're feeling and why. Use words, not actions. This is especially true for anger. Anger is one of the hardest emotions to manage because it's so strong—but everyone needs to learn how to express angry feelings without violence.

- **Know how to calm yourself down after you're upset.** Maybe you need to run around outside, listen to music, draw, or write poetry. Do whatever safe things you need to do to feel better.

- **When you have a problem, try to come up with a list of solutions.** Get someone else to help you if you can't think of at least three things to do. For each possible solution, ask yourself: "If I do this, what would happen next?"

- **Get some help from trusted adults** (someone like a parent, close relative, teacher, or neighbor). Know who you can count on to support and help you.

If You're Thinking Of Running Away

It might feel like there's no way to fix the problems that are making you think about running away. If you can, tell your mom or dad how you feel. They need to know that you're upset or that you're afraid they don't love you or want you around. It may be possible to work together as a family to change things for the better. Sometimes talking with a counselor as a family can help.

If the problem is as serious as abuse and a parent is involved, then talk to a teacher or counselor at school, a good friend's parent, a close relative, or another trusted adult. Let that person help you find somewhere safe to stay. It might be hard to share this secret because you may feel ashamed or afraid of getting someone in trouble, but remember that abuse is never your fault.

Another option is to call the National Runaway Switchboard at (800) 621-4000. It's open 24 hours a day and the call is free. The switchboard operators get thousands of calls each year, many from kids who have run away or know someone who has.

If Your Friend Wants To Run Away

If your friend is thinking about running away, warn him or her about how tough it will be to survive on the streets. Your friend is probably scared and confused. Try to be supportive and help your friend feel less alone.

Remind your friend that, whatever the problem is, there are other ways to deal with it, even if neither one of you can think of the ways right now. An adult will know how to help.

It takes courage to tell an adult that your friend is about to run away, but try to do this as soon as possible. Being a real friend doesn't mean keeping a secret when it can hurt someone. It means doing the best thing possible for your friend. And running away isn't a solution for either of you. It only leads to more problems and danger.

Chapter 64

Suicide Prevention

Suicide In America: Frequently Asked Questions

Suicide is a major public health concern. Around 38,000 people die by suicide each year in the United States. More people die by suicide each year than by homicide.

Suicide is tragic. But it is often preventable. Knowing the risk factors for suicide and who is at risk can help reduce the suicide rate.

Who is at risk for suicide?

Suicide does not discriminate. People of all genders, ages, and ethnicities are at risk for suicide. But people most at risk tend to share certain characteristics. The main risk factors for suicide are:

- Depression, other mental disorders, or substance abuse disorder

- A prior suicide attempt

- Family history of a mental disorder or substance abuse

- Family history of suicide

- Family violence, including physical or sexual abuse

- Having guns or other firearms in the home

About This Chapter: Excerpts from "Suicide in America: Frequently Asked Questions," March 2012, and "Many Teens Considering Suicide Do Not Receive Specialized Mental Health Care," October 2012, National Institute of Mental Health (www.nimh.nih.gov).

- Incarceration, being in prison or jail
- Being exposed to others' suicidal behavior, such as that of family members, peers, or media figures

The risk for suicidal behavior also is associated with changes in brain chemicals called neurotransmitters, including serotonin, which is also associated with depression. Lower levels of serotonin have been found in the brains of people with a history of suicide attempts.

Many people have some of these risk factors but do not attempt suicide. Suicide is not a normal response to stress. It is however, a sign of extreme distress, not a harmless bid for attention.

What about gender?

Men are more likely to die by suicide than women, but women are more likely to attempt suicide. Men are more likely to use deadlier methods, such as firearms or suffocation. Women are more likely than men to attempt suicide by poisoning.

What about children?

Children and young people are at risk for suicide. Year after year, suicide remains one of the top three leading causes of death for young people ages 15–24.

What about older adults?

Older adults are at risk for suicide, too. In fact, white males age 85 and older consistently have the highest suicide rate than any other age and ethnic group.

What about different ethnic groups?

Among ethnicities, American Indians and Alaska Natives tend to have the highest rate of suicides, followed by non-Hispanic Whites. Hispanics tend to have the lowest rate of suicides, while African Americans tend to have the second lowest rate.

How can suicide be prevented?

Effective suicide prevention is based on sound research. Programs that work take into account people's risk factors and promote interventions that are appropriate to specific groups of people. For example, research has shown that mental and substance abuse disorders are risk factors for suicide. Therefore, many programs focus on treating these disorders in addition to addressing suicide risk specifically.

Psychotherapy, or "talk therapy," can effectively reduce suicide risk. One type is called cognitive behavioral therapy (CBT). CBT can help people learn new ways of dealing with stressful experiences by training them to consider alternative actions when thoughts of suicide arise.

Another type of psychotherapy called dialectical behavior therapy (DBT) has been shown to reduce the rate of suicide among people with borderline personality disorder, a serious mental illness characterized by unstable moods, relationships, self-image, and behavior. A therapist trained in DBT helps a person recognize when his or her feelings or actions are disruptive or unhealthy, and teaches the skills needed to deal better with upsetting situations.

Some medications may also help. For example, the antipsychotic medication clozapine is approved by the U.S. Food and Drug Administration for suicide prevention in people with schizophrenia. Other promising medications and psychosocial treatments for suicidal people are being tested.

Still other research has found that many older adults and women who die by suicide saw their primary care providers in the year before death. Training doctors to recognize signs that a person may be considering suicide may help prevent even more suicides.

What Can Be Done To Prevent Suicide?

Getting help for mental illnesses can help prevent suicide. Because depression and substance abuse are linked to suicide, getting treatment for these disorders can help prevent suicide.

Stigma associated with mental illnesses can prevent people from getting help. Your willingness to talk about depression and suicide with a friend, family member, or co-worker can be the first step in getting help and preventing suicide. If you know someone whom you think may be suicidal, show that you care by:

Listening to them with sincere concern for their feelings. Do not offer advice, but let them know they are not alone.

Sharing your feelings with them. If you feel that they may make a reckless decision, tell that that you are concerned. They need to know that they are important to you and that you care.

Asking in a caring manner if they have had suicidal thoughts or if they have made a suicide plan. If you feel you cannot ask the question, find someone who can.

Calling the National Suicide Prevention Lifeline, 800-273-TALK (800-273-8255).

Source: Excerpted from "Preventing Suicide," Office on Women's Health (www.womenshealth.gov), March 2010.

What should I do if someone I know is considering suicide?

If you know someone who is considering suicide, do not leave him or her alone. Try to get your loved one to seek immediate help from his or her doctor or the nearest hospital emergency room, or call 911. Remove any access he or she may have to firearms or other potential tools for suicide, including medications.

What Are The Warning Signs Of Suicide?

Warning signs of suicide include:

- Ideation (thinking, talking, or wishing about suicide)
- Substance use or abuse (increased use or change in substance)
- Feeling purposeless (no sense of purpose or belonging)
- Anger
- Feeling trapped (feeling like there is no way out)
- Hopelessness (there is nothing to live for, no hope or optimism)
- Withdrawal (from family, friends, work, school, activities, hobbies)
- Anxiety (restlessness, irritability, agitation)
- Recklessness (high risk-taking behavior)
- Mood disturbance (dramatic changes in mood)

More warning signs of suicide include:

- Talking about suicide
- Looking for ways to die (Internet searches for how to commit suicide, looking for guns, pills, etc.)
- Talking about hopelessness, helplessness, or worthlessness
- Thinking about death a lot
- Suddenly acting happier, calmer
- Loss of interest in things one cares about
- Visiting or calling people one cares about, especially after a long absence
- Making arrangements or setting one's affairs in order
- Giving things away, such as prized possessions

Remember: A suicidal person needs to see a doctor or mental health professional right away.

Source: Source: Excerpted from "Preventing Suicide," Office on Women's Health (www.womenshealth.gov), March 2010.

Many Teens Considering Suicide Do Not Receive Specialized Mental Health Care

Most adolescents who are considering suicide or who have attempted suicide do not receive specialized mental health services.

Background

National survey data from the Centers for Disease Control and Prevention (CDC) notes that approximately 14 percent of high school students seriously consider suicide each year, 11 percent have a suicide plan, and six percent attempt suicide. Other research has suggested that less than half of teens who attempt suicide received mental health services in the year prior to their attempt.

Kathleen Merikangas, PhD, of the National Institute of Mental Health (NIMH) and colleagues analyzed data from the National Comorbidity Survey-Adolescent Supplement (NCS-A), a nationally representative, face-to-face survey of more than 10,000 teens ages 13–18. They asked teens whether they had any suicidal thoughts, plans, or actions (ideation) over a one-year period prior to the survey. They also completed a structured diagnostic interview regarding the full range of mental disorders including mood, anxiety, eating and anxiety disorders, and whether they had received treatment for emotional or behavioral problems in the past 12 months. Respondents were asked to differentiate between receiving care from a mental health specialist (such as, a social worker, psychiatrist, or other mental health professional) and receiving care from a general service provider (such as, a primary care physician).

Results Of The Study

The survey revealed that, within the past year, 3.6 percent of adolescents had suicidal thoughts, but did not make a specific plan or suicide attempt. In addition, 0.6 percent reported having a plan, and 1.9 percent reported having made a suicide attempt within the past year.

Suicidal behavior among youth was not only associated with major depression, but also with a range of other mental health problems including eating, anxiety, substance use, and behavior disorders, as well as physical health problems. Between 50 and 75 percent of those teens who reported having suicidal ideation had recent contact with a service provider. However, most only had three or fewer visits, suggesting that treatment tends to be terminated prematurely. Moreover, most teens with suicidal ideation did not receive specialized mental health care.

Significance

The results of this study suggest that depression and other mood disorders are not the only pathways to suicide. They also highlight the importance of integrating risk assessment for suicide into routine physical and mental health care for teens. Even if adolescents are in treatment, they should continue to be monitored for suicidal ideation and behaviors, the researchers concluded.

Part Eight
If You Need More Information

Chapter 65

Additional Reading About Mental Health And Mental Illness

Alcohol And Drugs

From Binge to Blackout

By Chris Volkmann, Toren Volkmann, Edward A. Malloy, and Cardwell C. Nuckols;
Published by NAL Trade, 2006

Getting Sober

By Kelly Madigan Erlandson; Published by McGraw-Hill, 2007

Teen HealthFX

Website: www.teenhealthfx.com/answers/alcohol,+smoking+drugs

TeenZeen

Source for teen drug abuse and alcohol prevention information; Website: www.teenzeen.org

Bullying And Cyberbullying

Bullying Under Attack: True Stories Written by Teen Victims, Bullies & Bystanders (Teen Ink)

By Stephanie Meyer, John Meyer, Emily Sperber, and Heather Alexander;
Published by HCI Teens, 2013

About This Chapter: The books and other items listed in this chapter were compiled from many resources. The list is far from comprehensive; it is intended to serve as a starting point for further research. Inclusion does not constitute endorsement, and there is no implication associate with omission. All website information was verified in September 2013.

The Bully Project

Stories of those who were bullies and resources for how to deal with and stop bullies.
Website: www.thebullyproject.com

STOMP Out Bullying

A national anti-bullying and cyberbullying program for kids and teens.
Website: stompoutbullying.org

Stop Bullying Now!

Website: www.stopbullying.gov

Teens Against Bullying

Created to help teens learn about bullying, how to appropriately respond, and how to prevent it.
Website: http://www.pacerteensagainstbullying.org/#/home

Youth Guide Blog—National Youth Advocacy Coalition

An advocacy organization for young people. Website: www.nyacyouth.org

Depression

Depression and Back: A Poetic Journey Through Depression and Recovery

By Susan Polis Schutz; Published by Blue Mountain Press, 2010

Facebook Depression

Website: www.yourlifeyourvoice.org/DiscoverIt/Articles/Pages/FacebookDepression.aspx

The 10 Best Ever Depression Management Techniques

By Margaret Wehrenberg; Published by W. W. Norton & Company, 2011

When Living Hurts

By Sol Gordon, PhD; Published by URJ Press, 2004. This is a what-to-do book for yourself
or someone you care about who feels discouraged, sad, lonely, hopeless, angry or frustrated,
unhappy, bored, depressed, or suicidal.

When Life Stinks: How to Deal With Your Bad Moods, Blues, and Depression

By Michel Piquemal; Published by Amulet Books, 2004

Eating Disorders

Food as Foe: Nutrition and Eating Disorders

By Lesli J. Favor; Published by Marshall Cavendish Benchmark, 2008

Hunger

By Jackie Morse Kessler; Published by Graphia Books, 2010

Life Beyond Your Eating Disorder: Reclaim Yourself, Regain Your Health, Recover for Good

By Johanna S. Kandel; Published by Harlequin, 2010

When the Mirror Lies Anorexia, Bulimia, and Other Eating Disorders

By Tamra Orr; Published by Franklin Watts, 2007

Grief And Loss

The Grieving Teen: A Guide for Teenagers and Their Friends

By Helen Fitzgerald; Published by Paw Prints, 2008

Healing Your Grieving Heart for Teens: 100 Practical Ideas

By Alan D. Wolfelt, PhD; Published by Companion Press, 2001

When a Friend or Loved One Dies: Grieving, Mourning, and Healing

By Alexandra Hanson-Harding; Published by Rosen Publishing Group, 2013

When Will I Stop Hurting? Teens, Loss, and Grief (It Happened to Me Series)

By Edward Myers; Published by Scarecrow Press, 2004

Weird Is Normal When Teenagers Grieve

By Jenny Lee Wheeler; Published by Quality Of Life Publishing Company, 2010

Homelessness And Runaways

Almost Home: Helping Kids Move from Homelessness to Hope

By Kevin Ryan and Tina Kelley; Published by Wiley, 2012

Covenant House: Meet Our Kids

Read the stories of how these kids rebuilt their lives with the support of the Covenant House.
Website: www.covenanthouse.org/homeless-kids

If You're Homeless or Need Help

Published by the National Coalition for the Homeless, Updated May 2013.
Website: www.nationalhomeless.org/need_help

Running Away

Website: nationalsafeplace.org/safe-place-teens/running-away

Street And Runaway Teens (Social Issues Firsthand)

By Cynthia A. Bily (Editor); Published by Greenhaven Press, 2007

What You've Got Wrong About Homeless Teens

Website: www.dosomething.org/tipsandtools/what-youve-got-wrong-about-homeless-teens

Mental Health

Asperger's Rules! How to Make Sense of School and Friends

By Blythe Grossberg; Published by Magination Press, 2012

The Aspie Teen's Survival Guide: Candid Advice for Teens, Tweens, and Parents, from a Young Man with Asperger's Syndrome

By J. D. Kraus; Published by Future Horizons, 2010

CopeCareDeal—Firsthand Accounts of Mental Illness

Free series of books with stories from teens and up-to-date information from experts on the illnesses, treatments, and tips for coping in everyday life. Website: www.copecaredeal.org/Articles.aspx?Theme=TheDeal&ArticleID=104 (Free book downloads)

Emotional Self-Help Toolkit: Bring Your Life Into Balance

A self-guided program to help teens relieve stress and take control of their life. Website: www.helpguide.org/toolkit/emotional_health.htm#toolkit_overview

Freaks, Geeks & Asperger Syndrome: A User Guide to Adolescence

By Luke Jackson; Published by Jessica Kingsley Publishers, 2002

Half of Us

Stories, videos, and information on dealing with mental illness. Website: www.halfofus.com

Healthy Place: America's Mental Health Channel

Comprehensive, trusted website providing information on psychological disorders and psychiatric medications from consumer and expert points of view; a mental health social network for support; online psychological tests; breaking mental health news; mental health videos; a live mental health TV and radio show; and more. Website: www.healthyplace.com

I'm Not Alone: A Teen's Guide to Living with a Parent Who Has a Mental Illness

By Michelle D. Sherman, PhD and DeAnne M. Sherman; Published by Beaver Pond Publishing

The Mind Zone—CopeCareDeal

Mental health website for teens that includes plenty of extremely helpful information. Website: http://www.copecaredeal.org/_MindZone.aspx

StrengthofUs.org

Online resource center/social networking website for teens living with mental health conditions. Website: www.StrengthofUs.org

Teen HealthFX

This site provides teens with answers to any and all of their questions regarding their mental and physical health, relationships, their body, and their sexuality. Questions are answered by a professional staff, and the site includes an "Emotional Health Quiz" and advice "For Teens by Teens." Website: www.teenhealthfx.com/answers/Emotional

Rape, Sexual Violence, And Domestic Violence

How Long Does It Hurt: A Guide to Recovering from Incest and Sexual Abuse for Teenagers, Their Friends, and Their Families

By Cynthia L. Mather; Published by Jossey-Bass, 2004

It Happened to Me: A Teen's Guide to Overcoming Sexual Abuse

By William Lee Carter; Published by New Harbinger Publications, 2002

Love Is Not Abuse

Website: www.loveisnotabuse.com

The Me Nobody Knows: A Guide for Teen Survivors

By Barbara Bean and Shari Bennett; Published by Jossey-Bass, 1997

School Violence

Hey, Back Off! Tips for Stopping Teen Harassment

By Jennie Withers and Phyllis Hendrickson; Published by New Horizon Press, 2011

School Violence (Current Controversies)
By Lucinda Almond (Editor); Published by Greenhaven Press, 2007

School Violence (Issues That Concern You)
By Peggy Daniels; Published by Greenhaven Press, 2008

Violence At School: What Can Teens Do To Stay Safe?
Website: http://mydoctor.kaiserpermanente.org/ncal/Images/011061-115%20Revised%20
3-11%20CL_tcm75-14769.pdf

Violence in Our Schools: Halls of Hope, Halls of Fear
By Tamra B. Orr; Published by Children's Press, 2003

Sexuality And Sexual Health

Maria Talks
A public health website containing medically accurate information about sexuality and sexual health for teens. Website: www.mariatalks.com

Stress And Anxiety

Anxiety In Teens Blog
A place where teens can connect and know they are not alone in their struggle.
Website: www.anxietyinteens.org

My Anxious Mind: A Teen's Guide to Managing Anxiety and Panic
By Michael A. Tompkins and Katherine A. Martinez; Published by Magination Press, 2009

Monkey Mind: A Memoir of Anxiety
By Daniel B. Smith; Published by Simon & Schuster, 2012

Stress Relief: The Ultimate Teen Guide
By Mark Powell; Published by Scarecrow Press, 2007

Too Stressed to Think? A Teen Guide to Staying Sane When Life Makes You Crazy
By Annie Fox; Published by Free Spirit, 2005

Suicide

Teen Suicide (Teen Mental Health Series)
By Lorena Huddle and Jay Schleifer; Published by Rosen Publishing Group, 2011

Chapter 66

Crisis Help And Hotlines

Note: All help and hotlines are available 24 hours a day, 7 days a week unless otherwise noted.

Alcohol And Drugs

Al-Anon/Alateen

Toll-Free: 888-425-2666
(8 a.m.–6 p.m. EST, M–F)
Website: www.al-anon.alateen.org/
for-alateen

Narconon

Toll-Free: 800-775-8750
Website: www.narconon.org

National Alcohol and Substance Abuse Information Center

Toll-Free: 800-784-6776
Website: www.addictioncareoptions.com
(Chat live 7 days/24 hours)

National Institute On Drug Abuse (NIDA) For Teens

Toll-Free: 800-662-HELP (800-662-4357)
Toll-Free TDD: 800-487-4889
Website: teens.drugabuse.gov

Bullying And Cyber-bullying

No More Bullying, Live Empowered (NOBLE)

Toll-Free: 800-231-1127
Phone: 248-809-5550 (Text)
Website: www.commongroundhelps.org
(Crisis Online Chat, 4p.m.–10p.m. EST, M–F)

About This Chapter: Information is excerpted from many sources deemed reliable. Inclusion does not constitute endorsement, and there is no implication associated with omission. All contact information was verified in September 2013.

Thursday's Child National Youth Advocacy Hotline

Toll-Free: 800-USA-KIDS (800-872-5437)
Phone: 818-893-4400 (Outside of the U.S.)
Website: www.thursdayschild.org

The Trevor Lifeline

Crisis intervention for lesbian, gay, bisexual, transgender, and questioning (LGBTQ)
Toll-Free: 866-4-U-TREVOR (866-488-7386)
Phone: 202-304-1200 or text TREVOR (4 p.m.–8 p.m. EST, Friday)
Website: www.thetrevorproject.org (Chat online 3 p.m.–9 p.m. EST, 7 days)

Depression

Crisis Call Center

Toll-Free: 800-273-TALK (800-273-8255) or text ANSWER to 839863
Phone: 775-784-8090
Website: crisiscallcenter.org/crisisservices.html

National Hopeline Network

Toll-Free: 800-SUICIDE (800-784-2433)
Toll-Free: 800-442-HOPE (800-442-4673)
Website: www.hopeline.com

Eating Disorders

National Association of Anorexia Nervosa and Associated Disorders

Phone: 630-577-1330 (9–5, CST, M–F)
Website: www.anad.org
E-mail: anadhelp@anad.org (E-mail helpline)

National Eating Disorders Association

Toll-Free: 800-931-2237 (9 a.m. to 9 p.m. EST, Mon.–Thurs.; until 5 p.m. on Fri.)
Website: www.nationaleatingdisorders.org (Chat online)

Grief And Loss

Tragedy Assistance Program for Survivors (TAPS)

Toll-Free: 800-959-TAPS (800-959-8277)
Website: www.taps.org

Homelessness And Runaways

Boys Town National Hotline

Serving all at-risk teens and children
Toll-Free: 800-448-3000
Website: www.boystown.org/hotline (Chat online 7:30 p.m.–12:00 a.m. CST, Monday–Thursday)

National Runaway Safeline

Toll-Free: 800-RUNAWAY (800-786-2929)
Website: www.1800runaway.org

National Safe Place

Toll-Free: 888-290-7233 or text SAFE and your current location (address/city/state) to 69866
Note: In seconds, a message with the closest Safe Place youth center location/contact number will be received. Text 2CHAT to continue texting with a mental health professional.
Website: nationalsafeplace.org/safe-place-teens

Mental Health

National Alliance on Mental Illness (NAMI) Information Helpline

Toll-Free: 800-950-NAMI (800-950-6264; 10 a.m.–6 p.m. EST, M–F)
Website: www.nami.org/Content/
NavigationMenu/Find_Support/Helpline/
NAMI_Information_HelpLine.htm

National Institute of Mental Health Information Center

Toll-Free: 866-615-6464 (8 a.m. to 8 p.m. EST, M–F)
Website: www.nimh.nih.gov/site-info/
contact-nimh.shtml

National Mental Health Association Hotline

Toll-Free: 800-273-TALK (800-273-8255)
Website: www.nmha.org

Rape, Sexual Violence, And Domestic Violence

Childhelp USA National Child Abuse Hotline

Toll-Free: 800-4-A-CHILD
(800-422-4453)
Website: www.childhelp.org/pages/
hotline-home

CyberTipline

Toll-Free: 800-843-5678
Website: www.cybertipline.com

loveisrespect.org

National teen dating abuse helpline
Toll-Free: 866-331-9474
or text LOVEIS to 22522
Toll-Free TTY: 866-331-8453
Website: www.loveisrespect.org
(Live online chat)

National Domestic Violence Hotline

Toll-Free: 800-799-SAFE (800-799-7233)
Toll-Free TTY: 800-787-3224
Website: www.thehotline.org/get-help/
contact-the-hotline

Rape, Abuse, and Incest National Network (RAINN)

Toll-Free: 800-656-HOPE
(800-656-4673)
Website: https://ohl.rainn.org/online
(Online hotline)

Safe Horizon's Rape, Sexual Assault, and Incest Hotline

Toll-Free: 800-621-HOPE (800-6214673;
Domestic Violence Hotline)
Toll-Free: 866-689-HELP (866-689-4357;
Crime Victims Hotline)
Toll-Free TDD: 866-604-5350
(for all hotlines)
Phone: 212-227-3000
(Rape, Sexual Assault, and Incest Hotline)
Website: www.safehorizon.org

SPEAK UP!

Toll-Free: 866-SPEAK-UP (866-773-2587)
Website: www.cpyv.org/programs/what-is
-speak-up-2/kids-and-teens

Sexuality And Sexual Health

Gay, Lesbian, Bisexual, and Transgender (GLBT) National Youth Talkline

Toll-Free: 800-246-PRIDE
(800-246-7743; 4 p.m.–12 p.m. EST, M–F;
12 p.m.–5 p.m. EST, Saturday)
Website: www.glnh.org/talkline
E-mail: youth@GLBTNationalHelp
Center.org

Planned Parenthood National Hotline

Toll-Free: 800-230-PLAN (800-230-7526;
for routing to local resources)
Website: www.plannedparenthood.org/
info-for-teens (Online chat)

Suicide

Hopeline

Toll-Free: 800-SUICIDE (800-784-2433)
Toll-Free: 800-442-HOPE (800-442-4673)
Website: www.hopeline.com

National Suicide Prevention Lifeline

Toll-Free: 800-273-TALK (800-273-8255)
Toll-Free TTY: 800-799-4TTY
(800-799-4889)
Website: http://www.youmatter.suicide
preventionlifeline.org/home/get-help
(Online chat available 5 p.m. to 1 a.m. EST,
M–F)

Suicide Hotline Listings by State

Website: http://www.suicidepreventionlife
line.org/getinvolved/locator

Youthline

Toll-Free: 877-YOUTHLINE (877-968-
8454; teen to teen peer counseling hotline)
Website: http://hopeline.com/
gethelpnow.html

Chapter 67

Directory Of Mental Health Organizations

National Mental Health Resources

Al-Anon Family Group Headquarters

1600 Corporate Landing Parkway
Virginia Beach, VA 23454-5617
Phone: 757-563-1600
Fax: 757-563-1655
Website: http://www.al-anon.alateen.org/for-alateen

American Academy of Child and Adolescent Psychiatry

3615 Wisconsin Avenue NW
Washington, DC 20016-3007
Phone: 202-966-7300
Fax: 202-966-2891
Website: www.aacap.org

American Art Therapy Association

225 North Fairfax Street
Alexandria, VA 22314
Toll-Free: 888-290-0878
Phone: 703-548-5860
Fax: 703-783-8468
Website: www.arttherapy.org
E-mail: info@arttherapy.org

American Association for Marriage and Family Therapy

112 South Alfred Street
Alexandria, VA 22314-3061
Phone: 703-838-9808
Fax: 703-838-9805
Website: www.aamft.org
E-mail: central@aamft.org

About This Chapter: Information in this chapter was compiled from various sources deemed reliable. All contact information was verified and updated in September 2013. Inclusion does not imply endorsement, and there is no implication association with omission.

American Association of Suicidology

5221 Wisconsin Avenue NW
Washington, DC 20015
Phone: 202-237-2280; Fax: 202-237-2282
Website: www.suicidology.org

American Counseling Association

5999 Stevenson Avenue
Alexandria, VA 22304
Toll-Free: 800-347-6647
TDD: 703-823-6862
Toll-Free Fax: 800-473-2329
Fax: 703-823-0252
Website: www.counseling.org
E-mail: webmaster@counseling.org

American Foundation for Suicide Prevention

120 Wall Street, 29th Floor
New York, NY 10005
Toll-Free: 888-333-AFSP (888-333-2377)
Phone: 212-363-3500; Fax: 212-363-6237
Website: www.afsp.org
E-mail: inquiry@afsp.org

American Psychiatric Association

1000 Wilson Boulevard, Suite 1825
Arlington, VA 22209-3901
Toll-Free: 888-35-PSYCH
(888-357-7924)
Phone: 703-907-7300
Website: www.psych.org
E-mail: apa@psych.org

American Psychological Association

750 First Street NE
Washington, DC 20002-4242
Toll-Free: 800-374-2721
Phone: 202-336-5500
TDD/TTY: 202-336-6123
Website: www.apa.org
E-mail: public.affairs@apa.org

American Psychotherapy Association

2750 East Sunshine Street
Springfield, MO 65804
Toll-Free: 800-205-9165
Phone: 417-823-0173
Fax: 417-823-9959
Website: www.americanpsychotherapy.com

Anxiety Disorders Association of America

8701 Georgia Avenue
Silver Spring, MD 20910
Phone: 240-485-1001
Fax: 240-485-1035
Website: www.adaa.org

Association for Applied Psychophysiology and Biofeedback

10200 West 44th Avenue, Suite 304
Wheat Ridge, CO 80033
Toll-Free: 800-477-8892
Phone: 303-422-8436
Website: www.aapb.org
E-mail: info@aapb.org

Association for Behavioral and Cognitive Therapies

305 7th Avenue, 16th Floor
New York, NY 10001
Phone: 212-647-1890
Fax: 212-647-1865
Website: www.abct.org

Balanced Mind Foundation

820 Davis Street, Suite 520
Evanston, IL 60201
Phone: 847-492-8510
Fax: 847-492-8520
Website: www.thebalancedmind.org
E-mail: info@thebalancedmind.org

Beyond Blue Ltd.

Website: www.beyondblue.org.au

Brain and Behavior Research Foundation

60 Cutter Mill Road, Suite 404
Great Neck, NY 11021
Toll-Free: 800-829-8289
Phone: 516-829-0091
Fax: 516-487-6930
Website: www.bbrfoundation.org
E-mail: info@bbrfoundation.org

Brain Injury Association of America

1608 Spring Hill Road, Suite 110
Vienna, VA 22182
Toll-Free: 800-444-6443
Phone: 703-761-0750
Fax: 703-761-0755
Website: www.biausa.org
E-mail: braininjuryinfo@biausa.org

Canadian Mental Health Association

Phenix Professional Building
595 Montreal Road, Suite 303
Ottawa, ON K1K 4L2
Fax: 613-745-5522
Website: www.cmha.ca

Canadian Psychological Association

141 Laurier Avenue West
Suite 702
Ottawa, ON K1P 5J3
Toll-Free: 888-472-0657
Phone: 613-237-2144
Fax: 613-237-1674
Website: www.cpa.ca
E-mail: cpa@cpa.ca

Caring.com

2600 South El Camino Real
Suite 300
San Mateo, CA 94403
Website: www.caring.com

Center for Mental Health Services

5600 Fishers Lane, Room 17C-20
Rockville, MD 20857
Phone: 240-276-1310
Fax: 240-276-1320
Website: mentalhealth.samhsa.gov
E-mail: info@mentalhealth.org

Center on Addiction and the Family

Website: www.coaf.org
E-mail: coaf@phoenixhouse.org

Depressed Anonymous

P.O. Box 17414
Louisville, KY 40217
Phone: 502-569-1989
Website: www.depressedanon.com
E-mail: info@depressedanon.com

Depression and Bipolar Support Alliance

730 North Franklin Street, Suite 501
Chicago, IL 60654-7225
Toll-Free: 800-826-3632
Fax: 312-642-7243
Website: www.dbsalliance.org
E-mail: info@dbsalliance.org

Eating Disorder Referral and Information Center

Website: www.edreferral.com

Families for Depression Awareness

395 Totten Pond Road, Suite 404
Waltham, MA 02451
Phone: 781-890-0220; Fax: 781-890-2411
Website: www.familyaware.org

Helpguide

Website: www.helpguide.org

International Foundation for Research and Education on Depression

P.O. Box 17598
Baltimore, MD 21297-1598
Fax: 443-782-0739
Website: www.ifred.org
E-mail: info@ifred.org

International OCD Foundation

P.O. Box 961029
Boston, MA 02196
Phone: 617-973-5801
Fax: 617-973-5803
Website: www.ocfoundation.org
E-mail: info@ocfoundation.org

International Society for the Study of Trauma and Dissociation

8400 Westpark Drive, Second Floor
McLean, VA 22102
Phone: 703-610-9037
Fax: 703-610-0234
Website: www.issd.org
E-mail: info@isst-d.org

International Society for Traumatic Stress Studies

111 Deer Lake Road, Suite 100
Deerfield, IL 60015
Phone: 847-480-9028
Fax: 847-480-9282
Website: www.istss.org
E-mail: istss@istss.org

Kristin Brooks Hope Center

1250 24th Street, NW, Suite 300
Washington, DC 20037
Toll-Free: 800-442-HOPE (800-442-4673)
Toll-Free Helpline: 800-SUICIDE (800-784-2433)
Toll-Free for Veterans: 877-VET-2-VET (877-838-2838)
Phone: 202-536-3200; Fax: 202-536-3206
Website: www.hopeline.com

Mautner Project

1300 19th Street NW
Suite 700
Washington, DC 20036
Toll-Free: 866-MAUTNER
(866- 628-8637)
Phone: 202-332-5536
Fax: 202-332-0662
Website: www.mautnerproject.org
E-mail: info@mautnerproject.org

Mental Health America (formerly National Mental Health Association)

2000 North Beauregard Street
6th Floor
Alexandria, VA 22311
Toll-Free: 800-969-6642
Toll-Free Crisis Line: 800-273-TALK
(800-273-8255)
Phone: 703-684-7722
Fax: 703-684-5968
Website: www.nmha.org
E-mail:
webmaster@mentalhealthamerica.net

Mental Health Minute

Website:
www.mentalhealthminute.info

Mind

15–19 Broadway
Stratford, London, UK E15 4BQ
Phone: +44 208-519-2122
Fax: +44 208-522-1725
Website: www.mind.org.uk
E-mail: contact@mind.org.uk

National Alliance on Mental Illness (NAMI)

3803 North Fairfax Drive
Suite 100
Arlington, VA 22203
Toll-Free: 888-999-NAMI
(888-999-6264)
Toll-Free: 800-950-NAMI
(800-950-6264 Helpline)
Phone: 703-524-7600
Fax: 703-524-9094
Website: www.nami.org
E-mail: info@nami.org

National Association of Anorexia Nervosa and Associated Disorders (ANAD)

800 East Diehl Road #160
Naperville, IL 60563
Phone: 630-577-1333
Phone: 630-577-1330 (Helpline)
Fax: 630-577-1323
Website: www.anad.org
E-mail: anadhelp@anad.org

National Association of School Psychologists

4340 East West Highway, Suite 402
Bethesda, MD 20814
Toll-Free: 866-331-NASP
(866-331-6277)
Phone: 301-657-0270
TTY: 301-657-4155
Fax: 301-657-0275
Website: www.nasponline.org
E-mail: center@naspweb.org

National Center for Child Traumatic Stress

Duke University
411 West Chapel Hill Street
Suite 200
Durham, NC 27701
Phone: 919-682-1552
Fax: 919-613-9898
Web site: www.nctsn.org
E-mail: info@nctsn.org

National Center for Posttraumatic Stress Disorder (NCPTSD)

U.S. Department of Veterans Affairs (VA)
810 Vermont Avenue NW
Washington, DC 20420
Toll-Free: 800-827-1000
Website: www.va.gov

National Center for Victims of Crime

2000 M Street NW, Suite 480
Washington, DC 20036
Phone: 202-467-8700
Fax: 202-467-8701
Website: www.ncvc.org
E-mail: webmaster@ncvc.org

National Council on Problem Gambling

730 11th Street NW, Suite 601
Washington, DC 20001
Toll-Free: 800-522-4700 (Hotline)
Phone 202-547-9204; Fax 202-547-9206
Website: www.ncpgambling.org
E-mail: ncpg@ncpgambling.org

National Eating Disorders Association

165 West 46th Street
New York, NY 10036
Toll-Free: 800-931-2237
Phone: 212-575-6200; Fax: 212-575-1650
Website: www.nationaleatingdisorders.org
E-mail: info@NationalEatingDisorders.org

National Federation of Families for Children's Mental Health

9605 Medical Center Drive, Suite 280
Rockville, MD 20850
Phone: 240-403-1901
Fax: 240-403-1909
Website: www.ffcmh.org
E-mail: ffcmh@ffcmh.org

National Institute of Mental Health

6001 Executive Blvd., Rm 8184, MSC 9663
Bethesda, MD 20892-9663
Toll-Free: 866-615-6464
Toll-Free TTY: 866-415-8051
Phone: 301-443-4513
TTY: 301-443-8431
Fax: 301-443-4279
Website: www.nimh.nih.gov
E-mail: nimhinfo@nih.gov

National Institute on Alcohol Abuse and Alcoholism

5635 Fishers Lane, MSC 9304
Bethesda, MD 20892
Phone: 301-443-3860
Website: www.niaaa.nih.gov
E-mail: niaaaweb-r@exchange.nih.gov

National Institute on Drug Abuse

6001 Executive Boulevard
Room 5213, MSC 9561
Bethesda, MD 20892-9561
Phone: 301-443-1124
Fax: 301-443-7397
Websites: www.nida.nih.gov and
www.drugabuse.gov
E-mail: information@nida.nih.gov

National Mental Health Information Center

Substance Abuse and Mental
Health Services Administration
P.O. Box 2345
Rockville, MD 20847
Toll-Free: 800-789-2647
Toll-Free TDD: 866-889-2647
Phone: 240-221-4021
TDD Phone: 240-221-4022
Fax: 240-221-4295
Website: mentalhealth.samhsa.gov
E-mail: nmhic-info@samhsa.hss.gov

National Women's Health Information Center (NWHIC)

Office on Women's Health
200 Independence Avenue SW
Room 712E
Washington, DC 20201
Toll-Free: 800-994-9662
Toll-Free TDD: 888-220-5446
Phone: 202-690-7650
Fax: 202-205-2631
Website: www.womenshealth.gov

Office of Minority Health

Resource Center
P.O. Box 37337
Washington, DC 20013-7337
Toll-Free: 800-444-6472
Phone: 240-453-2882
TDD: 301-251-1432
Fax: 301-251-2160
Fax: 240-453-2883
Website: minorityhealth.hhs.gov
E-mail:
info@minorityhealth.hhs.gov

Psych Central

55 Pleasant Street
Suite 207
Newburyport, MA 01950
Phone: 978-992-0008
Website: www.psychcentral.com
E-mail: talkback@psychcentral.com

Psychology Today

115 East 23rd Street
9th Floor
New York, NY 10010
Toll-Free: 888-875-3570
Phone: 212-260-7210
Website: www.psychologytoday.com

Schizophrenic.com

Website: www.schizophrenic.com
E-mail: info@schizophrenic.com

Social Phobia/Social Anxiety Association

Website: www.socialphobia.org

411

Substance Abuse and Mental Health Services Administration (SAMHSA)

1 Choke Cherry Road
Rockville, MD 20857
Toll-Free: 877-SAMHSA-7
(877-726-4727)
Fax: 240-221-4295
Website: mentalhealth.samhsa.gov
Mental Health Services Locator:
mentalhealth.samhsa.gov/databases

Suicide Awareness Voices of Education (SAVE)

8120 Penn Avenue South
Suite 470
Bloomington, MN 55431
Phone: 952-946-7998
Website: www.save.org

Suicide Prevention Resource Center (SPRC)

Education Development Center, Inc.
43 Foundry Avenue
Waltham, MA 02453-8313
Toll-Free: 877-GET-SPRC
(877-438-7772)
TTY: 617-964-5448
Fax: 617-969-9186
Website: www.sprc.org
E-mail: info@sprc.org

SupportGroups.com

Website: www.supportgroups.com
E-mail: info@supportgroups.com

State Mental Health Resources

Alabama

Division of Mental Health and Substance
Abuse Services
Alabama Department of Mental Health
P.O. Box 301410
Montgomery, AL 36130-1410
Toll-Free: 800-367-0955 (Hotline)
Phone: 334-242-3454; Fax: 334-242-0725
Website: http://www.mh.alabama.gov/sa
E-mail: Alabama.DMH@mh.alabama.gov

Alaska

Division of Behavioral Health
Alaska Dept. of Health and Social Services
P.O. Box 110620
Juneau, AK 99811-0620
Phone: 907-465-5808
Toll-Free: 877-266-4357 (Hotline)
Fax: 907-465-2185
Website: http://dhss.alaska.gov/dbh/
Pages/default.aspx

Arizona

Behavioral Health Services
Arizona Department of Health Services
150 North 18th Avenue, #200
Phoenix, AZ 85007
Phone: 602-364-4558
Fax: 602-364-4570
Website: http://www.azdhs.gov

Arkansas

Division of Behavioral Health Services
Arkansas Department of Human Services
305 South Palm Street
Little Rock, AR 72205
Phone: 501-686-9164
TDD: 501-686-9176
Fax: 501-686-9182
Website: http://humanservices.arkansas
.gov/dbhs/Pages/default.aspx

Colorado

Office of Behavioral Health
Department of Human Services
3824 West Princeton Circle
Denver, CO 80236-3111
Phone: 303-866-7400
Fax: 303-866-7428
Website: http://www.colorado.gov/cs/
Satellite/CDHS-BehavioralHealth/
CBON/1251578892077
E-mail:
cdhs.communications@state.co.us

Connecticut

Department of Mental Health
and Addiction Services
P.O. Box 341431
Hartford, CT 06134
Toll-Free: 800-446-7348
Phone: 860-418-7000
TDD: 860-418-6707
Website: http://www.ct.gov/dmhas

Delaware

Division of Substance Abuse and Mental
Health
Community Mental Health
and Addiction Services
1901 North DuPont Highway
New Castle, DE 19720
Toll-Free: 800-652-2929
(Helpline—Delaware Only)
Phone: 302-255-9399
Fax: 302-255-4427
Website: http://www.dhss.delaware.gov/
dsamh/index.html

District of Columbia

Department of Mental Health
64 New York Avenue NE
3rd Floor
Washington, DC 20002
Phone: 202-673-7440
TTY: 202-673-7500
Fax: 202- 673-3433
Website: http://dmh.dc.gov
E-mail: dmh@dc.gov

Florida

ACCESS Central Mail Center
P.O. Box 5200
Tallahassee, FL 32314-5200
Toll-Free: 866-762-2237
Toll-Free TTY: 800-955-8771
Website: http://www.myflfamilies.com/
service-programs/mental-health

Georgia

Division of Addictive Diseases
Department of Behavioral Health
and Developmental Disabilities
Two Peachtree Street NW
24th Floor
Atlanta, GA 30303-3171
Toll-Free: 800-715-4225 (Hotline)
Phone: 404-657-2331
Fax: 404-657-2256
Website: http://dbhdd.georgia.gov

Hawaii

Department of Health
Child and Adolescent Mental Health
Division
3627 Kilauea Avenue
Room 101
Honolulu, HI 96816
Phone: 808-733-9333
Fax: 808-733-9357
Website: http://health.hawaii.gov/camhd
E-mail:
camhdwebmaster@doh.hawaii.gov

Idaho

Division of Behavioral Health
Department of Health and Welfare
P.O. Box 83720
Boise, ID 83720-0036
Toll-Free: 800-922-3406
(Screening/Referral)
Phone: 208-334-6997
Website:
http://www.healthandwelfare.idaho.gov
E-mail: DPHInquiries@dhw.idaho.gov

Illinois

Division of Alcoholism and Addiction
Department of Human Services
401 South Clinton Street
Chicago, IL 60607
Toll-Free: 800-843-6154 (Help Line)
Toll-Free TTY: 800-447-6404
(Help Line)
Phone: 312-814-5050
TTY: 312-793-2354
Website: http://www.dhs.state.il.us/
page.aspx?item=29728
E-mail: DHSWebBits@illinois.gov

Indiana

Division of Mental Health and Addiction
Family and Social Services Administration
P.O. Box 7083
Indianapolis, IN 46207-7083
Toll-Free: 800-901-1133
Toll-Free: 800-662-4357 (Hotline)
Phone: 317-233-4454
Fax: 317-233-4693
Website: http://www.in.gov/fssa/
dmha/index.htm

Iowa

Division of Behavioral Health
Department of Public Health
Lucas State Office Building
321 East 12th Street
Des Moines, IA 50319-0075
Toll-Free: 866-227-9878
Phone: 515-281-4417
Fax: 515-281-4535
Website: http://www.idph.state.ia.us/bh/
substance_abuse.asp

Kansas

Community Services and Programs
Department for Aging and Disability
Services
New England State Office Building
503 South Kansas Avenue
Topeka, KS 66603-3404
Phone: 785-296-4986
Fax: 785-296- 0557
Website: http://www.dcf.ks.gov/Pages/
Default.aspx

Kentucky

Cabinet for Health and Family Services
Department for Behavioral Health,
Developmental, and Intellectual
Disabilities
100 Fair Oaks Lane, 4E-B
Frankfort, KY 40621
Phone: 502-564-4527
TTY: 502-564-5777
Fax: 502-564-5478
Website: http://dbhdid.ky.gov/kdbhdid/
default.aspx

Louisiana

Office of Behavioral Health
Department of Health and Hospitals
P.O. Box 629
Baton Rouge, LA 70821-0629
Phone: 225-342-9500
Fax: 225-342-5568
Website: http://www.dhh.louisiana.gov/
index.cfm/subhome/10/n/6

Maine

Substance Abuse and Mental
Health Services
Department of Health and
Human Services
41 Anthony Avenue
#11 State House Station
Augusta, ME 04333-0011
Phone: 207-287-2595
Fax: 207-287-4334
Website: http://www.maine.gov/
dhhs/samhs/osa
E-mail: osa.ircosa@maine.gov

Maryland

Department of Health
and Mental Hygiene
201 West Preston Street
Baltimore, MD 21201
Toll-Free: 877-463-3464
Phone: 410-402-8300
Website: http://dhmh.maryland.gov/
bhd/SitePages/Home.aspx
E-mail: healthmd@dhmh.state.md.us

Massachusetts

Health and Human Services
Office of Children, Youth, and Family
Services
One Ashburton Place
11th Floor
Boston, MA 02108
Phone: 617-573-1600
Website: http://www.mass.gov/eohhs/
consumer/behavioral-health/
mental-health

Michigan

Department of Community Health
Capitol View Building
201 Townsend Street
Lansing, MI 48913
Phone: 517-373-3740
Website: http://www.michigan.gov/mdch

Minnesota

Department of Human Services
Mental Health Division
P.O. Box 64981
St. Paul, MN 55164-0981
Phone: 651-431-2225
Fax: 651-431-7418
Website: http://mn.gov/dhs

Mississippi

Mississippi Department of Mental Health
1101 Robert E. Lee Building
239 North Lamar Street
Jackson, MS 39201
Toll-Free: 877-210-8513 (Helpline)
Phone: 601-359-1288
TDD: 601-359-6230
Fax: 601-359-6295
Website: http://www.dmh.ms.gov

Missouri

Division of Behavioral Health
Missouri Department of Mental Health
P.O. Box 687
Jefferson City, MO 65102
Toll-Free: 800-575-7480
Phone: 573-751-4942
Fax: 573-751-7814
Website: http://www.dmh.mo.gov/ada
E-mail: dbhmail@dmh.mo.gov

Montana

Addictive and Mental Disorders Division
Department of Public Health
and Human Services
P.O. Box 202905
Helena, MT 59620-2905
Phone: 406-444-3964
Fax: 406-444-9389
Website: http://www.dphhs.mt.gov/amdd
E-mail: hhsamdemail@mt.gov

Nebraska

Division of Behavioral Health
Department of Health and
Human Services
P.O. Box 95026
Lincoln, NE 68509-5026
Toll-Free: 888-866-8660 (Helpline)
Phone: 402-471-8553
Fax: 402-471-9449
Website: http://www.dhhs.ne.gov/
Behavioral_Health
E-mail:
DHHS.BehavioralHealthDivision@
Nebraska.gov

Nevada

Department of Health and
Human Services
Division of Mental Health
and Development Services
4126 Technology Way, 2nd Floor
Carson City, NV 89706
Phone: 775-684-4190
Fax: 775-684-4185
Website: http://mhds.state.nv.us
E-mail: MHDS@mhds.nv.gov

New Hampshire

Department of Health and
Human Services
105 Pleasant Street
Concord, NH 03301
Toll-Free: 800-804-0909
Phone: 603-271-6738
Fax: 603-271-6105
Website:
http://www.dhhs.nh.gov/index.htm

New Jersey

Department of Human Services
Division of Mental Health
and Addiction Services
222 South Warren Street
Trenton, NJ 08625
Toll-Free: 800-238-2333 (Hotline)
Phone: 609-292-5760
Fax: 609-292-3816
Website: http://www.state.nj.us/
humanservices/das/home
E-mail: dmhas@dhs.state.nj.us

New Mexico

Behavioral Health Services Division
Human Services Department
P.O. Box 2348
Santa Fe, NM 87504
Toll-Free: 800-362-2013
Phone: 505-476-9266
Fax: 505-476-9277
Website:
http://www.hsd.state.nm.us/bhsd

New York

State Office of Mental Health
44 Holland Avenue
Albany, NY 12229
Toll-Free: 800-597-8481
Website: http://www.omh.ny.gov

North Carolina

Department of Health
and Human Services
Division of Mental Health,
Developmental Disabilities,
and Substance Abuse Services
3007 Mail Service Center
Raleigh, NC 27699-3007
Toll-Free: 800-662-7030
Phone: 919-733-4670
Fax: 919-733-4556
Website: http://www.dhhs.state.nc.us/
mhddsas

North Dakota

Division of Mental Health
and Substance Abuse Services
Department of Human Services
Prairie Hills Plaza
1237 West Divide Avenue
Suite 1C
Bismarck, ND 58501-1208
Toll-Free: 800-755-2719
(North Dakota only)
Phone: 701-328-8920
Fax: 701-328-8969
Website: http://www.nd.gov/dhs/
services/mentalhealth
E-mail: dhsmhsas@nd.gov

Ohio

Department of Mental Health
and Addiction Services
30 East Broad Street
36th Floor
Columbus, OH 43215-3430
Toll-Free: 877-275-6364
Toll-Free TTY: 888-636-4889
Phone: 614-466-2596
TTY: 614-752-9696
Fax: 614-752-9453
Website: http://mha.ohio.gov
E-mail: askODMH@mh.ohio.gov

Oklahoma

Department of Mental Health
and Substance Abuse Services
P.O. Box 53277
Oklahoma City, OK 73152-3277
Toll-Free: 800-522-9054
Phone: 405-522-3908
TDD: 405-522-3851
Fax: 405-522-3650
Website: http://ok.gov/odmhsas

Oregon

Addictions and Mental Health Division
Oregon Health Authority
500 Summer Street NE
Salem, OR 97301-1079
Toll-Free TTY: 800-375-2863
Phone: 503-945-5763
Fax: 503-378-8467
Website: http://www.oregon.gov/
oha/amh/Pages/index.aspx
E-mail: Amh.web@state.or.us

Pennsylvania

Department of Health
02 Kline Plaza, Suite B
Harrisburg, PA 17104-1579
Phone: 717-783-8200
Fax: 717-787-6285
Website:
http://www.health.state.pa.us/bdap

Rhode Island

Department of Behavioral Healthcare
Developmental Disabilities
and Hospitals
Barry Hall Building
14 Harrington Road
Cranston, RI 02920
Phone: 401-462-2339
Fax: 401-462-3204
Website:
http://www.bhddh.ri.gov/SA

South Carolina

Department of Mental Health
Administration Building
2414 Bull Street
Columbia, SC 29202
Phone: 803- 898-8581
TTY: 864-297-5130
Website: http://www.state.sc.us/dmh

South Dakota

Division of Community
Behavioral Health
Department of Social Services
c/o 700 Governor's Drive
Pierre, SD 57501
Toll-Free: 800-265-9684
Phone: 605-773-3123
Fax: 605-773-7076
Website: http://dss.sd.gov/
behavioralhealthservices/community
E-mail: infoMH@state.sd.us

Tennessee

Department of Mental Health
and Substance Abuse Services
601 Mainstream Drive
Nashville, TN 37243
Toll-Free: 800-560-5767
Toll-Free: 855-274-7471 (Hotline)
Phone: 615-532-6500
Website: http://www.tn.gov/mental
E-mail: OC.TDMHSAS@tn.gov

Texas

Mental Health and
Substance Abuse Division
Department of State Health Services
P.O. Box 149347
Austin, TX 78714-9347
Toll-Free: 866-378-8440
Phone: 512-206-5000
Fax: 512-206-5714
Website:
http://www.dshs.state.tx.us/MHSA
E-mail: contact@dshs.state.tx.us

Utah

Division of Substance Abuse
and Mental Health
Utah Department of Human Services
195 North 1950 West
2nd Floor
Salt Lake City, UT 84116
Phone: 801-538-3939
Fax: 801-538-9892
Website: http://www.dsamh.utah.gov
E-mail: dsamhwebmaster@utah.gov

Vermont

Department of Mental Health
Redstone Building
26 Terrace Street
Montpelier, VT 05609-1101
Toll-Free: 888-212-4677
Phone: 802-828-3824
Fax: 802-828-3823
Website: http://mentalhealth.
vermont.gov/contact

Virginia

Department of Behavioral Health
and Developmental Services
P.O. Box 1797
Richmond, VA 23218-1797
Phone: 804-786-3906
TDD: 804-371-8977
Fax: 804-786-9248
Website:
http://www.dbhds.virginia.gov

Washington

Division of Behavioral Health
and Recovery Services
Department of Social and Health Services
P.O. Box 45330
Olympia, WA 98504-5330
Toll-Free: 877-301-4557
Toll-Free: 866-789-1511 (Help Line)
Toll-Free TTY: 800-833-6384
TTY: 206-461-3219 (Help Line)
Fax: 360-586-0341
Website: http://www.dshs.wa.gov/dbhr
E-mail: DASAInformation@dshs.wa.gov

West Virginia

Bureau for Behavioral Health
and Health Facilities
Department of Health and
Human Resources
350 Capitol Street, Room 350
Charleston, WV 25304
Phone: 304-356-4811
Fax: 304-558-1008
Website: http://www.dhhr.wv.gov/bhhf/
Pages/default.aspx

Wisconsin

Department of Health Services
1 West Wilson Street
Madison, WI 53703
Phone: 608-266-1865
Website: http://www.dhs.wisconsin.gov/
MentalHealth/INDEX.HTM
E-mail: DHSwebmaster@wisconsin.gov

Wyoming

Behavioral Health Division
Mental Health and Substance Abuse
Services
Department of Health
6101 Yellowstone Road
Suite 220
Cheyenne, WY 82002
Toll-Free: 800-535-4006
Phone: 307-777-6494
Fax: 307-777-5849

Index

Index

Page numbers that appear in *Italics* refer to tables or illustrations. Page numbers that have a small 'n' after the page number refer to citation information shown as Notes. Page numbers that appear in **Bold** refer to information contained in boxes within the chapters.

A